YOUNGER FOR LONGER

How You Can Slow the Ageing Process
and Stay Healthy for Life

Dr Duncan Carmichael

A How To book

ROBINSON

ROBINSON

First published in Great Britain in 2018 by Robinson

1 3 5 7 9 10 8 6 4 2

A CIP catalogue record for this book
is available from the British Library.

ISBN: 978-1-47214-249-8

Typeset in Whitman by Hewer Text UK Ltd, Edinburgh
Printed and bound in Great Britain by CPI Group (UK), Croydon CR0 4YY

Papers used by Robinson are from well-managed forests and other responsible sources.

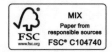

Robinson
An imprint of
Little, Brown Book Group
Carmelite House
50 Victoria Embankment
London EC4Y 0DZ

An Hachette UK Company
www.hachette.co.uk

www.littlebrown.co.uk

How To Books are published by Robinson, an imprint of Little, Brown Book
Group. We welcome proposals from authors who have first-hand experience
of their subjects. Please set out the aims of your book, its target market and
its suggested contents in an email to howtobooks@littlebrown.co.uk

Contents

It is not that we have a short time to live, but that we waste a lot of it. Life is long enough, and a sufficiently generous amount has been given to us for the highest achievements if it were all well invested. But when it is wasted in heedless luxury and spent on no good activity, we are forced at last by death's final constraint to realise that it has passed away before we knew it was passing. So it is: we are not given a short life but we make it short, and we are not ill-supplied but wasteful of it.

Seneca, c. 5 BCE – 65 CE

The doctor of the future will give no medication, but will interest his patients in the care of the human frame, diet and in the cause and prevention of disease.

Thomas Edison

To Megan

My wife, my partner, my muse, my fellow adventurer.

May we continue exploring new worlds together.

Introduction

The chief object of education is not to learn things, but to *unlearn* things.

G. K. Chesterton

In 1992, when I was a young and eager medical student, one of my professors told our class that within five years we would need to unlearn around half of what we were being taught. Medicine, he explained, was moving so far and so fast that some of today's perceived wisdom would appear much less worthy tomorrow.

Fast-forward five years: I was a young and eager doctor, and the medical world understood that the essential factor in preventing heart attacks was the level of cholesterol in your blood. Five years after that, we doctors had flow-charts on our desks showing us the link between your cholesterol level and the recommended treatment to decrease that level using low-fat diets and statin tablets. Eggs were off your 2002 breakfast menu, and were replaced by cereals such as Kellogg's Special K, which was low in fat and high in carbohydrates.

Moving ahead another five years to 2007, and the emphasis on how best to lower your heart attack risk had shifted away from lowering cholesterol and was now focused on cutting inflammation.[1] Five years after that and our knowledge had improved to such an extent that we knew low-fat diets did *not*, in fact, help to lower your heart attack risk.[2] Instead, a major culprit in the

1 Ridker, P. M. et al. 'C-Reactive Protein Adds to the Predictive Value of Total and HDL Cholesterol in Determining Risk of First Myocardial Infarction.' *Circulation* (1998): 97: 20: 2007–11.
2 Hooper, L. et al. 'Reduced or Modified Dietary Fat for Preventing Cardiovascular Disease.' *The Cochrane Library* (2012).

obesity and heart-attack epidemic was the high sugar content of low-fat foods.[3]

As I write these words in 2018 we know that, for many people, low-fat diets can be a health catastrophe. Why? Because most low-fat items are high in sugar in order to make the food taste at least half-reasonable. The problem is that sugar is inflammatory and it unequivocally heightens your heart-attack risk.[4] Today, more than fifteen years after eggs were taken off our breakfast menu for being too fatty, they have returned with a full pardon from the US Food and Drug Administration.[5] Talk about coming full circle.

I should say that, as medical students, most of us did not pay much heed to our sage professor. However, having worked for more than two decades as a doctor and then as an anti-ageing specialist, it turns out he was right. Every five years we doctors have had to unlearn a surprising amount of what we had thought was true – as the story of cholesterol shows. In the same way, much of what we learned in other areas of medicine and health has moved on, been disproven or simply gone in new and interesting directions. The professor's point was that a lot of knowledge is not set in stone, and that is certainly true of medicine. My profession is by nature conservative – which is usually a good thing – but as professionals we have the difficult obligation of being open to new research while retaining a healthy degree of scepticism for fads. Like much in life, this requires a balance that is easier to preach than to achieve.

When it comes to anti-ageing, which is my particular interest, I am astounded at how much we have learned in the past few years. Anti-ageing medicine has benefited tremendously from research into hormones, stem cells and genetics, to name just three areas, and I am excited at the prospect of how much more we will find out in the coming years.

3 Lustig, R. *Fat Chance: The Hidden Truth About Sugar*, Penguin (2014).
4 US Department of Health and Human Services and US Department of Agriculture. '2015–2020 Dietary Guidelines for Americans.' 8th Ed. (December 2015). [See Chapter 6: Cross-cutting Topics of Public Health Importance.] Full guideline available at http://health.gov/dietaryguidelines/2015/guidelines/
5 Ibid.

The advances of science mean we now have a much more rigorous understanding of the causes and consequences of ageing. These are exciting times and, although we can expect to improve our knowledge in the coming years, we already know more than enough to live a *Younger for Longer* life.

We are far from being the first generation to seek to live a longer, healthier life: 2,200 years ago, China's first emperor Qin Shi Huang – the famous Terracotta Army depicts his warriors – sent troops to seek out the island of Penglai (known to the Japanese as Horai), which was home to the Eight Immortals and where fruits grew that cured all illness and conferred eternal youth. Qin Shi Huang was obsessed with immortality; ironically he died from poisoning from the mercury prescribed to him by his physicians, who assured him the toxic metal would ensure he lived forever.

A century earlier and a long way further west (or east, depending on which way you travel) it had been the turn of another emperor, Alexander the Great, who reputedly discovered a river with healing powers. It did Alexander little good – he died aged thirty-three. And fast-forward nearly two millennia to 1513 when Spanish explorer Juan Ponce de Léon and his conquistadors landed in Florida; if you believe the fable, they were there to find the Fountain of Youth, although there is little evidence to suggest this is true. A few decades later, the British scientist Francis Bacon wrote on the possibility of humans living to 1,000 – as Adam and his ilk reputedly had done.

In other words, there is nothing new about the quest for eternal youth, and there remains little chance of success – at least in my lifetime – though that will not stop people seeking it. With that said, it is worth explaining briefly what else this book is *not* about. It is not a gushing tribute to the cleverness of hormone injections that claim to keep us virile, healthy and young. Some practitioners argue that if you look good on the outside then you must be strong on the inside, and that powerful daily injections are the solution. That is not the case; anti-ageing is a far more subtle science.

Similarly this book is not an ode to the old boys' medical club that views anti-ageing doctors as heretics blindly following pioneering pathways with insufficient evidence. (When I hear that, I am reminded of the German philosopher Arthur Schopenhauer's comment that: 'All truth passes through three stages. First, it is ridiculed. Second, it is violently opposed. Third, it is accepted as being self-evident.') Among them are those who reject the idea that injections of Botox or testosterone have a place in modern medicine, and who decry these innovations as mere symptoms of greed and vanity over-powering medical values.

Others argue – not without justification – that we should spend our time and money on ridding the world of malaria, malnutrition and AIDS before pandering to the needs of the wealthy in their pursuit to look younger or to age more slowly. Still others say change will come through politics, not medicine, so those looking to make a difference should hang up their white coats and pursue that path.

What this tells me is that medicine is as dispute-ridden and full of moral conundrums as ever, yet that is how it should be. The world is big enough to accommodate all of these opinions, and our inability to agree on them does not necessarily render them invalid.

What is important is to keep an open mind and to try to assess new information fairly. And *that* is what this book is about.

With that established, let me tell you what you *will* find out. This book will lead you through the fascinating minefield that is modern medicine, through the profound changes of the last two decades when practitioners began revising a millennia-old view: instead of medicine being solely about how best to treat illness, it has widened to incorporate the concept of 'wellness' that targets health today and longevity tomorrow. Along the way it will explain how medicine arrived at its present state so that you can understand the angry battle lines that some medical groups have taken in defending their positions.

Most importantly, *Younger for Longer* will tell you what you can do to maximise your health, and will explain why bio-identical hormones, nutrition and liver detoxification constitute the three key steps.

Medicine is racing ahead with research on topics as diverse as genetic manipulation, stem-cell therapy and hormone cocktails; at the same time aesthetics has evolved into a huge industry that can tighten, tuck and make the skin glow like that of a twenty-year-old. The effect on medical professionals is immense: Hervé Raspaldo, a respected French plastic surgeon whom I met at an anti-ageing conference in Cape Town in 2008, told me surgery comprised just 20 per cent of his business, down from nearly 100 per cent five years earlier; the rest of his time was spent on what we call aesthetic procedures: Botox, fillers and laser therapy. Technology has changed so fast that, despite training as a surgeon, Raspaldo felt he could achieve more on most patients with fillers and lasers than he could with a scalpel. Besides, he said, many patients prefer the convenience of a half-hour procedure in their lunch break to the inconvenience of an operation.

At the same time as these medical advances, a cultural shift is also under-way as populations in developed countries age. These days sixty-five is no longer seen as the time to retire (and given the pensions time bomb ticking in Europe and the US, my generation will need to keep working later than that). It is of little surprise nowadays that Barack Obama became the fifth-youngest U.S. president at forty-seven, followed by Donald Trump who became the oldest president at seventy.

On the other side of the Atlantic, in the United Kingdom, the Queen Mother lived healthily to 101. At the time of writing, her daughter Elizabeth, ninety-two, is still on the throne and was until recently regularly accompanied by her ninety-six-year-old husband Prince Philip. Their eldest son Charles is sixty-nine and has not yet ascended the throne at an age when most people would have retired. This is a family that has successfully practised healthy ageing for three generations.

During that time, life expectancy in the developed world has risen steadily, and many of us assume that people in rich countries will continue to lead ever-longer lives. Not everyone agrees: some scientists argue that we are on the cusp of a reversal thanks to the effects of obesity.[6] Indeed, the success of the likes of Britain's royal family is far from universal. In the US, one in nine children has asthma, and late onset diabetes is no longer restricted to people in their sixties but is reported in overweight teenagers.

6 Olshansky, S. J. et al. 'A Potential Decline in Life Expectancy in the United States in the 21st Century.' *N Engl J Med* (2005): 352: 1138.

The modern world offers us the chance of excellent health or of early debilitating illness. What is abundantly clear is that our health is, for most of us, largely in our hands. The question is: how can we find out what will help us and what will harm us? There are so many changes taking place so quickly in so many areas of medicine that yesterday's cure might be tomorrow's curse (and that is without worrying about whether someone is merely a snake-oil salesman in a white coat). Finding reliable information without being swamped in this internet age is no easy matter.

My task is to map out a useful path for you, which is something I started doing around the turn of the millennium. Back then I was working as a doctor in the United Kingdom's National Health Service. While I remain passionate about the NHS and its pledge of free treatment for all, I was frustrated that the ten-minute consultation periods with my patients meant I could do little more than treat the illness in front of me. I remember being particularly exasperated when treating a patient for his eighth chest infection that winter. Many of the people I saw wanted much more than merely to get treatment for what ailed them; they wanted to know how to *maintain* their health.

But that is not something the NHS focuses on so I began to look elsewhere for the answers. My search led me to an emerging health-related speciality called anti-ageing hormone balancing, and I was so impressed by a lecture on the topic by Belgian endocrinologist Thierry Hertoghe that I went to Brussels to study under him. Not long after that, the American actress Suzanne Somers published a book on how bio-identical oestrogen had helped her to overcome breast cancer; her celebrity status propelled public interest in the subject of hormones.

Since 2008 I have worked and lectured on hormones full time.

More recently, researchers have turned their attention to determining what goes on inside the cell, and this has become the latest branch of wellness medicine: examining the different nutrients and how these affect our cells and our DNA. One key area is working out how nutrients and chemicals penetrate the cell membrane; the logic is that if we can improve getting certain elements into our cells and getting others out, we can improve our wellbeing. (Researchers use the term 'epigenetics' to describe the study of how nutrients and toxins affect our DNA.) As we will see later, there is also much talk about so-called cellular messengers, which also have an impact on our DNA. In the US the entire field – from hormone balancing to epigenetics – has grown in stature under the banner of 'Functional Medicine'.

Rest assured, if some of these terms sound confusing, they will make sense in due course. For now, the point is this: just as we were beginning to get comfortable looking at the body in relation to hormones, much of the research shifted to another horizon, and by the time you read this it might be focusing on another. That is all to the good, because none of this discounts the hormonal model of understanding how our bodies work; instead it enhances it. Every few years a new layer of medicine appears on our horizon, and we need to examine it, take what is useful and apply it to what we already know. For my money, the next layer looks likely to incorporate DNA manipulation and stem-cell treatments.

This ongoing accumulation of knowledge is fascinating and, I believe, will help move us to a place where we can slow the deleterious effects of ageing. It might seem like a complex mix of interminable scientific terms, but I promise you it has logic and simplicity. Throughout this book you will see how this diversity of subjects – such as detoxification, hormone treatments and cellular medicine – work smoothly together, just as an orchestra's range of instruments combines to create a symphony.

I would take this one step further and suggest that, if we want to benefit from these treatments of the future, we must ensure we are optimising our health today. For example, studies show that stem-cell treatments using cells harvested from smokers are far less effective than those from non-smokers, and this is because smoking significantly lowers the ability of stem cells to regenerate. And so, by optimising our health – our sleep, our hormones, and our nutrition, while minimising stress and toxins – we are putting ourselves in a position where we can benefit much more comprehensively from the fascinating stem-cell and gene treatments that are being prepared for tomorrow.

I will close by explaining how the book is laid out. The chapter on the theories of ageing will explain not only why we age but that we really have just two health choices: either live a life of excess and sloth, and spend our last twenty years in declining health, or take care of ourselves and maximise our chances of living a full and energetic life until the end. Anti-ageing medicine is currently focused on helping us to live healthy lives but some researchers believe that in the future, once we are able to manipulate our genes, we could live healthily for several hundred years. Pie in the sky? Possibly, but we can agree or disagree about that later.

The chapter on inflammation and obesity, which looks at what goes on at the level of our cells, explains why it is far harder to clear the simple sugar known as glucose from our arteries when they are inflamed. That is important because if we cannot process glucose in the way that we should, then our body will store it as fat. This eventually leads to obesity, diabetes and heart attacks, and is one of the main causes of premature ageing.

The chapter on adrenal health examines stress and explains why this is our biggest killer. Chronic stress either causes us to end up overweight and at risk of heart attacks and strokes, or thin and sickly and at risk of cancer. In the modern world, and certainly in the rich world, managing stress is our main challenge.

Other chapters explore the damage done by synthetic hormones, and will show what evidence we have to explain how liver damage stagnates our natural sex hormones, contributing to baldness and weight gain. Yet we can prevent this in men and women by looking after our livers. Supporting a tired liver is done with a detoxification programme – and that is so important a process that I have devoted an entire chapter to it. There are also chapters on nutrition, the brain, the skin and, of course, hormones.

That is a taster for now. The book has much else too, including specific chapters on men's and women's health. I hope that by the end you will have as sound a grasp of anti-ageing medicine as is currently possible. A fervent curiosity is a basic requirement for a healthy, productive life, as Albert Einstein knew well. Near the end of his life he described himself in a letter to his biographer Carl Seelig as having 'no special talents. I am only passionately curious.'

I believe that the best education is the one that breeds inquisitiveness, and I am also convinced there is no such thing as a boring topic, only poor teaching. With that in mind, I hope my writing style is lucid enough to make this variety both interesting and memorable. And do not be intimidated by the medical words; I will explain them all in due course and, in cases where they appear in different chapters, I will do so several times. (You can also look at the Glossary for simple definitions.)

Within a few years I will surely have to refine what is written here; I might even need to discard some of it. That is the welcome price of moving forward, and for that reason this book will not be the last word on anti-ageing. But having spent much of my professional life immersed in the subject, I believe that what is within these pages will give you the tools to live as healthily as possible based on the current evidence.

Finally, please use this book as a springboard to improve your knowledge about anti-ageing. It is up to you to listen to your inner voice to decide which truths resonate for you and which do not. Question everything and, like Einstein, retain an insatiable curiosity. Understanding what is written here will give you the best possible basis for evaluating what you learn elsewhere, whether online, in the media or from your doctor. After all, it is your health that this book is aimed at improving, and I cannot think of a better goal than that.

DMC

Cape Town, July 2018

Chapter 1

THE BEGINNING – A VERY GOOD PLACE TO START

It ain't what you don't know that gets you into trouble;
it's what you know for sure that just ain't so.

Attributed to Mark Twain, probably incorrectly

When it comes to dispensing advice we doctors have a mixed track record, and that is putting it kindly. On the plus side, we long ago stopped recommending what passed for first-rate treatment in medieval times – a course of leeches to suck out bad blood and thereby balance your four humours. Yet that pales next to our worst recommendation: that smoking was a healthy way to cut stress. While the slogan 'More Doctors Smoke Camels Than Any Other Cigarette' was a marketing triumph, it remains a toe-curling embarrassment for my profession.[1]

That sort of bad advice is pretty easy to spot – it is simply wrong. It is far harder to see where my profession errs in giving second-rate advice, or even in failing to know *what* to tell our patients. It is not that we are being obstructive; it is just that knowledge evolves quickly, and medical bodies can be slow to change what they advise. Perhaps the most obvious example of this is our failure to recognise the importance of 'enhancing health'. As doctors, we have become very good at treating illness. However, treating an illness without optimising your health is like emptying water out of your boat without fixing the leaks. For example, for years we promoted low-fat eating to help

1 Gardner, M. 'The Doctor's Choice is America's Choice.' *Am J Public Health* (2006): 96: 222–32.

heart-attack patients, but what we failed to see is that this advice often resulted in higher sugar consumption, which promoted more heart attacks. We are good at treating heart attacks, but we could do much better at optimising health to prevent a heart attack in the first place.

That, very briefly, is what this book is about – giving the reasons and showing the advice that will optimise your health, to make you the healthiest you that you can be.

This seems to me to be the logical approach. After all, it makes little sense to think about our health only when something goes wrong; instead it is wiser to be proactive, to strive to avoid illness and to maximise our health. Yet rising global obesity rates show the world has been going in the opposite direction. The danger is that if we do not fix this problem then society will pay dearly, and in more than just financial terms.

None of which is to say that the focus on treating illness is a bad idea; indeed, it is essential. Take, for example, the United Kingdom's National Health Service (NHS), which provides free healthcare for anyone who needs it. Before the Clement Attlee government set up the NHS in 1948, those who could not afford to pay a doctor simply did not see one, and that could be fatal, as my maternal great-grandfather, Albert Russell, found. Albert contracted pneumonia while out seeking work in London during the Great Depression. He lacked the necessary sixpence for a doctor's visit, and died shortly afterwards leaving behind a widow and two young children with all of the impoverishment and misery that entailed. Less than two decades later Albert Russell would have been treated for free and he might well have lived.

The NHS remains largely a world-class health facility despite having its grand vision pared back by budget cuts. As you might expect, the mix of ailments it treats has changed. When the NHS opened, 15 per cent of deaths in England were caused by pneumonia and tuberculosis; today those account for less than 5 per cent.[2] Deaths from cancers, on the other hand, have nearly doubled.

2 See, for instance: 'The NHS in Numbers: Then and Now.' BBC (2008). Accessed at: http://news.bbc.co.uk/2/hi/health/7475035.stm

Treating illness, then, is only half the battle; the other half is working to stay healthy for as long as we can. And if you are wondering how we are doing on *that* score, the answer is: not very well. We will see in the chapter on inflammation that most of today's deaths in the developed world (and increasingly in the developing world) are linked to inflammation. What contributes to inflammation, you ask? Some of the most important aspects are lifestyle factors such as consuming too much sugar and alcohol; smoking and stress; and a lack of exercise. All conspire to leave our bodies inflamed and unhealthy, which for most people will culminate in their needing medical treatment.

Ignoring our health, as so many people do, typically results in a slow and sometimes tortuous decline in the final decade, characterised by reduced mobility, lethargy, medication, depression and perhaps an operation or two. Yet with a little luck and a fair amount of effort, all of that can be avoided. As we shall see, taking care of our health today brings lifelong benefits.

OPTIMISING YOUR HEALTH

The purpose of this book is to give you the tools to live as healthily as possible; in short, to optimise your health. Should you choose to follow this philosophy – and I hope, having come as far as buying this book, that you will – then this comprehensive guide will help you get there.

There is plenty to learn, but perhaps the most important aspect revolves around understanding our pillars of health, and how to maintain them. Directly linked to those pillars are what I refer to as the Three Horsemen of the Health-pocalypse: sugar, toxins and stress, the dark riders that conspire to undermine us. On that note the book will show us:

- Why sugar lurked in our blind spot for decades, and how 'Big Food' has been damaging our health in ways similar to the deceits practised by Big Tobacco.[3]

---

3 See, for example: 'Former Advertising Executive Reveals Junk Food-pushing Tactics' by Sarah Boseley, *The Guardian* (2 January 2018).

- How our modern world is flooded with toxins, and why in many cases it is so hard to prove they are unhealthy.
- Why stress is arguably the most damaging factor in our modern, ever-busy world, and what it does to our brain and immune system.

On the plus side, we will learn how to deal with sugar, remove toxins and minimise stress. We will also look at balancing our hormones, which are the numerous chemical messengers that regulate our body's myriad functions. Our hormone balance can easily be upset by the Three Horsemen, even in people in their twenties and thirties, but the good news is that it can be reset.

Some of the hormones we encounter later in the book will sound familiar (adrenalin, testosterone, progesterone, serotonin, insulin); others might not (glucagon and somatomedin). But what really counts is how influential our hormones are, and to that end here is a snapshot that shows some of their power:

- Hormones influence whether the human embryo develops into a boy or a girl.
- Hormones drive puberty, and account for teenage mood swings that have plagued parents for millennia.
- The changes in certain hormones are associated not only with a poorer quality of life, but also with illness and death.[4]
- In the chapter on the theories of ageing, we will learn how a high insulin level switches on genes that shorten our lives; the chapter on inflammation will show why that might affect up to 80 per cent of us.
- We will see in the chapter on stress that, as the levels of our hormones produced by the adrenal glands diminish, so too does our immune system and our ability to rebuild muscle.
- And the chapter on women's health will explain why shifting hormone levels during menopause are associated with worsening health and the risk of an earlier death.

4 Brown-Borg, H. M. 'Hormonal Regulation of Longevity in Mammals.' *Ageing Res Rev* (2007): 6: 28–45.

We will find out much more besides, but for now it is enough to know that hormones are literally vital: they define us from before birth to death and, in many ways, determine our quality of life. We will also find out how some hormones can provide us with a second shot at youth, a possibility that was not available to previous generations as they smoked their way through their stresses and who, when they reached their fifties and became tired and forgetful, accepted that as a natural part of getting older.

And although we cannot avoid the passage of the years, the exciting truth about being alive today is that we no longer need to view many of the aspects we associate with ageing as inevitable. Indeed, we have an array of opportunities to maximise our health. For instance:

- We can correct hormone imbalances to reboot vitality. My clinic regularly measures the hormones of men and women in their forties (and sometimes younger), and works to rebalance them in order to boost what the French call joie de vivre or 'the joy of being alive'.
- There is a vast amount we can do to rejuvenate the skin, and by that I mean genuinely turning back the clock.
- Looking to the future, stem cells show great promise. Currently we can use them for healing and rebuilding, but their full potential is still to be unlocked. In the final chapter we will see that stem cells could one day be used to rejuvenate failing organs.

THE EVOLUTION OF HEALTHY-AGEING MEDICINE

That, then, outlines some of the path we will travel with this book, but before we get going it is useful to see how we got to where we are today. To my mind, the world of anti-ageing medicine – or, as I prefer to call it, healthy-ageing medicine – is the combination of an unlikely alliance of sports medicine, natural medicine and aesthetic medicine (which uses products such as Botox).

These subjects might seem worlds apart, but they have grown closer over the years, with the internet being the glue that has helped to bind them. Indeed, it strikes me that the internet has had an impact on society similar to that which the development of the printing press had in the 1400s. Credit for that generally goes to Johannes Gutenberg, whose method allowed books to be mass-produced where previously they had been written out by hand. As literacy spread, more people could read the Bible, as well as any number of pamphlets and tracts, and decide for themselves what was right or wrong. The spread of information on the printed page upended medieval society.

There are clear parallels with our world. Until the 1980s, many people would fall back on the venerable *Encyclopaedia Britannica*, the bulky, multi-volume set of the accumulated knowledge that sat proudly in the living rooms of those who could afford it, and which eager schoolchildren would consult for their homework. Now anyone with a smartphone can find out anything they want, including the most arcane details of any medical topic.

Indeed, someone going online has more knowledge at their fingertips than any doctor had thirty years ago. This access to information has allowed people to cast a wider net in their search for information than ever before – not always for the better, mind you, but I suspect there were similar grumbles centuries ago about the effects of publishing. One consequence has been a schism in medicine, with people turning to a booming number of practition-ers who provide a message different to that of conventional medicine.

Sports medicine

Sports medicine is perhaps the closest of the three to healthy-ageing medicine. In the early 1980s, sports medicine had a keen and understandable interest in maximising health. It was less interested in how to prevent a heart attack, and much more interested in working out health parameters that could help to answer:

- How to use science to achieve your personal best in a race.
- If you became 2 per cent dehydrated during a race, how would that affect your performance?
- The psychology behind why no runner could break the four-minute mile until Roger Bannister did in 1954, and why a flurry of runners have since done so.

Sports medicine looked at a range of aspects including nutrition, fluid intake and exercise programmes, and in that way was the first to provide the average person with easy access to scientific advice that would enhance their health. That caught people's imagination, got them off the couch and down to the track or the gym. And, instead of winning or (more likely) losing, participation became more a matter of competing against yourself and beating your personal best. That meant it did not overly matter if you lumbered along at the back of the field and crossed the finishing line long after the sponsors' banners had been cleared away. If you managed that ten seconds faster than before, then yours was a worthy victory.

In addition, the science was no longer confined to medical journals. Books were published to inspire anyone to tackle sports such as running, cycling or weightlifting. Sports magazines became far more popular too and skipped out of the shops. Many who grew up in the 1980s will remember Jane Fonda exercise videos, along with the leg warmers and the fluorescent bandannas that kept the decade's big hair in order. These were symbols of a societal change of attitude towards health – in the West at least.

In the following decade, this can-do attitude spread to other areas of our lives, helped in large part by the spread of the internet, which allowed people to take control over aspects that had previously been the domain of experts – personal finance and investing, for instance, and, most importantly for our purposes, their health.

Natural medicine

At the same time, natural medicine began its inexorable rise. What do I mean by natural medicine? Well, if you live in the US, Europe, Australia or even in my somewhat poorer nation South Africa, you will have noticed how much the products on the pharmacy shelves have changed, and how many health shops there are now, both online and on the high street. That was not the case thirty years ago. Back then your choices would be limited to a multivitamin of questionable potency, calcium tablets and some severe-looking bottles of cod liver oil. Today you can choose from multiple brands of alpha-lipoic acid, rosehip oil and echinacea, to name just three.

Natural medicine has flourished, helped in part by the information revolution. The two have worked together to generate a significant and long overdue reassessment by patients of the advice they received from their doctors. This meant patients not only felt free to question the need to take drugs for treatments, but that they could seek answers elsewhere including from friends, from the media and online. Over time, natural medicine has gained much greater credibility with the public as a relevant alternative to conventional medicine.

Natural medicine has also benefited from studies reported in the media outlining the benefits of specific compounds. One study, for example, showed how a compound called lecithin, which is a fatty substance that is found naturally in the body, could help with weight loss; others demonstrated that an amino acid (the building blocks of proteins) called L-glutamine could help to build muscle and yet another that omega acids could help limit arthritis and improve brain function.

It strikes me that this new approach, with the individual taking responsibility for his or her health, is the most significant event in medicine since the advent of the contraceptive pill. That is not to say this avalanche of information and opportunity is without its flaws; there are, after all, plenty of snake-oil salesmen out there. But it is broadly positive.

Evidence-based medicine – a side note

At the same time as patients were becoming more discerning towards their doctors, my profession was engaged in its own revolution: one known as 'evidence-based medicine'. What this term means is that, as a doctor, we can advise a patient to take a tablet only if there is enough evidence in enough high-quality studies to support doing so. The laudable idea is to standardise treatments worldwide.

You might assume that, prior to the 1990s, doctors routinely prescribed only those medicines that had been proven to work. You would be wrong. Before the advent of evidence-based medicine, this process was much more hit and miss. But today, using a huge database called the Cochrane Library, which is completely independent, and that amalgamates the results of reliable research, doctors can see what has been proven to work and can prescribe the most appropriate treatment for a particular condition.

In areas of emergency medicine and obstetrics this has brought significant clarity. Take, for example, a heart-attack patient. If you were rushed to the emergency room of your local hospital in 1985, the treatment you received would likely depend upon the whims of the consultant on duty. One might put you on a magnesium drip because he liked the study that supported that intervention. Another might make a different choice because he felt the study supporting treatment by magnesium drip was flawed.

With evidence-based medicine those personal whims are irrelevant, because the Cochrane Library has assessed every serious scientific study on the use of magnesium drips after heart attacks and made a standardised decision based on all the available evidence. The way it works is simple: the Cochrane Library's researchers conclude that the evidence is 'strongly for', 'strongly against' or 'not clear'. If the evidence is strongly for or against a particular treatment, then the doctor's decision is simple. Where the evidence is not clear, the doctor will tend to steer clear of that treatment until such time as more evidence becomes available.

In the case of magnesium drips, the researchers concluded that there was not enough benefit to recommend it after a heart attack and too much risk that it would cause low blood pressure.[5] In many countries, the Cochrane Library database is freely available, and you can search for standardised evidence on any number of topics: from whether vitamin C helps the common cold (only in huge doses) to how useful beta-blocker medication is for lowering blood pressure (quite useful).

5   Li, J. et al. 'Intravenous Magnesium for Acute Myocardial Infarction.' Cochrane (2007). Accessed at: http://www.cochrane.org/CD002755/VASC_intravenous-magnesium-for-acute-myocardial-infarction

That, then, is the good news about evidence-based medicine. Less positively there are conditions such as allergies, arthritis, asthma, fatigue and depression for which treatments are much more difficult to prove to the required standard, and where the evidence is listed as 'not clear'. Compared to the progress seen in cardiology and genetics in recent decades, the treatments for allergies and arthritis have moved slowly. As a result, we doctors have rejected natural treatments for these conditions in part because the evidence is not 'strongly positive'.

The topic is more complicated still because there is generally no cure for chronic or long-lasting conditions such as arthritis. Instead there is a plethora of treatments from acupuncture to nutrition that will help some sufferers but not others. For afflictions like arthritis and others, there are simply too many variables to reach conclusive yes or no answers. These sit in a grey zone, a place that evidence-based medicine cannot resolve. And it is in fields like that – in which many doctors hold fast to the approach that, 'If it has not been proven, we should not use it' – where we see division.

Aesthetic medicine

Aesthetic medicine is the third element in the alliance that I see as having formed healthy-ageing medicine, and it took off in the 1990s with the advent of Botox. This chemical, which is derived from the clostridium bug, freezes the muscle tissue for a few months and, in so doing, lessens wrinkles. Overnight Botox changed the way people approached cosmetic surgery. No longer was plastic surgery the exclusive domain of the rich and famous, and no longer was it a process that required days or weeks of recovery out of sight. You could pop into a clinic for a Botox injection at lunch and be back at your desk by two o'clock.

After Botox came gels called fillers, which could be injected under the skin to fill the lines that we know as wrinkles, boost sagging jowls and revitalise the skin. The principle was not new: a century ago the rich were doing much the same thing, but with toxic petroleum and injections of silicone. The difference is that modern fillers, known as hyaluronic acid fillers, are actually good for the skin, which means the more you inject (within reason), the more your skin rejuvenates.

The floodgates opened and other treatments began to find favour: mesotherapy for fine lines, sclerotherapy for thread veins, and a product known as Lipostabil, which dissolves fatty areas. Other processes designed to make the skin look younger include skin peels, carboxytherapy and laser therapy. Before long, the informal speciality called aesthetic medicine started to threaten traditional cosmetic surgery.

As with conventional medicine, this new way of doing things increasingly appealed to people who wanted to exert control over an area of their health. In a world increasingly focused on beauty and youth, aesthetic medicine provided solutions that were affordable and that did not require the permission of one's doctor.

By now the sports medicine lobby was also changing, and doctors who had become interested in the effects of hormones and nutrients on a healthy body began to share ideas. They had noticed that people were interested not only in improving their exercise performance, but that baby boomers – who by the turn of the millennium were in their fifties – were willing to pay good money to stay younger for longer.

That demand drove the industry as doctors examined different theories on the causes of premature ageing and offered treatments to tackle those causes. Key among what came next was sharp disagreement about whether to treat declining hormone levels as we age. Some practitioners felt we should support hormone levels using bio-identical supplements (hormones that are not synthetic, in other words). Others, more conventional in their views, felt equally strongly that our declining hormone levels were a natural part of growing old, and should be left to diminish naturally.

The birth of healthy-ageing medicine

Within a decade, practitioners in the fledgling field of healthy-ageing medicine had formed the A4M association in the US and EuroMediCom in Europe. Today these associations have a combined membership of more than 12,000 physicians in sixty-five countries.

The demand for healthy-ageing medicine had consequences in other areas too. Take pathology laboratories, which until then typically tested for markers of disease such as evidence of cancer. A new field opened up as people wanted to know about markers of health in their blood. Before long you could get your hormone levels tested or have a laboratory check the level of toxins in your blood. And should you want an antioxidant stress test or to find out whether you are lacking certain nutrients, well they can do that too.

Where industries go, conferences follow and by 2017 there were at least two international anti-ageing congresses a month. The 2017 EuroMediCom in Monaco drew over 11,000 delegates, many of them doctors, who came to hear talks on subjects as varied as Botox, growth hormone, heavy metal toxins and laser therapy.

Healthy-ageing medicine, which many practitioners call anti-ageing medicine, has become a fast-moving industry driven by public demand, the internet and the sheer pace of development. It is a fascinating field in which to work, though that does not mean it is all sweetness and light. Take hormones, for instance: these extraordinarily powerful substances are not fully understood, and that breeds disagreement. After all, is it even healthy to take testosterone, oestrogen or growth hormone? It is worth pointing out that some anti-ageing practitioners have been found guilty of doping charges for allowing their patients to take testosterone and human growth hormone at dangerously high levels in their quest for perfect bodies.

Given the amount of money people are prepared to spend in their quest for youth, it is not surprising that anti-ageing medicine has its share of duplicitous individuals and of rancour. In 2006, for example, a prominent US medical journal called *JAMA* published an article that claimed anti-ageing medicine was a dangerous medical group led by charlatans, and called for the doctors practising it to be struck off. The A4M hit back in the press. That anti-ageing medicine was riling some in the world of conventional medicine was hardly a surprise, but there were raised eyebrows at the public spat that ensued as the latex gloves came off.

All of this might make you wonder where matters are headed. For my part, I would like to see health medicine combine the best of conventional, natural and healthy-ageing medicine, and that is what this book is about. All three have their flaws, but together they can shape a better reality for us all.

In the meantime, change keeps coming. We have seen how fast technology has moved in the past decade with smartphones and tablets dominating our lives in ways that are both beneficial and controversial. The various medical fields have made great strides too and, if nothing else, you can bet that in the coming decade there will be benefits and controversies aplenty. Indeed, I am certain that arguments we see around, say, doping scandals in sports will pale next to the practical and ethical considerations in the fields of stem cells and genetic manipulation.

Take stem cells, for example: these are the foetal cells that build every structure in our bodies and that, in the right hands, can be extracted from our fat cells and injected into any diseased organ we hope to repair. Today's technology sees scientists working to direct stem cells to rebuild the specific organ we want to heal:[6] the ambition is that the modified stem cells that they inject migrate to the muscles, heart, liver or brain where they can carry out their repair work.

The potential to heal is immense, and so are the prospects for abuse. The off-season on the sporting calendar could easily see athletes visiting private clinics to rebuild their bodies in superhuman directions, which would make the doping scandal that surrounded disgraced US cyclist Lance Armstrong seem of little significance. And although we have come a long way in our understanding of stem-cell therapy, we are still learning about the mechanisms that tell them where to go, and we do not understand quite how they evolve into the differentiated cells that we need to rebuild organs.

6   Daoud, J. et al. 'Pancreatic Islet Culture and Preservation Strategies: Advances, Challenges and Future Outlooks.' *Cell Transplant* (2010): 19 (12): 1523–35.

So, while many developments are inspiring and although the speed of change is breathtaking, the dangers are there. The best way to face them is to arm ourselves with knowledge, and that is in part what this book is about. None of what you read here, however, will help you to avoid the inevitable. So before we find out how best to live a healthy (and hopefully long) life, it is worth considering the inescapable marker that stands at the end of all of our roads.

THE UNYIELDING REAPER

Man has always had a fascination with immortality, and that makes it a subject worthy of a brief detour with a good guide. Stephen Cave, a British philosopher, is that guide: someone who has tangled with this toughest of questions and wrote an excellent book about it.[7]

As Cave puts it, humankind has four immortality stories, and they go something like this.

First up is what he calls the 'elixir story', which is common to every culture. This is a narrative about some or other fountain of youth or magic potion that, if we could only find it, would assure eternal life. But, as he points out, every elixir-drinker in history is now dead, so we need 'a back up plan'.

That brings him to our second immortality story: physical resurrection. In this version, we understand that we will one day die, but we know too that at some point we will rise up again and live. As Cave notes, this story has translated well in the technology age – some people believe that with cryogenics (freezing themselves), a scientist will one day be able to revive them. Just as soon as humankind has the knowledge.

The third group favours the possibility of spiritual resurrection – the soul will live on into eternity even as the body crumbles to dust. This is a popular approach: in 2012, the Pew Research Center found around eight people in ten worldwide hold some form of religious belief.[8]

7   Cave, S. *Immortality: The Quest to Live Forever and How It Drives Civilization.* Crown (2012).
8   The Global Religious Landscape. Pew Research Center. 2012: http://www.pewforum. org/2012/12/18/global-religious-landscape-exec/

The fourth kind, he says, is legacy. Cave cites the Greek warrior Achilles who was killed in battle at Troy, yet whose story of heroism remains known to millions. We cannot all be Achilles, but the less heroic among us might live on through our nation or children, we might endow a library or write music, or undertake any number of feats to ensure something outlasts the physical presence. Not everyone is convinced, Cave admits, citing film-maker and comedian Woody Allen, who said: 'I don't want to live on in the hearts of my countrymen; I want to live on in my apartment.' But that approach, Cave says, merely takes us back to needing an elixir.

Cave's solution is to consider our lives as a book whose covers mark our birth and death. When we read a novel, the characters created by the writer are not aware of anything outside their own story, and that does not change when the book is closed. As a result, those characters do not fear the moment when the reader reaches the end.

'The only thing that matters (for your happiness in life),' Cave wrote, 'is that you make it a good story.'

If you ask me, Cave is right, but that does not stop many of us from going to great lengths to dye our telltale grey hairs, pluck our nose hairs and conceal our wrinkles, ultimately all in a deep-seated bid to dodge death. Those external signs of ageing are what we fear and what our culture abhors: we live in a society that venerates the young and the beautiful, and negates the old.

Other cultures see matters differently. In his book *The Metabolic Plan*, American nutritional biochemist Stephen Cherniske writes of when he worked among tribal peoples in Papua New Guinea, and his question, 'How old are you?' drew the response, 'Fine, wonderful.' It was not a matter of being lost in translation; it was simply that they saw life and death differently, with the latter, in Cherniske's words, 'something that happens in the course of events, like rain'.

The perception by young people of their tribal elders was different too, with the words 'wise, respected, venerable, beloved, experienced' commonly used. In our culture, Cherniske notes, people generally describe senior citizens with words such as 'grizzled, old, grey', which is hardly positive.

With views like that it is no wonder we spend a lot of money hiding the signs of ageing or keeping ourselves so busy that we have no time to worry about it. Yet although it is logically impossible to separate our impending death from our current life, few of us feel comfortable thinking deeply about it until it is much too late. The Lebanese writer Kahlil Gibran tackled that in his classic *The Prophet*, in which he wrote:

> *You would know the secret of death,*
> *But how shall you find it unless you seek it in the heart of life?*
> *. . . If you would indeed behold the spirit of death, open your heart wide*
> *   unto the body of life.*
> *For life and death are one, even as the river and the sea are one.*

Gibran's point is that if we are in touch with life and are living it fully then we will develop a comfortable understanding of death. Yet our society is arguably further from being in touch with death now than at any time. Commonly when a loved one dies, they are whisked off to a mortuary before anyone has the opportunity to sit with the body, mourn their passing and start the process of moving on. Previous generations laid out the deceased at home, allowing friends and relatives, including children, to pay their last respects, and experience the circle of life.

Today many elderly people die in nursing homes, not the family home. Death has become a remote and sterile event. Yet if we do not see death, then we are not forced to confront it, and in that case how can we hope to understand it? Our fear of death is natural, but our avoidance of its reality is, I would submit, unhealthy.

Native Americans were afraid not of death but of a dishonourable death, and so they planned how they would react in certain circumstances to ensure honour in death. Facing the concept takes some of the fear out of it and, as Cave points out, the solution is to face up to its reality: make a will; decide whether you want to be buried or cremated and, if the latter, then where you would like your ashes scattered. It is a small start, but it begins to bring the concept of death into our consciousness. If we can achieve our death with minimal suffering, having achieved our life's purpose and having said goodbye to our loved ones, then that in my view would qualify as an honourable death.

The Roman senator Seneca, whose classic work *On the Shortness of Life* contains hours of wisdom still relevant 2,000 years after he penned it, was not short of advice on life's purpose to his fellow citizens, most of whom, in his view, frittered away their lives inconsequentially.

'You are living as if destined to live forever: your own frailty never occurs to you,' Seneca wrote in scolding fashion. 'You act like mortals in all that you fear, and like immortals in all that you desire. You hear many people saying: "When I am fifty I shall retire into leisure; when I am sixty I shall give up public duties."'

Seneca chastised busy people for regarding the art of living as their 'least important activity'.

'Yet there is nothing which is harder to learn,' he wrote. 'But learning how to live takes a whole life, and, which might surprise you more, it takes a whole life to learn how to die. So you must not think a man has lived long because he has white hair and wrinkles: he has not lived long, just existed long . . . He did not have a long voyage, just a long tossing about.'

And so, with the waspish words of Seneca ringing in our ears, it is time to turn away from the compelling topic of death to the theories of ageing because, while there are many books that cover the subject of death, and while I would encourage you to read widely on it, this book's lessons are concerned with the years you have ahead of the Grim Reaper's inevitable arrival.

To that end, the next chapter will look at some of the different theories of ageing. The bad news is that there is no elixir of life – not yet, at any rate. And so, as Cave suggests, it makes sense to have a backup plan.

My backup plan, which you are welcome to adopt, is to live a Younger for Longer life: a way of living that should bring a long and healthy life and then a peaceful death after a rapid decline. As we shall see in the next chapter, disregarding our health generally leads to a worse outcome: a long decline, with the last decade spent in pain and unhappiness.

And even though it is much too late to ask him, I feel confident that my backup plan is one that even the grumpy Seneca would have agreed is worth striving for.

Chapter 2

THEORIES OF AGEING – GREAT MINDS DON'T THINK ALIKE

I told you I was ill.

The inscription on the grave of British-Irish comedian Spike Milligan

There is little new in the quest for immortality. Take the philosopher's stone, for example – a substance believed to turn base metals into gold, and perhaps to convey the ultimate prize: everlasting life. To seek out the philosopher's stone was a noble calling, and evidence of this search goes back millennia. The Arabic phrase *al-'iksir* refers to the preparation that supposedly could do either of those things, and is the source of the English word 'elixir'. There are references to it in Buddhism, Taoism and Hinduism, evidence of a widespread fascination for immortality.

The search for the stone in physical form may have ended, but its spirit lives on. Today's alchemists wear lab coats and enjoy the funding of Silicon Valley billionaires: Google's Larry Page, for instance, was involved in setting up Calico, a biotech company focused on preventing ageing, and which has employed top scientists such as Cynthia Kenyon whom we will meet later. Microsoft's Bill Gates and Paul Allen have donated vast sums to medicine, including towards the issue of longevity. And Facebook's Mark Zuckerberg and his wife have pledged billions towards curing all disease by the end of the century.

But perhaps my favourite modern-day alchemist is a Briton whose magnificent beard would have made the druids proud. Aubrey de Grey used his inheritance to start a regenerative medicine non-profit organisation in California called the SENS Research Foundation. De Grey revels in shaking things up, and has made statements that both thrill and appal, including saying that "the first person to live to be a thousand might be sixty already".[1] De Grey's view is that ageing is merely a disease that can be cured, a view he outlines in his theory called Strategies for Engineered Negligible Senescence, or SENS. So controversial is this that in 2005 the *MIT Technology Review*, a prestigious US publication, offered a $20,000 prize to any qualified molecular biologist who could prove that de Grey's SENS theory was 'so wrong that it is unworthy of learned debate'. To date the prize remains unclaimed.

Some regard de Grey as a provocateur, others as someone ahead of his time. He seems unfazed either way, simply saying that it takes 'a certain amount of guts to aim high'.

That is certainly true, so with that sentiment in mind let us suspend what we believe to be true and aim high. Is ageing merely a disease – a curable condition? And is it necessary for us to age? Or to age as fast as we do? After all, nature does not restrict every creature to our arguably short lifespan:

- Sturgeon fish, for instance, can live to 150 years without appearing to age, and then die with no apparent damage to their organs; bowhead whales can live to 200.
- The so-called immortal jellyfish (*turritopsis dohrnii*) that is found in the Mediterranean and off Japan is only 4.5mm at full height, but it never dies, unless eaten by a predator. Instead it divides to make offspring. In tough times it retreats back to being a polyp.
- Other creatures that might display immortality are hydra – which are tiny creatures found in freshwater ponds – as well as planarian flatworms and some fungi and bacteria.
- And then there is my favourite: an ocean quahog clam nicknamed Ming, which was caught in 2006 and was thought to have been 507 years old. (Unfortunately for Ming, 2006 was also its final year.)

Even within orders of animals there are huge discrepancies. Rats live for about two years, but a fellow rodent called the naked mole rat, which we will meet later, does not get cancer and can reach thirty.

---

1 'We will be able to live to 1,000.' *BBC News* (2004). Accessed at: http://news.bbc.co.uk/2/hi/uk/4003063.stm

As we shall see in this chapter, many theories try to describe the ageing process. One of the most basic reckons that our cells can divide only a fixed number of times before they become what is known as 'senescent', which in cellular terms means the cell can no longer divide and grow. That happens because the ends of the DNA strands – called telomeres, which are often likened to a cap like the tag on the end of a shoelace, and which protect our genetic code – shorten each time the cell divides, and eventually run out of length. At that point, the cell can no longer divide.[2] Studies have shown that the accumulation of senescent cells leads to inflammation and then cancer and degenerative diseases.[3]

Figure 1: A DNA chromosome showing at its end the telomeres, which shorten each time the cell divides

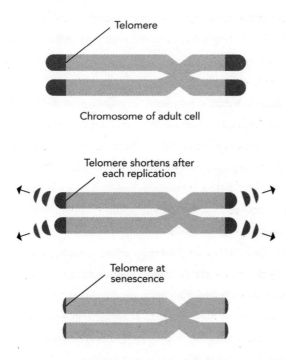

2 Bekaert, S. et al. 'Telomere biology in mammalian germ cells and during development.' *Develop Biol* (2004): 274: 15–30.
3 Campisi, J. 'Aging, cellular senescence and cancer.' *Annu Rev Physiol* (2013): 75: 685–705. Accessed at: https://www.ncbi.nlm.nih.gov/pmc/articles/PMC4166529/

Linked to this is the concept of entropy, which is all around us: a garden, for instance, will become overgrown and wild if left to its own devices, and a car will eventually rust into a heap. This gradual slide into disorder also happens to us as we age – our cells become senescent, which accounts for the body's general weakening and decay.

Oddly, though, parts of us *do* avoid entropy. By the time we reach our mid-thirties we have accumulated a significant amount of damage, but we can still create a baby that has no signs of entropy. Called 'negative entropy', it refers to the fact that some of our cells never stop dividing: for example, the germ cells in the testes that can divide continuously to form sperm. An enzyme in those cells (called telomerase) protects the telomeres on their DNA from shortening, and that makes them immortal.[4] And on the subject of telomeres, scientists in 2017 were able to reactivate senescent cells, lengthen their telomeres and get them to start dividing again.[5] That is an exciting development, and the hope is that this could help to counter the degenerative diseases associated with ageing.

In other words, our bodies contain cells that do not follow the rules of entropy and that will divide repeatedly for as long as we live; and we have found a way to reactivate senescent cells and allow them to divide again. All of this means there is growing evidence that we can do quite a lot about the ageing process. Could modern-day alchemists be closing in on the philosopher's stone?

Perhaps they are, but that day remains some way off. In the meantime, to understand ageing better we need to look at some of the theories of ageing and the research that has led us this far, and that is the purpose of this chapter. And while the likes of de Grey are perfectly entitled to consider the possibility of immortality, we will try to work with what has already been discovered.

4 Ozturk, S. 'Telomerase activity and telomere length in male germ cells.' *Biol Reprod* (2015): 92: 53.
5 Latorre, E. et al. 'Small molecule modulation of splicing factor expression is associated with rescue from cellular senescence.' *BMC Cell Biol* (2017): 18: 31. Accessed at: https://bmccellbiol.biomedcentral.com/articles/10.1186/s12860-017-0147-7

LIFESPAN AND HEALTHSPAN

Our expected lifespan is seventy-eight years, give or take. But to my mind a more important measure is our Healthspan, which is the number of years we are healthy; after all, the longer we are healthy, the better our quality of life. And although there is currently not much we can do to extend our lifespan – attaining the spectacular age of Ming the quahog clam looks out of reach – there are plenty of steps we can take to improve our Healthspan.

Indeed, of the multitude of theories proposed to explain why we age, only two have been proven to help us live longer – in other words, to extend our lifespan. Those are calorie restriction and lowering our basal temperature, and we will meet them both. Antioxidants, which were once the great hope, have so far failed to extend lifespan convincingly, as we shall see.

Before we launch into the different anti-ageing theories, you might be surprised to learn just how hard it is to increase lifespan. If we cured all cancers, for instance, one study suggests that we would increase the population's average lifespan by just over three years (in other words, we could expect to live to eighty-one).[6] It is the same story for heart attacks – preventing every death from that cause would add just three more years.[7] That tells us that a healthy ageing treatment that would extend the population's *lifespan* significantly would need to be very special indeed.

And so to the theories that purport to describe ageing, and of which there are many. On the grounds that they cannot all be correct, I have outlined some of the most interesting and credible. The point is that once we understand why we think we age, we should be able to look more critically at what we are told will help us. And that is what much of the rest of the book will tackle.

6 Arias, E. et al. 'United States life tables eliminating certain causes of death 1999–2001.' *National Vital Statistics Reports* (2013): 61: 9. https://www.cdc.gov/nchs/data/nvsr/nvsr61/nvsr61_09.pdf
7 Ibid.

THE THEORIES OF AGEING

At the most basic level, any satisfactory theory should provide the following:

- A reasonable explanation as to why its proponent believes it to be true; and,
- A study, which is usually carried out on animals, to prove that the theory is true, and which can be repeated.

Without those elements, any theory's outcome could be down to chance and skewed statistics. Yet even with them, as we shall see, it is common to encounter scientific rebuttals explaining why a theory might be nonsense. It is in this way – assertion, debate, counter-assertion, and so on – that theories evolve.

For our purposes, following the threads of these evolving theories brings us through the labyrinth of competing ideas to the current sum of knowledge today, rather in the manner that the Greek hero Theseus used a ball of wool to find his way back through the subterranean labyrinth after slaying the half-bull, half-man Minotaur. Usefully, this process will also arm us to decide for ourselves which of the myriad supplements that are advertised for our health are any use. After all, although the ball of wool was essential for Theseus to guide himself, he still needed that sword.

The theories we will look at can be divided into two groups: Random Theories of ageing and Genetic Theories of ageing, and at their most basic level they consider how much of the ageing process is caused by environmental factors and how much is due to genetic causes. A renowned study carried out in 1996 on Danish twins shows that both factors count, with 75 per cent of ageing attributed to environmental causes and the remaining 25 per cent due to genetic reasons.[8]

So there, upfront, is the good news. Our lifestyle, which we obviously can influence, seems to be much more important than our genes in determining our health and how we age. Armed with that piece of information, let us look in a bit more detail at these two groups.

Random Theories: these revolve around preventing premature ageing or

8 Herskind, A. M. et al. 'The heritability of human longevity: a population-based study of 2872 Danish twins born 1870–1900.' *Human Genetics* (1996): 97: 319–23.

improving our Healthspan. Any factor from sunburn to smoking, and plenty in between, that causes inflammation in the body will cause us to age before our time. In other words, if our genes are designed to get us to 100 but our lifestyle means we die at seventy-eight, then the potential improvement is obvious. When we start removing damaging factors from our bodies, we allow ourselves to live each day to its full potential.

Genetic Theories: these are equally fascinating and – like the Minotaur – a potentially far more dangerous beast. Some scientists believe that if we could determine what causes our genetic DNA to stop dividing then we could ensure that people could extend their lifespan and live forever. (And if that sounds too much like science fiction, you will be interested to hear that a 2016 study on mice showed that manipulating their genes extended their lifespan by 25 per cent. By splicing in a bit of genetic code, the mice were much more effective at removing senescent cells, which meant they were healthier and lived longer.)[9]

The two classes of theory also suggest a host of ethical, societal and moral dilemmas that lie beyond the scope of this book, including: at what age should we retire, given that the longer we work the more easily we could afford expensive organ-rebuilding procedures? Could governments fund pensions and health costs for citizens who live for several hundred years? Do we stop at manipulations that prolong life, or should we use genetics to customise an entire body? And at what stage of this process have we started to play God?

Should these possibilities become a reality, it is likely that the world would be pushed even further into a two-tier existence where those with money and the time to pursue medical interventions would live much longer, while the poorer majority would live shorter lives, eat worse food, and not have access to these medical advances. In the US today, nearly two-thirds of men aged sixty-two to seventy-four with a professional degree are still working versus just one-third of their peers who have a high-school certificate. The 'haves'

---

9   Baker, D. J. et al. 'Naturally occurring p16ink4a positive cells shorten healthy lifespan.' *Nature* (2016): 530-184-89. https://www.nature.com/articles/nature16932

earn more, stay healthier for longer and work far longer than the 'have nots'. In Europe the pattern is similar.[10]

But for now we will leave the amazing (and possibly horrifying) possibilities of genetic manipulation, and instead look at some of the Random Theories of ageing that have evolved over the past century or so.

Wear and Tear Theory

Allow me to introduce you to August Weismann, a rather severe-looking German gentleman with glasses and a beard who concluded his professional life in 1910 as professor of zoology at the venerable University of Freiburg in the south-western corner of Germany, tucked up to the Black Forest near the borders of Switzerland and France.

Weismann, relatively unknown today, was a giant of the period: he was one of the most important evolutionary theorists of the nineteenth century, second only to Charles Darwin. Like much in the realm of scientific endeavour, Weismann's work was derived from studies he carried out on animals – in his case on the humble sea urchin between 1896 and 1910. His defining work came at the end of a life in which he had been a researcher, a medical doctor and an academic.

Weismann derived his Wear and Tear Theory after observing that a horse grinds down its teeth through the duration of its life, and that once this happens it can no longer eat, and it wastes away. That theory is useful today in helping us to understand degeneration in three areas of the body: the liver, the cells and our DNA. Take the liver, one of our most important organs. Its role is to remove toxins and hormones from the body, but as we get older the liver becomes damaged and no longer works as well. Once hormones such as oestrogen, for example, are not properly processed through the liver, they become rancid and can cause cancer, cellulite formation and fat accumulation.

The same problem of wear and tear also takes place on a cellular level as the organelles (the tiny organs of life inside each cell) become damaged from use. In the end the cell's repair system fails and the damaged cell dies, an outcome known as apoptosis.

10 'A billion shades of grey'. *The Economist* (26 April 2014).

This theory is also useful to describe how wear and tear happens every time a cell divides – at the level of DNA, the genetic coding of chromosomes that lies in a double helix inside each cell. Earlier we encountered the telomeres, the small protective casings at the end of each DNA strand that prevent the ends of those strands from fraying. But every time the DNA divides to form two new cells, this telomere casing shortens. Once the telomere is gone, the DNA can no longer divide and, as we saw earlier, the cell becomes senescent. Too many of those leaves us susceptible to inflammation and degenerative disease.

Weismann's Wear and Tear Theory was regarded as a pillar of ageing for decades, and it was not until the 1950s that British Nobel laureate Peter Medawar came up with the first reasonable challenge to it. Medawar proposed a randomness to ageing that is particularly notable in our DNA. He suggested that it is not just wear and tear that damages genes, but that the longer they are around, the greater the chance that they will suffer damage at some point. He found that DNA damage in older people is more accelerated than one would expect.

Also around that time the American academic George C. Williams noted how strange it was that many species were vibrantly virile in their youth, reproducing extensively, but that this ability declined rapidly before they became old. Williams theorised an 'antagonistic pleiotropic (AP) effect', which in plain English means that those factors that contribute to our youthful vibrancy can turn around and accelerate our decline when we age. In other words, Mother Nature finds us useful when we are young and fertile, but speeds up the process of getting rid of us once we are past our reproductive years. One example, seen in both humans and mice, is growth hormone: those with naturally high levels of this are stronger, more virile and more attractive as young adults, but they tend to age more quickly and die younger than their low-level peers.[11]

11 Masternak, M. M. et al. 'Growth hormone, inflammation and aging.' *Pathobiol Aging Age Relat Dis* (2012): 2: 10. Accessed at: https://www.ncbi.nlm.nih.gov/pmc/articles/PMC3417471/

Speed of Life Theory

The next theory was developed in 1908 by the German scientist Max Rubner. His theory, which is also known as the Rate of Living Theory, holds that animals that live quickly and whose hearts race, die younger. Compare mice and elephants, for instance. The average mouse clocks around 1 billion heartbeats in a couple of years before it dies, but it takes an elephant its lifespan of sixty to seventy years to reach that number of heartbeats.

There is a size versus lifespan ratio that most animals fit neatly into: mice, for example, are tiny and live just a year or two; rabbits can reach ten in captivity while lions can make it to thirty. Elephants can live to seventy.

There is a simple relationship of Size:Lifespan that these animals follow and it gives them a Lifespan Quotient of 1 (LQ=1). However other creatures – including humans – function differently:

- Humans who live to 100 defy this formula and have an LQ of 4.5
- Naked mole rats cheat death on many levels. They live to thirty and also enjoy an LQ of 4.5.
- Best of all are the tiny Hagrid's bats, which clock in with a staggering 9.8 LQ, twice as impressive as any centenarian human. Then again, they do have to survive in Siberia's tough climes, so perhaps we should not envy them too much.

Waste Accumulation Theory

Animals become senescent, which as we have seen is medical-speak for 'worn out', because they accumulate more waste than they can comfortably get rid of. If our cells fill with toxins faster than they can be removed, then those cells stop functioning efficiently and start to malfunction. You might recognise that this is similar to how the Wear and Tear Theory applies to liver damage.

Lysosomes are our cells' garbage-collecting system and so, under this theory, improving lysosomal functioning should improve the cell's longevity. Studies have shown this to be true: the healthier the lysosome, the longer that particular cell lives.[12]

12 Carmona-Gutierrez, C. et al. 'The crucial impact of lysosomes in aging and longevity.' *Ageing Res Rev* (2016): 32: 2–12.

Failing Endocrine System Theory

Our hormone system is also known as our endocrine system, and in later chapters we will see that the levels of many of our hormones decrease with age. This involves not just the sex hormones (oestrogen, progesterone and testosterone), but the *entire hormone system* including melatonin, growth hormone and serotonin (the happiness hormone made in the brain), thyroid hormone, insulin from the pancreas, and DHEA (a welcome abbreviation for dehydroepiandrosterone), which is manufactured by the adrenal glands.

For growth hormone (GH) this decrease is probably a good thing, because high levels of GH are associated with cancer and an early death.[13] Similarly, high insulin levels in otherwise healthy adults, a condition known as insulin resistance, is a key driver for heart attacks, cancer and an early death.[14] (In the chapter on nutrition we will see how to keep this level low as we age.)

So although lower insulin and GH levels *are* healthy as we age, the fact that our sex hormones tend to decline is generally not. In later chapters we will explore how boosting the levels of these hormones can be beneficial provided it is done correctly. For example:

- Elderly men with naturally high levels of DHEA, which is a hormone that among other things boosts our immune system, tend to live longer than elderly men with low levels of DHEA.[15]
- Replacing oestrogen and progesterone in menopausal women is healthier than not replacing it.[16]

13 Bartke, J. 'Growth hormone and aging: A challenging controversy.' *Clin Interv Aging* (2008): 3: 659–65.
14 Zhang, X. et al. 'Fasting insulin, insulin resistance and risk of cardiovascular or all-cause mortality in non-diabetic adults: A meta-analysis.' *Biosci Rep* (2017): 37. Accessed at: https://www.ncbi.nlm.nih.gov/pubmed/28811358
15 Ravaglia, G. et al. 'Determinants of Functional Status in Healthy Italian Nonagenarians and Centenarians: A Comprehensive Functional Assessment by the Instruments of Geriatric Practice.' *J Am Geriatr Soc* (1997): 45: 10: 1196–202.
16 Sarrel, P. M. et al. 'The mortality toll of oestrogen avoidance: An analysis of excessive deaths among hysterectomized women aged 50 to 59 years.' *Am J Public Health* (2013): 103: 1583–8.

- Replacing testosterone in men – if done correctly – is associated with improving their immune system and lowering their risk of a heart attack.[17]

Our hormones are fascinating indeed, and my work has shown me that optimising these levels can make a huge difference to the quality of life of middle-aged men and women.

Free Radical Theory

When patients come to see me for the first time, they sometimes arrive with a bag of supplements. Most are antioxidants like vitamins C, E and A, and they work, in theory, by neutralising the damaging molecules in the body that we call free radicals. The Free Radical Theory has been *the* anti-ageing theory for decades and has earned health shops a lot of money. But is there any truth to it?

When Denham Harman proposed the Free Radical Theory in 1954, nobody took him seriously. He had started out as a scientist working in the oil industry, but went back to university at thirty-eight to study medicine. He became fascinated with ageing and, instead of going into private practice, took a job at a laboratory to work out why we age. He came up with his now famous theory that cells become damaged when free radicals – which are atoms or molecules that lack an unpaired electron on their oxygen element – bounce around the cell like unstable magnets causing havoc. The most common free radical is an unstable form of oxygen called superoxide (O_2-). Given that oxygen is used extensively in every cell in the body to make energy, the fact that superoxide is so prevalent is not surprising.

Today Harman's proposals are widely accepted, but in 1954 this was revolutionary stuff. It took a decade before his theory was recognised as a central component of ageing, and that happened only after scientists discovered an antioxidant known as superoxide dismutase, or SOD, that lives inside cells. The presence of this intracellular antioxidant meant there *had* to be free

---

17 Hanke, H. et al. 'Effect of testosterone on plaque development and androgen receptor expression in the arterial vessel wall.' *Circulation* (2001): 103: 1382–5.

radicals there for the SOD to neutralise – otherwise, why would it be there in the first place? And indeed, tackling antioxidants in the cells is exactly what it does: one of SOD's key jobs is to remove the unstable superoxide O2- that we met earlier.[18]

Any joint or muscle or area of skin that is warm, swollen or red is probably inflamed, and that means there are too many free radicals bouncing around. We know these free radicals cause an increase in the levels of an inflammatory messenger called NFϰB, which if left unchecked can cause DNA damage.[19] What the antioxidants do is act as firefighters, putting out these free radical flames.

Antioxidants get their name because they calm down the free radicals' unstable molecule by donating an electron to the oxygen element; this provides stability, which stops the damaging oxidation process. The body makes its own antioxidants, of course, but there are plenty of supplements available including vitamins C, E, A, coenzyme Q10, melatonin, testosterone and oestrogen.[20] The protective effects of antioxidants are borne out by numerous studies that show, for example, that vitamin A and C reduce sun damage, DNA damage and skin cancer.[21]

In short order, the Free Radical Theory became the most widely quoted theory of ageing, and vitamin C and other antioxidants became popular supplements. The understanding behind the theory was this: the more antioxidants we take, the quicker they will snuff out inflammation before it starts and the less damage we will suffer. It seemed logical, and there are plenty of studies that show we do accumulate more oxidative damage as we age.[22] But three cracks eventually appeared:

18 Fukai, T. et al. 'Superoxide dismutases: Role in redox signaling, vascular functioning and diseases.. *Antioxid Redox Signal* (2011): 15: 1583–606.

19 Morgan, M. J. et al. 'Crosstalk of reactive oxygen species and NFkB signaling.' *Cell Res* (2011): 21: 103–15.

20 Reiter, R. J. et al. 'Melatonin as an anti-oxidant: Under-promises but over-delivers.' *J Pineal Res* (2016): 61: 253–78.

21 Dreher, F. 'Topical antioxidants protect against UVA & UVB sun damage.' *Curr Probl Dermatol* (2001): 29: 157–64.

22 Stadtman, E. R. 'Review: Protein oxidation and aging.' *Science* (1992): 257: 1220–4.

- Firstly, free radicals do not *always* harm us. Experiments on worms show that if the main antioxidant mechanism in their cells (the SOD system) is switched off, then the worms do not die at a young age from damage caused by free radicals, and some even live longer.[23] That is contrary to what we would expect with the Free Radical Theory, which tells us that the free radicals should have caused irreparable damage.

- Secondly, it turns out that free radicals can boost the protective capacity of our SOD system – which is a good thing.[24] However, that is not what the Free Radical Theory says; it tells us that exercise leads to a release of free radicals, which causes inflammation and potential damage to the muscle cells[25] – which is a bad thing. But it turns out that this exercise-induced inflammation can be beneficial because it wakes up the cell's antioxidant system by increasing SOD activity in the cell, and that gives enhanced protection from free radical damage.[26] In other words, some short-term pain for some long-term cellular gain.

- Lastly, we now know that free radicals actually *encourage* muscle repair and cell growth. So, although too many free radicals damage our cells, a certain level is necessary to stimulate a process involving the inflammatory messenger NFκB, which we met earlier, and which repairs cells and encourages cell growth.[27] This inflammatory pathway

---

23   Van Raamsdonk, J. et al. 'Deletion of the mitochondrial Superoxide dismutase SOD-2 extends life in *Caenorhabditis Elegans*.' *PLoS Genetics* (2009). Accessed at: http://journals. plos.org/plosgenetics/article?id=10.1371/journal.pgen.1000361

24   Sun, J. et al. 'Sequential Upregulation of Superoxide Dismutase 2 and Heme Oxygenase 1 by tert-Butylhydroquinone Protects Mitochondria during Oxidative Stress.' *Mol Pharmacol* (2015): 88 (3): 437–49.

25   Davies, K. J. et al. 'Free radicals and tissue damage produced by exercise.' *Biochem Biophys Res Commun* (1982): 107: 1198–205.

26   Hitomi, Y. et al. 'Acute exercise increases expression of extracellular superoxide dismutase in skeletal muscle and the aorta.' *Redox Rep* (2008): 13 (5): 213–16.

27   Morgan, M. J. et al. 'Crosstalk of reactive oxygen species and NFκB signalling.' *Cell Res* (2011): 21: 103–315.

is stimulated by exercise such as running or lifting weights to make our muscles stronger.

All of which means that although free radicals are part of the problem when it comes to accumulating toxins and damage within our cells, we do need them in order to grow and repair our cells. (Not for the last time I will tell you that a Younger for Longer life is about balance.) That is why flooding the body with antioxidants is probably counterproductive. And we know this because research showed that, for example, giving antioxidants to either rats or mice did not make them live longer.

Take the studies on mice, which Harman and others worked on in the 1960s and 1970s, giving them different antioxidants and measuring their effects. Frustratingly, it was a case of one step forward and two steps backwards. For example, although cancer-prone mice seemed to benefit for a time from having antioxidants, other mice did not live any longer. And although antioxidants saw the *average* lifespan improve (more mice lived to an expected old age), the *maximum* lifespan did not rise beyond what was expected.[28] In other words, antioxidants seemed to reduce disease but not to increase lifespans.

Researchers also found the same effect in rats: giving them antioxidants did not help them to live longer. They had wondered whether naked mole rats lived up to fifteen times longer than normal rats because they have less cellular stress caused by free radicals; instead they found that antioxidants did not account for that.[29]

Cyanide, anyone?

Free radicals are charged particles, and these are essential to life. If we were to remove all free radicals from the body, then our nerves would not conduct signals, and we would die.

28 Harman, D. 'Free radical theory of aging: dietary implications.' *Am J Clin Nutr* (1972): 839–43.
29 Andziak, B. et al. 'Antioxidants do not explain the disparate longevity between mice and the longest living rodent, the naked mole-rat.' *Mech Ageing Dev* (2005): 126: 1206–12.

That is how cyanide works. Indeed, cyanide is the ultimate anti-oxidant, removing all charged particles and so stopping the nerves from conducting. It is, of course, *not* recommended.

By 2000, we had learned a lot about antioxidants: we knew free radicals could be damaging, and that antioxidants could protect us from that damage; we knew free radicals harm our cells and in particular the mitochondria in our cells;[30] and we knew that the older we are, the more protein-scarring we have from free radical damage.[31]

We also knew that antioxidants are protective:

- The SOD system inside our cells protects those cells from free radical damage.
- Fruit flies that have a stronger antioxidant system live longer than other fruit flies.[32]
- Antioxidant supplements in humans reduce the chances of skin cancer by protecting DNA found in the skin.[33]

By then we had also learned that free radicals are important to life, and that antioxidants are not as beneficial as we had hoped. Naked mole rats, for example, are extensively scarred from free radical damage yet this does not cause them to die early.[34] And although exercise causes free radical damage to cells, this stimulates the cell's SOD system and encourages cell repair. We also found that antioxidant supplements do not increase the lifespan of mice or rats.

30 Ozawa, T. 'Mitochondrial DNA Mutations and Age.' in *Towards Prolongation of the Healthy Lifespan: Practical Approaches to Intervention*. Eds D. Harman, R. Holliday. New York Academy of Sciences (1998).

31 Stadtman, E. R. 'Protein oxidation and aging.' *Science* 257 (1991): 1220–4.

32 Zuo, Y. et al. 'Black rice extract extends the lifespan of fruit flies.' *Food Funct* (2012). Accessed at: http://pubs.rsc.org/-/content/articlelanding/2012/fo/c2fo30135k/unauth#!div Abstract

33 Dreher, F. 'Topical antioxidants protect against UVA & UVB sun damage'. *Curr Probl Dermatol* (2001): 29: 157–64.

34 Andziak, B. et al. 'Antioxidants do not explain the disparate longevity between mice and the longest living rodent, the naked mole-rat'. *Mech Ageing Dev* (2005): 126: 1206–12.

With progress stalling, the once-favourable opinions on antioxidant supplements began to swing in the opposite direction, with suggestions that the supplements might even be harmful. While low-dose multivitamins with antioxidants were seen as being a good idea, particularly given the nutrient-depleted foods many people eat, it was felt that the use of very high-dose vitamin C could be counterproductive. That position was further supported in 2005 by the results of four major clinical trials suggesting that supplementing with vitamin E, another antioxidant, not only failed to protect from cancer, but also slightly increased the chance of premature death.[35]

It was a puzzle. After all, if we know free radicals damage DNA *and* we know SOD is the intra-cellular antioxidant that prevents this from happening, then why would vitamin E have a harmful effect? The best theory we have to explain this is that swamping the cells with antioxidants switches off the natural SOD protective process, and this leaves cells susceptible to damage when the next batch of free radicals arrives.

In summary, then, free radicals damage cells, and our SOD system prevents this harm. Some free radical damage from daily exercise appears to stimulate our cells and wake up our SOD system, and is therefore beneficial. Too much free radical damage appears to be harmful.

If for example we are sunburned – which is basically lots of free radical damage on the skin – and our SOD system is unable to cope with that, then applying an antioxidant like vitamin C serum to the skin is beneficial, as we shall see in the chapter on the skin. But taking *daily* high-dose antioxidants probably does more harm than good.

The future of the Free Radical Theory will be in studies that look to stimulate our SOD system.

The rise and demise of EUK-8

By the turn of the millennium, after companies had spent millions

---

35 Guallar, E. et al. 'An editorial update: Annus horribilis for vitamin E.' *Ann Intern Med* (2005): 143: 143–5.

trying to find an antioxidant that could extend life, a small firm called Eukarion came up with a result that made global headlines. Rather than trying to remove free radicals using antioxidant supplements, Eukarion decided to support the SOD system in our cells.

It developed an antioxidant called EUK-8 that was not only a super-efficient mimic of SOD, but which also performs something called catalase activity – removing a harmful product of SOD and turning it into water. In a famous study on worms, Eukarion extended their lifespan by half by giving them EUK-8.[36]

Not surprisingly, the medical world took notice. At last, to the relief of anti-ageing practitioners, the study of ageing, known as gerontology, was being viewed as a serious medical speciality. They could even show off the proof, as carried in one respected peer-reviewed journal, that a tablet could extend lifespan, even if it could only do so in a worm.

Sadly, that turned out to be EUK-8's highpoint. Another study two years later showed that EUK-8 could not do the same in house-flies or in other types of worms, and the excitement dissipated.[37] But the search goes on for supplements that will stimulate the SOD system, rather than flood it with antioxidants taken in supplement form.

Gerontogenes Theory

Until the early 1970s, it was widely assumed there was very little we could do about ageing, and that any anti-ageing quest was doomed to failure. Broadly speaking, the consensus was that we just wear out, and that therefore our hope was to take antioxidants to try to slow the damage. The idea that certain

36 Melov, S. et al. 'Extension of life-span with superoxide dismutase/catalase mimetics.' *Science* (2000): 289: 1567–9.
37 Bayne, A. C. et al. 'Effects of superoxide dismutase/catalase on lifespan and oxidative stress resistance in the housefly, Musca domestica.' *Free Radic Biol Med* (2002): 32: 1229–34.

genes might be able to play a part in helping us to live longer was not a serious consideration.

Some scientists, though, did wonder whether there were genes that oversee the ageing process, and they christened this class of (then-theoretical) genes 'gerontogenes'. In research involving long-lived fruit flies, evolutionary biologist Michael Rose showed about 2 per cent of their genes were involved in controlling ageing.[38] That raised the questions: what are those genes and can they be turned off and on?

In the 1990s Cynthia Kenyon, then the leading light in the field of worm gene research, 'got lucky' (in her words) and discovered that disabling a gene known as Daf-2 could double a worm's lifespan.[39] Even more amazing was how lifestyle affected that gene: give the worm sugar and the gene turned on, stimulated insulin and resulted in the worm dying younger. Remove sugar and the gene turned off, resulting in no insulin spikes and long-living worms.

Kenyon then showed that switching off another longevity gene, known as Daf-16, saw the worms live even longer. Because Daf-16 normally shortens life, it was predictably enough nicknamed the 'Grim Reaper'. Before long, the FOXO gene was discovered – and nicknamed the 'Sweet-16 gene' as it keeps even humans looking younger for longer – and has been linked to longevity.[40]

Next it was the turn of resveratrol, the antioxidant found in the skin of grapes that gives us the excuse to enjoy a glass of red wine guilt-free. Researcher David Sinclair found that resveratrol could extend the life of the humble yeast by turning on a gene called SIR.[41] Studies of flies and worms showed they too

---

38 Rose, M. R. *The Long Tomorrow: How Advances in Evolutionary Biology Can Help Us Postpone Aging.* Oxford University Press, USA (2005).

39 Kenyon, C. et al. 'A C elegans mutant that lives twice as long as wild type.' *Nature* 366: 1993: 404–5.

40 Martins, R. et al. 'Long live FOXO: unravelling the role of FOXO proteins in aging and longevity.' *Aging Cell* (2016): 15: 196–207.

41 Sinclair, D. A. et al. 'Small molecule activators of sirtuins extend Saccharomyces cerevisiae lifespan.' *Nature* (2003): 425: 191–6.

lived longer when given resveratrol to spark their SIR gene,[42] all of which made resveratrol the first antioxidant proven to extend life. Sadly, though, that is where this fairy tale ends: research has not shown any longevity benefits in mammals,[43] and a 2014 Italian study found that elderly people with high levels of resveratrol lived no longer than anyone else.[44]

Wine-lovers of the world should not despair, however. There are a couple of good reasons to enjoy a glass of red wine in the evening: firstly, scientists recently showed that mild consumption of wine improves the clearing of toxins from the brain when we sleep,[45] which lowers damage to the brain and reduces the chance of illnesses such as Alzheimer's; and secondly, resveratrol might have failed as a life-extender, but it has been shown to inhibit one of our genes called the mTOR gene, and in plain terms that means it encourages the removal of cancerous cells.[46]

Cynthia Kenyon now has all the technology that Silicon Valley's deep pockets can offer, and she remains determined to convert what she has learned about longevity genes into a pill that one day can help us live healthier and longer lives.[47] Year by year, scientists are getting closer to this philosopher's stone.

Already we know much more about this important mTOR gene. For a start, it is essential for athletes because it switches on to build muscle during times of plenty. On the other hand, if it is left on for too long it can cause

42   Sinclair, D. et al. 'Sirtuin activators mimic caloric restriction and delay ageing in metazoans.' *Nature* (2004): 430: 686–9.

43   Khushwant, S. 'Lifespan and healthspan extension by resveratrol.' *BBA Mol Basis Dis* (2015): 1852: 1209–18.

44   Semba, R. D. et al. 'Resveratrol levels and all-cause mortality in older community-dwelling adults.' *JAMA* (2014): 174: 1077–84.

45   Nedergaard, M. et al. 'Beneficial effects of low alcohol exposure, but adverse effects of high alcohol intake on glymphatic function.' *Nature Res* (2018): 8: 2246. Accessed at: https://www.nature.com/articles/s41598-018-20424-y

46   Park, D. et al. 'Resveratrol induces autophagy by directly inhibiting mTOR through ATP competition.' *Nature* (2016): 6: 21772. Accessed at: https://www.nature.com/articles/srep21772

47   'Cynthia Kenyon: "The idea that ageing was subject to control was completely unexpected."' *The Guardian* (2013)

obesity and even cancer. We also know that a drug called rapamycin switches off mTOR and, when given to mice in later life, helped them to live longer.[48]

In other words, mTOR is useful in small bursts for building muscle after exercise, but if left on continuously can lead to problems like cancer. The hope is that studies in humans will show that giving rapamycin to older people will switch off mTOR, decrease the likelihood of cancer and help us live longer. Whether or not that works remains to be seen, but studies around gerontogenes are a big hope for the future.

Lowered Temperature Theory

Your core body temperature varies naturally; for most of us it runs at between 35 and 37°C. However, some people are able to drop their core temperature, and that has long intrigued researchers. They have studied, for instance, how the hunter-gatherer San people of southern Africa are able to lower their core temperature at night without any ill effects and raise it the next morning.[49]

The Lowered Temperature Theory surmises that if we could drop our core body temperature to 32°C every night for the eight hours that we sleep, our body clock would slow, our body's processes would be slowed and we should be able to extend our lifespan. Lowering our core temperature would, it goes on, slow cell activity, and that would reduce toxin production, cut cell damage and allow cells to function longer.

Most studies show that it does not matter whether you are a tiny freshwater invertebrate or a fish, a fly or a mouse, moderate lowering of your core temperature can increase your lifespan by at least one-quarter.[50] Human studies are harder, because it takes decades to get the results. That said, an

48 Ehninger, D. et al. 'Longevity, aging and rapamycin.' *Cell Mol Life Sci* (2014): 71: 4325–46.

49 Hammel, H. T. et al. 'Thermal and metabolic responses of the Kalahari bushmen to moderate cold at night.' *Researchgate* (1963). Accessed at: https://www.researchgate.net/publication/235016637_Thermal_and_metabolic_responses_of_the_Kalahari_bushmen_to_moderate_cold_exposure_at_night

50 Keil, G. et al. 'Being cool. How body temperature influences ageing and longevity.' *Biogerontology* (2015): 16: 383–97.

excellent piece of research called the Baltimore study showed that lower basal body temperature in older adults is associated with healthy ageing.[51]

The theory is all well and good, but few of us are likely to sleep in a nightly ice-bath to get our temperature down, even if doing so could mean we would easily reach 100. It has been suggested that we would sleep best if the bedroom temperature was between 18 to 20°C, but to get our core temperature down to 32°C would require a much colder room than that – near-freezing conditions, and our chattering teeth would surely keep us awake.

A more practical solution is to immerse ourselves in a bath of ice for a time once a day, and many people do that. An icy bath improves our blood pressure, our hormones and our mood.[52] (Its benefits as a recovery from exercise are much less certain.)[53]

The flip side of this theory is potentially more interesting: how damaging is it to *raise* our core body temperature? Humans struggle with heat, and for the sick and the elderly and the very young, a heatwave can be a killer – even up to a year later.[54] Raising our core temperature, then, can be extremely damaging.

Even though I am a fan of daily exercise, I get very concerned when I see marathon runners collapsing from heat exhaustion. Exercise is, of course, profoundly beneficial: it reduces insulin-resistance, switches on our longevity genes, breaks down our stress hormones, switches on our mTOR muscle-building pathways, and helps to reduce our likelihood of developing inflammation-related illnesses such as heart attacks and cancer. But – and this is an important 'but' – the Baltimore study showed an association between lower body temperature and healthy ageing, and my concern is that exercising to the point that our core body

51   Simonsick, E. M. et al. 'Basal body temperature as a biomarker of healthy aging.' *Age* (2016): 38: 445–54.
52   Mooventhan, A. et al. 'Scientific evidence-based effects of hydrotherapy on various systems of the body.' *N Am Med J Sci* (2014): 6: 199–209.
53   Peake, J. M. et al. 'The effects of cold water emersion and active recovery on inflammation and cell stress responses in human skeletal muscle after resistance exercise'. *J Physiol* (2017): 595: 695–711.
54   Semenza, J. C. et al. 'Heat-related deaths during the July 1995 heat wave in Chicago.' *N Engl J Med* (1996): 335: 84–90.

temperature goes up for prolonged periods could risk real damage. Noël Coward was not far off when he wrote that only mad dogs and Englishmen go out in the midday sun. The rest of his song also contains good advice: most other people, he wrote, use that time for a snooze.

Caloric Restriction Theory

The final theory I want to look at is Caloric Restriction (CR), because out of all of the competing theories for promoting healthy longevity this has the most evidence of success. For that we have the American researcher Clive McCay to thank. In the 1930s, McCay showed that a calorie-restricted diet allowed rats to live significantly longer,[55] and for nearly a century since, his is the theory with the potential to be 'the big one'.

So has it delivered? I would have to say yes. Researchers have produced overwhelming evidence that restricting by 20–40 per cent the amount of food normally eaten helps flies, worms, rodents, monkeys – and even humans – to live longer.[56] Scientists have worked out that if a human cut their calorie intake by 30 per cent from the age of thirty, they would add seven years to their life.[57] As someone who studies ageing for a living, that is an astonishing result and, by way of comparison, is about the same that the world would get by eliminating all forms of cancer and all heart disease.

CR is increasingly accepted as being the most useful proven tool to ensure that people, whether overweight or of normal weight, can live longer and healthier.

Earlier I said that for a theory to be successful, it needs a good reason to explain it and then studies to show it works. It turns out that some of the other theories of ageing that we have encountered go a long way to explaining why CR works.

55 McCay, C. M. et al. 'The effect of retarded growth upon the length of life span and upon the ultimate body size' (1935). *Nutrition* (1989): 5: 155–71.
56 Lee, C. et al. 'Dietary restriction with and without calorie restriction for healthy aging.' *MC* (2016): 5. Accessed at: https://www.ncbi.nlm.nih.gov/pmc/articles/PMC4755412/
57 Speakman, J. R. et al. 'Starving for life: What animal studies can and cannot tell us about the use of Caloric Restriction to prolong human Lifespan.' *J Nutr* 137: (2007): 1078–86.

Free Radical Theory: studies on rats show CR decreases the formation of free radicals and protects against oxidative damage.[58]

Gerontogenes Theory: studies on yeast show CR switches on the SIR gene, which is good for living longer.[59] And in worms it has been shown to switch off Daf-16, which is the one we call the Grim Reaper.[60]

Lowered Temperature Theory: CR has been shown to lower core temperature in rodents, monkeys and humans. And, as this theory tells us, a lower temperature is seen as a mechanism for longer life.[61]

Failing Endocrine System Theory: CR reduces insulin resistance and, as we will see in the chapter on inflammation, this is very important when it comes to ageing. For now I will keep it brief and tell you that insulin is the hormone that pushes excess glucose into our fat cells where that glucose stays until we need it. However, if we become insulin-resistant, then this process of shoving glucose into fat cells gets harder, which means the body has to pump out more insulin to do that job. That is not a good thing; as we shall see, insulin resistance means a greater risk of heart attacks, cancer, diabetes and a host of other inflammatory diseases. CR has been shown to be very effective at reducing insulin resistance in humans, and that means less illness and a longer life.[62]

Over the years, CR's effect on reducing insulin resistance has become the leading explanation as to why this theory works so well in practice.

58 Gredilla, R. et al. 'Caloric restriction decreases mitochondrial free radical generation at complex 1 and lowers oxidative damage to mitochondrial DNA in the rat heart.' *FASEB Journal* (2001). Accessed at: http://www.fasebj.org/doi/10.1096/fj.00-0764fje.

59 Lin, S. J. et al. 'Calorie restriction extends Saccharomyces by cerevisiae lifespan by increasing respiration.' *Nature* (2002): 418: 344–8.

60 Greer, E. L. et al. 'Different dietary restriction regimens extend lifespan by both independent and overlapping genetic pathways in C. elegans.' *Aging Cell* (2009): 8: 113–27.

61 Soare, A. et al. 'Long-term calorie restriction, but not endurance exercise lowers core body temperature in humans.' *Aging* (2011): 374–9.

62 Larson-Meyer, D. E. et al. 'Effect of calorie restriction with or without exercise on insulin sensitivity, B-cell function, fat cell size and ectopic lipid in overweight subjects.' *Diabetes Care* (2006): 29: 1337–44.

Mice fed a CR diet showed low levels of glucose and a protein called IGF-1 (low levels of which are associated with low body fat), as well as decreased rates of cancer and inflammation. The result: the mice lived longer.[63]

Not only that, but Cynthia Kenyon has shown that not only does a CR diet reduce glucose, IGF-1 and inflammation, it also turns important genes on or off. For instance, a gene that makes insulin was turned off, while a gene that controls cell repair was turned on.[64] The importance of Kenyon's study goes well beyond one gene being turned off and another turned on: it is important because it shows our lifestyle is an essential component of a Younger for Longer life. When it comes to our genes we all have some that are better than others, but a healthy lifestyle can turn on good genes and switch off bad ones.

What to eat on a CR diet?

I am often asked which macronutrients (the proteins, carbohydrates and fats) we should cut out when fasting or trying to follow a CR approach. The fact that we have only three to choose from makes this decision a little easier.

It was long thought that fats should go, because they have twice as many calories per gram as carbohydrates. But, as we shall see in the chapter on inflammation, research has shown the opposite is true: in mice a very high-fat, very low-carbohydrate diet (known as a ketogenic diet), for example, reduces insulin resistance, lowers weight and extends life.[65] The fats, of course, need to be healthy.

63 Longo, V. D. et al. 'Evolutionary medicine: from dwarf model systems to healthy centenarians?' *Science* (2003): 299: 1343–6.

64 Guarente, L. and Kenyon, C. 'Genetic pathways that regulate ageing in model organisms.' *Nature* (2000): 408: 255–62.

65 Roberts, M. N. et al. 'A ketogenic diet extends longevity and healthspan in adult mice.' *Cell Metabolism* (2017): 26: 539–46.

In practical terms – and if you have ever eaten a diet that is very high in fat, then you will know this – a high-fat diet makes you feel full quite quickly, and that means you tend not to eat large helpings of anything. In other words, a high-fat diet will help to correct insulin abnormalities (because we will eat less carbohydrates and sugar) *and* it provides its own limit on the number of calories we do eat.

A second approach, which works well, is to cut back on both fats *and* carbohydrates, which means eating a relatively higher amount of protein. Chicken breast and broccoli have long been the backbone of many a successful weight-loss plan.[66]

The third approach is to reduce all three macronutrients equally. In my experience this is the hardest to keep to, and that is because protein and fats fill you up; therefore, cutting back on these means you feel hungry a lot of the time.

Whichever way you go, though, if you want to stick to a CR diet then you need to cut out about one-third of your normal calorie intake. Or, to put it in nutrition-speak, you must consume less than 1,200 kilocalories per day.

So is CR good news all the way? Well, despite what looks like an avalanche of awesomeness, it is important to stress the following: although CR *might* be the brightest star in our firmament of healthy ageing treatments, and although it *has* shown a number of mechanisms that are important in maintaining our health, it has not yet been conclusively proven in humans. But there are positive signs: the residents of Japan's Okinawa Island practise moderate CR – their calorie intake is just 83 per cent of the Japanese average – and live-

---

66 Johnston, B. C. et al. 'Comparison of Weight Loss Among Named Diet Programs in Overweight and Obese Adults: A Meta-analysis.' *JAMA* (2014): 312: 923–33.

significantly longer than the rest of us. They also have fewer cancers and heart attacks.[67]

It is also true that reducing our food intake by 20–40 per cent is a big ask. Happily, though, two easier habits have been shown to be useful in moving us towards the benefits of CR. The first habit is intermittent fasting, an example of which is eating normally one day and fasting the next day. If that sounds too much, then an alternative is to eat nothing until midday, and then eat healthily but have nothing after 8pm. That will give a 2:1 fasting:eating ratio (sixteen hours of not eating and eight hours in which you do eat), which is healthy.[68] Intermittent fasting reduces insulin resistance without having to restrict calories. It also reduces inflammation, switches on healthy genes and extends lifespan.[69]

The second habit is a form of exercise known as HIIT, which stands for high-intensity interval training. This is typically twenty minutes of exhaustive exercise that mixes cardiovascular and anaerobic exercise (like lifting weights) with short recovery periods. It has been shown to reduce insulin resistance for between one and two days,[70] which is very important for the 30 per cent of society that suffers from insulin resistance and the damage it brings. In addition, aerobic exercise has been shown to switch on healthy genes in experiments in mice. Notably, in older mice, exercise switched off some of the bad genes that had been switched on as the mice had aged.[71] In short, on its own HIIT does not extend lifespan, but when added to CR it does enhance CR's effects.[72]

67   Chan, Y. C. et al. 'Calorie restriction in the Okinawa people of Japan.' *J Cell Nutr* (1997).

68   Anson, R. M. et al. 'Intermittent fasting dissociates beneficial effects of dietary restriction on glucose metabolism and neuronal resistance to injury from calorie intake.' *Proc Natl Acad Sci USA* (2003): 100: 6216–20.

69   Martin, B. et al. 'Caloric restriction and intermittent fasting: two potential diets for successful brain aging.' *Ageing Res Rev* (2006): 5: 332–53.

70   Keshel, T. E. et al. 'Exercise training and insulin resistance: a current review.' *J Obes Weight Loss Ther* (2015): 5: S5–003.

71   Kohman, R. A. et al. 'Voluntary wheel-running reverses age-induced changes in hippocampal gene expression.' *PLOS One* (2011): 6: e22654.

72   Davis, R. A. H. et al. 'High-intensity interval training and calorie restriction promote remodeling of glucose and lipid metabolism in diet-induced obesity.' *Am J Physiol Endocrinol Metab* (2017): 313: E243–56.

Gene-mapping

In recent years there was a lot of attention on the Human Genome Project, which mapped every human gene, an undertaking as vast as it seems. Scientists have mapped the sequences of other organisms too: in 2012, for example, the gene sequence of the humble tomato was put together thanks to the collaboration of 300 scientists.[73]

One interesting point from that exercise was the realisation that splicing a gene fifty years earlier on a breed of large tomatoes in a bid to keep them red for longer had inadvertently switched off the sweet taste gene.[74] So if you ever wondered why big red tomatoes in supermarkets do not taste of much, now you know why – with the important lesson that fiddling with one gene can inadvertently affect another.

The healthier, or perhaps less risky approach, to working with genes is to measure individual gene nucleotides to see which are deficient, and then, in that particular individual, to replace that deficiency with a specific supplement. Down that road lies precision medicine, and we will meet that in the final chapter when we look at CRISPR technology, which involves manipulating our genes by cutting out and inserting bits of DNA.

Summary

I find the theories of ageing fascinating, not least because each holds some important truths. De Grey talks about attacking ageing on seven fronts, and it seems sensible to do more than one thing to minimise the damage of ageing and get us closer to our genetic potential of 100 or 110 years.

73 Zamir, D. et al, open letter. 'The tomato genome sequence provides insights into fleshy fruit evolution.' *Nature* (2012): 485: 635–41.
74 Kupferschmidt, K. 'How tomatoes lost their taste.' *ScienceNOW* (28 June 2012). Accessed at http://news.sciencemag.org/sciencenow/2012/06/how-tomatoes-lost-their-taste.html

These theories give us some other interesting pointers too:

- We should minimise the wear and tear in our DNA, our cells and our liver if we want to optimise our health. To that end the chapter on toxins will look at detoxification in greater detail.

- It is important to support our hormones. The chapter on nutrition will examine why we should balance our insulin level, while the chapters on men's health and women's health will show how to support testosterone, progesterone and oestrogen to help us move better through middle age.

- Free radicals are damaging, and there is a movement towards supporting our powerful SOD antioxidant system rather than flooding our bodies with the likes of vitamin C. Stimulating our SOD system has been shown to be useful, and we can do that with supplements like wheat-sprouts, melon, magnesium and zinc.

- Gerontogenes are genes that extend healthy life and these are the hope for the future. Until science comes up with a safe pill, we can help ourselves with daily exercise, cutting out sugar, and drinking small amounts of red wine (or eating grapes).

- Lowering our body temperature will extend life, but is difficult in practice. Daily cold baths, however, do help. In addition we should avoid overheating the body; that means exercising during cooler times of the day.

- Calorie restriction will help you live longer; the problem is that it is highly restrictive. Other options include practising intermittent fasting, which means eating only between, say, midday and 8pm, cutting out refined carbohydrates and sugar, and exercising every day.

Unlike de Grey, our goal is not to live to 1,000 but to work with what we already know. In the final section of this chapter we will look at two approaches to life, and how the approach we choose will determine a lot about how we die.

LIVE FAST, DIE YOUNG?

I would like you to meet Steve. Although Steve does not exist, we all know him: the guy with a lot of friends, but who does not take much care of himself. We see him in his twenties, as he starts his first job and lives a pressured, unhealthy life. We have all done it for a while – work hard, play hard, plenty of socialising, less exercise than before, late nights, increasing stress levels. Steve has lots of energy, and is proud that he can cope with this fast life while others have already dropped by the wayside.

Soon enough, Steve gets promoted, gets married, buys a house and has a couple of children. Life is good, as it should be.

A decade later, Steve is still burning the candle at both ends, and is getting ahead. He knows he will never be able to afford that yacht he once dreamed of and, despite being divorced, is unlikely to marry his movie-star crush from twenty years ago. Worryingly he is starting to put on a bit of weight – not too much, he tells himself, but as he looks at photographs of himself from his early twenties he notices that he looked better then.

He presses on with the life he knows, seeing the kids every other weekend, and still working and playing hard. In his early forties his doctor gives him his first warnings: his blood pressure and cholesterol have crept up. In gentle GP fashion, that message is tempered by advising Steve that this is mainly stress-related, and that as long as he loses some weight and starts exercising he should be fine. Steve assures his doctor that he will make those lifestyle changes; it turns out that now is not quite the right time, but he will get to it just as soon as this particular high-pressure period is over.

By the time he is in his fifties, still putting work ahead of his health (after all, there is just a decade of work to go, the children are in university and there are still those alimony bills), Steve is decidedly overweight. He lacks the time for enough exercise, and when he does work out it is no longer fun. Instead he enjoys relaxing after a long day with a couple of beers and a cigarette. By now he is taking an array of tablets on a regular basis to counter the joint aches, over-the-top cholesterol and some stubbornly high blood pressure. He does not sleep well these days, his libido is shot and he gets irritated with the traffic, which is far busier than it used to be. He yearns for those heady student days where the weekends were for partying. Now that two-day break is barely enough to recover from the ravages of the working week.

By sixty, Steve is starting to feel old and depressed, which scares him. He is embarrassed by what he sees in the mirror and wonders just what he achieved by working so hard for so long. And, now that you mention it, where *did* those years go? Steve cuts back on sugar, as per the GP's orders, because nothing else seems to help combat his weight. He is paring back coffee too because the hypertensive headaches it brings are not worth it. In desperation Steve tries to follow the advice he was given twenty years earlier, but each time he exercises he feels light-headed and ill, so he decides sport is not good for him. The middle-aged spread that has wrapped itself firmly around his waist is easily ignored by staying away from the full-length mirror.

By sixty-five, Steve has retired, but freedom from work has coincided with the fact that physical movement is painful. The world has become a more limited place, and our once-sociable friend is not living in the land of adventure he dreamed of. Instead he is depressed and angry, and that is not what he recalls he was promised when he signed up as the bright young hope in the company four decades ago. He spends his final eight or nine years in declining health swallowing packs of tablets, sleeping poorly, struggling to wake up and not having the energy to organise much more than a trip to the GP's surgery. His final years are spent in an old-age home where his kids seldom visit. And so, by the time the Grim Reaper makes his rounds, Steve might well echo the final lines of Winston Churchill, who reportedly said: 'I'm so bored of it all.'

If it all sounds depressing, it need not. Had Steve made only a few changes in his 30s or 40s, things would have been quite different. The good news is that this is not hard to do. A 2009 study showed that if Steve stuck to four basic principles, he could significantly reduce the risk of that miserable demise.[75] These two dos and two don'ts for men and women should come as no surprise:

75   Ford, E. et al. 'Healthy living is the best revenge. Findings from the European prospective investigation into cancer and nutrition – the Potsdam study.' *Arch Intern Med* (2009): 169: 1355–62.

- Eat healthily.
- Exercise for three and a half hours a week.
- Do not smoke.
- Do not become obese.

Following those four principles would cut Steve's risk of diabetes by 93 per cent, his heart attack risk by 81 per cent, his stroke risk by half, and his cancer risk by about one-third.[76] Steve could expect to have the vitality in his fifties and sixties similar to that which he enjoyed in his twenties.

Figure 2: The two walks of life we can choose

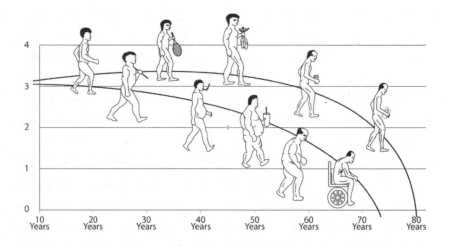

The figure above shows the two walks of life: Steve's unhealthy life, in which he is obese by fifty, in pain at sixty, in a wheelchair by seventy, and dead shortly after that; and the other one that, had he followed the four rules, would have seen him feeling healthy and vigorous at fifty, still active at seventy, and dead at eighty after a short illness.

It is not that the healthier choice sees us living much longer; more that the quality of life in our final decades is far better.

76 Ibid.

In addition to the four principles, there is plenty of evidence to suggest that most of us would also benefit from the following four approaches:

Gentle hormone balancing: after forty, many people feel tired, sluggish and not as vital as they once were. A blood test followed by some mild hormone balancing often corrects this.

Moderate vitamin and mineral support: 'Not too much and not too little' should be the mantra of vitamin support. What we need to do is supplement what we lack in our food, but we do not want to take so many vitamins that we switch off our own SOD system. A good multivitamin taken three times a week should suffice.

Liver support: in the chapter on toxins we will see that our bodies are flooded by toxins, and that our liver – our key detoxification organ – struggles to clear everything. A good-quality detox supplement is one solution to help the liver get rid of toxins; my preference is for a glutathione drip a few times a year.

Stress management using meditation and regular exercise: the modern world stimulates us far more than is healthy and, as we shall see in the chapter on the brain, mindful meditation is essential to allow the brain to hear the state of the body.

To that mix of mainly physical remedies I would add this pearl from Albert Einstein who, when asked in his later years whether he thought of himself as very intelligent, replied that he was not, but 'just very, very inquisitive'. To my mind, people who are still inquisitive in their old age are on the right track. A good sense of humour and an optimistic nature are also useful.

If we get our health right then there is no reason we should not walk in the mountains in our seventies, sleep well each night, and be happy from the moment the sun comes up each day. Current statistics suggest that we could expect one year of bad health and a peaceful death at eighty, although many of us could likely live healthily for much longer than that.

Not that there is anything wrong with following Steve's fast-and-loose life-style, of course, provided we understand how it will probably end: badly. The 'live fast, die young' mantra generally does not hold; typically we keep living, but in a lifestyle that chips away at our Healthspan leaving us with a grim last decade or two.

For me, the absence of healthy years was highlighted when I visited the frail-care facility where my father lived out his final years, and where many of the residents had ended up because they had not taken the best care of themselves when they were younger. Some were simply unlucky to have lost their health, but for many their condition was in large part down to their own choices.

What was most apparent during the hours I spent at the facility was that modern medicine has become particularly good at keeping us alive, but not very good at optimising our health.

The simple truth is that it is our choice as to which path we will walk, and having a realistic idea of the consequences of our decisions should help us to choose. The rest of this book will focus on helping you to identify which choices are best for you.

THE HUNDRED CLUB

Before we close this chapter, you might be curious to know what traits are useful in making it to 100. A survey done in the UK shows that people who get that far have a number of characteristics in common:[77]

- Most are active into their eighties or nineties.
- Most are lean, not obese.
- Most are mentally acute into their nineties.
- They tend not to have suffered from the modern chronic illnesses of diabetes or heart attacks.
- They tend to deal well with stress.
- Spirituality is important, and most have an active religious life.
- They are generally not heavy smokers or heavy drinkers.
- They live in non-toxic environments.
- Longevity is a family trait.

Clearly, then, lifestyle choices make a big difference. And on that note it seems apt to end with the words of the world's oldest recorded human,

---

77 Goodman, S. 'Commonalities amongst centenarians.' *The Centenarian* (2015).

France's Jeanne Calment, who turned twenty-one in the year that August Weismann began his work on sea urchins.

Calment, who met the artist Vincent Van Gogh in her youth (describing him as 'very ugly, ungracious, impolite, sick – I forgive him, they called him loco'),[78] had a number of factors in her favour: she played several sports in her youth, her parents lived to a ripe old age, she cycled until her 100th birthday, kept active, and was, according to her biographer, 'immune to stress'.

Calment did not move into a nursing home until she was 110, and she kept puffing cigarettes for another seven years (thereby giving hope to countless smokers around the world). She retained her health until her final weeks in 1997, and throughout her life seems to have been blessed with a sharp sense of humour: when one visitor commented on leaving, 'Until next year, perhaps,' she replied: 'I don't see why not! You don't look so bad to me.'

78 'Jeanne Calment, World's Elder, Dies at 122.' *The New York Times* (5 August 1997).

Chapter 3

Inflammation and Obesity – Because You Aren't What You Eat

There is no love sincerer than the love of food.

George Bernard Shaw

Does it really matter if we are overweight or obese? After all, those are not illnesses, so how important can they be? Well, the one-word answer is: *extremely*. As we will see over the course of the next two chapters, these conditions are generally accompanied by low-grade inflammation in the body, and it is inflammation that contributes to the chronic diseases from which we in the modern era suffer.[1]

As we saw in the previous chapter, people who live healthily to 100 are typically not overweight or obese and they do not suffer from inflammation-related illnesses.[2] That is no coincidence.

Around the time that today's centenarians were babies, the range of illnesses in the developed world was quite different. In 1900, for example, when industrialisation and smoke stacks were at their peak, it was ailments such as influenza, tuberculosis and stomach infections that killed most Americans.[3]

---

1 Lumeng, C. et al. 'Inflammatory Links Between Obesity and Metabolic Disease.' *J Clin Invest* (2011): 121: 2111–17.
2 Santos-Lozano, A. et al. 'Implications of Obesity in Exceptional Longevity.' *Ann Transl Med* (2016): 4: 416.
3 Centers for Disease Control and Prevention. 'Top 10 Causes of Death in the United States from 1900–2010.'

Those killers have largely dropped off the rich world's radar, and they are dropping off the radar of much of the rest of the world too. These days fewer people die from communicable diseases and – logically enough – more are succumbing to non-communicable diseases. While on the one hand that means people are living longer, it also means that their quality of life in their last ten years is often poor, and their medical costs high.

Take India, for example. There, the fastest-growing causes of disease in the last quarter-century were diabetes (its rate nearly doubled) and heart disease (up around one-third). In 1990, some 38 per cent of deaths in India were due to non-communicable diseases; by 2016 that figure had climbed to 60 per cent.[4]

The developing world is following the developed world in many ways, including how people die. In the US, for example, about six out of every ten deaths in 2015 were caused by a chronic illness,[5] with the most important of those being:

- Heart disease
- Cancers
- Chronic lung diseases such as asthma, emphysema and bronchitis
- Strokes
- Alzheimer's
- Diabetes

These days nearly one in two American adults has at least one chronic illness.[6] The pattern is largely the same in other developed nations. Aside from the individual tragedy of each death, there is a wider problem – these diseases are expensive, not least because they take a long time to

---

4 'Comprehensive Health Study in India Finds Rise of Non-communicable Diseases.' IHME (2017). See: http://www.healthdata.org/news-release/comprehensive-health-study-india-finds-rise-non-communicable-diseases

5 Heron, M. 'Deaths: Leading Causes for 2015.' *National Vital Statistics Reports* (2017): 66 (5).

6 Bauer, U. E. et al. 'Prevention of Chronic Disease in the 21st Century: Elimination of the Leading Preventable Causes of Premature Death and Disability in the USA.' *The Lancet* (2014): 384: 45–52.

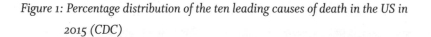

Figure 1: Percentage distribution of the ten leading causes of death in the US in 2015 (CDC)

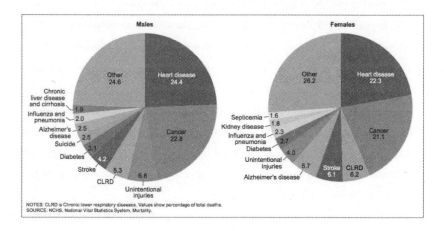

kill. Compare influenza with cancer: the former either kills us within a few days or we recover completely. Cancer is of an entirely different order.

As these paragraphs show, the trends in the world's health are moving fast and the news is often not encouraging. The *Global Burden of Disease Study*, which is funded by the Bill & Melinda Gates Foundation, covers health trends across nearly 130 countries. Among its findings:

- The percentage of people who died from a chronic disease increased from 57 per cent in 1990 to 71 per cent by 2015.
- The biggest risk factors for chronic illness are *not* genetics. They are lifestyle choices, among which we can include smoking, obesity, lack of exercise, stress and – as we will see – consuming too much sugar.
- Someone with a chronic illness can expect to spend the final ten years of their life in poor health.

More positively, global life expectancy has risen from mid-sixties to early seventies. However, set against that is the unenviable fact that a higher percentage of people are dying from chronic illnesses and, as noted earlier, that means many will spend the last decade of their lives in a miserable way, often with substantial medical bills. In other words, although living into our seventies sounds like a boon, it could be seen as a step backwards if it comes with ill-health attached. That is not the goal of healthy ageing.

This chapter will explore the common threads behind the global pandemic of chronic illness. We will see how consumption of sugar and processed carbohydrates is closely tied to rising obesity rates, and that the failure to act against both of these is behind the increasing prevalence of diseases such as diabetes, heart attacks and cancer. There is also evidence that links obesity with diabetes and other illnesses. A 2014 report in the *British Medical Journal* found the proportion of British adults surveyed who were on the cusp of becoming diabetic trebled from nearly 12 per cent to 35 per cent between 2003 and 2011.[7] The study also noted that half of British adults who were overweight had pre-diabetes, and that diabetes was costing the NHS one-tenth of its budget.

At the centre of this nutritional maelstrom is inflammation: it drives our chronic illnesses and, as we shall see, it is sugar that drives inflammation. That makes it vital to understand what inflammation is and how it works.

WHAT IS INFLAMMATION?

When an area of the body gets damaged, the immune system releases a cascade of products to start the healing process. This healing response might be felt as a warming of the area, and is what we call inflammation.

Take one common example: sunburn. Too much exposure to the sun damages the skin cells and, in response, the immune system takes action to heal the skin. What we see and feel is a red, warm patch of skin. This is inflammation in action; it is simply our body's response to damage. Pimples are another example. What we see as inflamed pustules is not damage caused by the bacteria under the skin; rather it is our immune system's response to kill and expel the bacteria.

---

7 Mainous, G. et al. 'Prevalence of Prediabetes in England from 2003 to 2011: Population-based, Cross-sectional Study.' *BMJ Open* (2014): Vol 4: Issue 6.

Inflammation is inextricably linked with our immune system. Indeed, the fact that our immune system is so efficient is – for most of us, most of the time – a very good thing. However, that is not the case when it causes continuous, or ongoing, inflammation, because inflammation is at the centre of every chronic illness, as the following examples show:

- Asthma is an inflammation of the lungs. It makes sense that our airways tighten to protect us from breathing in soot; however, with asthma this tightening is so severe that we can suffocate.
- Arthritis is an inflammation of the joints.
- Sugar causes inflammation of the arteries, which can lead to diabetes and obesity.[8]
- Heart attacks and strokes are caused primarily by inflamed arteries – we will go into this in much greater detail later in the chapter.
- Cancer genes can stimulate an inflammation cascade that triggers cancer.[9]
- An inflamed brain contributes to Alzheimer's in susceptible people.[10]

In addition, studies have shown that once we have one inflammatory disease we are at a higher risk of developing another:

- Researchers have shown that people with rheumatoid arthritis double their risk of a heart attack.[11]
- Children with irritable bowel disease (inflamed intestines, where the immune system attacks the bowel) have twice the risk of developing cancer.[12]

8 Endemann, D. H. et al. 'Nitric Oxide, Oxidative Excess and Vascular Complications in Diabetes Mellitus.' *Curr Hypertens Rep* (2004): Vol 6: 2: 85–9.

9 Liu, J. et al. 'A Genetically Defined Model for Human Ovarian Cancer.' *Cancer Res* (2004): 64: 1655–63.

10 Heppner, F. L. et al. 'Immune Attack: The Role of Inflammation in Alzheimer's Disease.' *Nat Rev Neurosci* (2015): 16: 358–72.

11 De Busk, L. M. 'Tie2 Receptor Tyrosine Kinase, a Major Mediator of TNFa Induced Angiogenesis in Rheumatoid Arthritis.' *Arthritis Rheum* (2003): 48: 9: 2461–71.

12 Olen, O. et al. 'Childhood Onset of Inflammatory Bowel Disease and Risk of Cancer: A Swedish Nationwide Cohort Study 1964–2014.' *BMJ* (2017): doi:10:1136/bmj.j3951.

- Someone whose blood test shows raised inflammatory markers such as C-reactive protein (known as CRP, and which we will come back to later) are at greater risk for heart disease. They are also at risk of a second inflammatory problem: blindness from macular degeneration.[13]

In summary: inflammation is our body's healing response to injury, and most chronic illnesses are caused by *ongoing* inflammation in the body.

Because inflammation drives chronic disease, tackling it at source is a smart move. But before we talk about how best to do that, I want to tell you what we know about the illness that remains most likely to carry us off: heart attacks. Our chance of dying from a heart attack or stroke is around 40 per cent, so reducing that risk would be a great start.[14]

THE QUEST FOR HEALTHY HEARTS

There has been plenty of debate over the years around what causes heart attacks and, logically enough, what might be useful in preventing them. Until a few years ago we thought the problem was primarily that fat blocks arteries. It seemed straightforward: the more fat you ate, the more cholesterol you accumulated, and the more your arteries clogged up until you suffered a heart attack or stroke. Eating fat was likened to pouring lard down a drain: it clogged the arteries. Bad cholesterol (there is a good cholesterol, thus the distinction) is called Low-Density Lipoprotein (LDL), and is seen as the main cause of this problem.

This 'lard down a drain' image is easy to visualise and it certainly seems logical, so it is not surprising that it caught on. It is, however, fundamentally wrong, and it has taken us the best part of seventy years to work that out.

13 Vine, A. K. et al. 'Biomarkers of Cardiovascular Disease as Risk Factors for Age-related Macular Degeneration.' *Opthalmology* (2005): 112: 2076–80.
14 Fuster, V. and Kelly, B. B. 'Promoting Cardiovascular Health in the Developing World: A Critical Challenge to Achieve Global Health.' See: https://www.ncbi.nlm.nih.gov/pubmed/20945571

The theory behind the 'fat is bad' thesis is known as the lipid hypothesis of heart disease. It originated in the 1800s, but was taken seriously only a century ago when rabbits that were fed a high-fat diet were shown to develop fatty streaks in their arteries.[15] In the 1950s, American researcher Ancel Keys added to that hypothesis when he commenced his Seven Countries Study in which he assessed nearly 13,000 men across seven countries in four regions of the world to see whether a diet high in saturated fat (which is predominantly animal fat, but also includes coconut oil and palm oil) was associated with an increased risk of heart disease.

Keys published his results in the 1970s, and suggested that a high-fat diet was indeed associated with an increased heart-attack risk. This was a profound moment in the history of public health: on the back of Keys' research, the world moved towards low-fat eating to prevent heart disease.[16]

This theory that blood cholesterol causes heart attacks was accepted by the medical community in 1984 when the now-famous Coronary Primary Prevention Trial showed that swallowing a medication for bile acid was able to cut blood cholesterol levels and also reduce the incidence of heart attacks.[17] Measuring and then treating blood cholesterol levels became a national priority.

In 1987 the first statin tablet came out. What do statin tablets do? They block a pathway in the liver that makes cholesterol. With this pathway blocked, the level of cholesterol in the blood drops.

With that, it seemed, we had the final piece in the lipid hypothesis puzzle:[18]

- We had a seemingly sensible theory that eating fat caused fatty arteries.
- We knew that high cholesterol was associated with heart attacks.

---

15 Anitschkow, N. N. and Chatalov, S. 'Über experimentelle Cholesterinsteatose und ihre Bedeutung für die Entstehung einiger pathologischer Prozesse.' *Zentralbl Allg Pathol* (1913): 24: 1–9.

16 Keys, A. 'Coronary Heart Disease in Seven Countries.' *Circulation* (1970): 41(4S1): 1–198.

17 'The Lipid Research Clinics Coronary Primary Prevention Trial results. I. Reduction in incidence of coronary heart disease.' *JAMA* (1984): 251: 351–64.

18 Endo, A. 'A Historical Perspective on the Discovery of Statins.' *Proc Jpn Acad Ser B Phys Biol Sci* (2010): 86: 484– 93.

- And we had a tablet that lowered cholesterol levels and reduced the incidence of heart attacks.

The handful of statin tablets on the market end in the suffix 'statin' or the letters 'or': among them are simvastatin (marketed as Zocor), atorvastatin (Lipitor) and rosuvastatin (Crestor). It was true in 1987 when they were launched, and it remains true today: statins lower cholesterol levels and cut the incidence of heart attacks.[19]

So there it was. A huge amount of work and a few Nobel Prizes later and the medical world had shown that a high-fat diet was associated with an increased heart-attack risk. We also had proof that statin tablets reduced our heart-attack risk and lowered our cholesterol levels.

Unfortunately an unproven conclusion underpinned the overall hypothesis: *that a low-fat diet would reduce our heart attack risk.* What got researchers' attention was that – despite the developed world's fifty-year love of low-fat food – heart disease has not plummeted; it has merely declined slightly. At the same time, obesity and diabetes rates have sky-rocketed.[20]

It took many more years to prove that sugar – not fat – in our diet was the *root cause* of heart disease. (If you take the fat out of foods, the easiest way to make it palatable is to add sugar: thus, low fat equals high sugar by default.) Worse still, the low-fat advice that we doctors had been dishing out resulted in a glut of high-carbohydrate eating and the associated global obesity epidemic.

Associating sugar consumption with obesity, however, does not prove that one *causes* the other. We made that mistake with low-fat eating, and look where we ended up. What we needed was to prove causation: that a high-sugar, high-carbohydrate diet *causes* heart disease. Can we prove that? Let us take a look.

19 Strandberg, T. et al. 'Cholesterol Lowering after Participation in the Scandinavian Simvastatin Survival Study 4S.' *European Heart Journal* (1997): 18: 11: 1725–7.
20 To see the Centers for Disease Control's maps of trends in diagnosed diabetes and obesity as of April 2017, see: https://www.cdc.gov/diabetes/statistics/slides/maps_diabetesobesity_trends.pdf

The inflammation model of heart disease

Many writers have speculated as to whether Keys cherry-picked the results in his Seven Countries study. What is true is that he started with twenty-two countries, but in the end used just seven in his results.[21] For our purposes it is worth noting that his report was only an *observational* study: the high-fat diets of those seven countries were *associated* with a higher heart attack risk. His study in no way proved *causation* of a heart attack. In other words, Keys never proved that eating saturated fats *causes* heart disease.

If that sounds confusing, consider this analogy: the association between ambulances and car accidents. It is true that whenever there is an accident, there is generally an ambulance. To the uninformed observer, it might appear that ambulances *cause* accidents because they are always at the scene. But that is merely an association. It does not prove that ambulances cause accidents.

This is why, although studies of association are interesting, they do not prove anything. In our debate over fats and heart attacks, proving this one way or the other would require putting one group of people on a high-fat diet, another on a low-fat diet, and recording the outcome. Eventually that very study was completed, but it took until 2017.

We will get to its results shortly. Before that, however, we need to look again at the subject of this chapter: inflammation. The past half-century has seen numerous theories to explain what causes heart attacks, and the evidence we have now from an impressive array of studies is that inflammation is to blame. That is so important that I will say it again: the evidence suggests that *inflammation is in large part responsible for heart attacks and strokes.*

The person at the centre of the Inflammation Theory is Paul M. Ridker, a medical researcher from Brigham University in the US. In my view, there are three key reasons why Ridker is the most important figure in cardiac research in decades. Firstly, he showed how inflammation of the arteries is a much better predictor of heart disease than cholesterol levels are. Secondly, he showed that statin tablets work primarily by reducing inflammation of the

21   Yerushalmy, Y. and Hilleboe, H. E. 'Fat in the Diet and Mortality from Heart Disease: A Methodologic Note.' *NY State J Med* (1957): 57: 2343–54.

arteries. And thirdly, Ridker showed that a powerful anti-inflammatory medication that *only* reduces inflammation of the arteries is superior to statins that cut both inflammation and cholesterol levels.

In short, Ridker has shown that inflammation – not cholesterol – is the root cause of heart disease.

It started back in 1998, when it was suggested that inflammation rather than cholesterol was the key to understanding cardiovascular disease. This discussion entails once again meeting something called CRP (it stands for C-reactive protein). CRP is the protein in your blood that is a very useful marker for inflammation: the higher the level of inflammation in your body, the higher your CRP reading will be. In 1998, Ridker found that healthy middle-aged men with the highest CRP levels were three times more likely to suffer a heart attack than those with the lowest CRP levels.[22] The CRP blood test has since been proven to be a highly sensitive marker of heart disease across all populations in the world.[23]

Ridker's research was big news and it caused many in the medical world to rethink what we had understood to be the root cause of atherosclerosis, or hardening of the arteries.

It also caused many people to wonder where that left statin tablets. In the face of Ridker's findings, did statins even have a place? A landmark study in 2000, aptly called the LIPID study, showed that they do. It demonstrated that statin tablets *do* lower heart-attack rates even for people who had not previously had a heart attack and were suffering only from angina, which is the term for poor blood flow to the heart that causes pain during exercise.[24] In other words, statin tablets work.

Earlier we saw that statins lower cholesterol levels; the LIPID findings caused researchers to wonder whether statins work primarily by reducing

22 Ridker, P. M. 'C-Reactive Protein Adds to the Predictive Value of Total and HDL Cholesterol in Determining Risk of First Myocardial Infarction.' *Circulation* (1998): 97: 20: 2007–11.

23 Fonseca, F. A. H. et al. 'High-Sensitivity C-Reactive Protein and Cardiovascular Disease Across Countries and Ethnicities.' *Clinics* (2016): 71: 235–42.

24 Tonkin, A. M. et al. 'Effects of Pravastatin on 3,260 Patients with Unstable Angina: Results from the LIPID Study.' *The Lancet* (2000).

arterial inflammation rather than by lowering cholesterol. They went to work on a study known as the JUPITER trial, a catchy acronym that disguised a much more laborious title ('Justification for the Use of Statins in Primary Prevention: An Intervention Trial Evaluating Rosuvastatin').

Ridker was the lead researcher, and JUPITER, which was spread across twenty-six countries, assessed nearly 18,000 people whose LDL levels were low or normal, yet whose CRP levels were high. Its results, presented in 2008, found that statins lower cholesterol (which we already knew), and that statins also reduce inflammation.[25]

Yet as much of a landmark as the JUPITER trial was, there was still not enough evidence to determine whether the improvement in heart-attack risk from statins was because they lowered cholesterol or because they reduced inflammation. Given that it took decades to prove that smoking is bad for our health, perhaps it was no great surprise that it was taking even longer to determine the root cause of arterial blockages.

We will come back to that conundrum shortly, but on the heels of the JUPITER study another question raised its head: given that statins reduce inflammation, and given that inflammation is central to chronic illnesses, perhaps we would all benefit from taking statins?

The JUPITER study went on to look at this too, but its conclusions were mixed. Although inflammation did indeed decrease, the incidence of diabetes, for example, increased.[26] A blizzard of meta-analyses (studies that review the results of many different studies) followed trying to decide whether the public should take statin tablets – or, as one doctor put it, 'add it to the drinking water'. A large UK observational study helped to knock that idea on the head, showing that you would need to give statins to 1,429 *healthy* people who did not have heart disease before one would be saved from a heart attack; set against that, doing so would cause two cases of kidney failure, nine cases of liver dysfunction and fourteen cases of muscle

25 De Rao, A. 'To JUPITER and Beyond: Statins, Inflammation and Primary Prevention.' *Critical Care* (2010) 14: 310.
26 Ibid.

damage.[27] Common sense prevailed and statins were not added to the drinking water.

By now, though, many people in medicine and beyond were intrigued by the idea that inflammation might be central to the formation of arterial plaque. The next logical question was: 'If inflammation is so important in reducing heart-attack risks, then could natural anti-inflammatories do the job just as well?'

It so happened that around the time of the JUPITER study, another group of scientists was looking at that. They found that, for middle-aged men like me who have a medium-to-low risk of a heart attack, half an aspirin a day is effective in reducing inflammation and preventing heart attacks. Only once our heart-attack risk increases to 10 per cent (i.e. we are now considered to have a moderate risk), does the addition of a statin become more useful than half an aspirin.[28]

With renewed kudos to aspirin (the drug derived from the bark of the willow tree, and whose patent expired a century ago), other researchers chose to focus their efforts on the natural anti-inflammatory properties of fish oil on heart attacks. Again it was shown that for *healthy people* who are not on heart medication, taking fish oil every day is more effective than taking statins to reduce arterial inflammation and heart-attack risk.[29] Yet another study has shown that alpha-lipoic acid, an antioxidant that is integral to maintaining healthy arterial walls, reduces arterial inflammation and cardiovascular disease.[30]

In other words, by this time the medical world knew that inflammation lay at the core of the problem, and that reducing inflammation was a sensible way to lower the risk of having a heart attack.

27 Hippisley-Cox, J., Coupland, C. 'Unintended Effects of Statins in Men and Women in England and Wales: Population-based Cohort Study Using the QResearch database.' *BMJ* (2010): 340: c2197.

28 Pignone, M. et al. 'Aspirin, Statins or Both Drugs for the Primary Prevention of Coronary Heart Disease Events in Men: A Cost-utility Analysis.' *Ann Intern Med* (2006): Vol 144, 5: 326–36.

29 Tavazzi, L. 'Rationale and Design of the GISSI Heart Failure Trial: A Large Trial to Assess the Effects of N-3 Polyunsaturated Fatty Acids and Rosuvastatin in Symptomatic Congestive Heart Failure.' *Eur J of Heart Fail* (2004): 6: 635–41.

30 Harding, S. V. et al. 'Evidence for Using Alpha-lipoic Acid in Reducing Lipoprotein and Inflammatory-related Atherosclerotic Risk.' *J Diet Suppl* (2012): 9: 116–27.

However, that is not quite the end of the story; for that, you will need to bear with me a little longer as I introduce you to a version of cholesterol called 'oxidised LDL'. We met LDL earlier: it is the so-called 'bad cholesterol' (as opposed to HDL or 'good cholesterol').

The theory goes like this: once our arteries have become inflamed, it is not ordinary LDL that burrows into the damaged walls and initiates blockages in the arteries; rather it is this version of LDL that we call oxidised LDL that causes blockages.[31]

What exactly is oxidised LDL? Simply put, it is *inflamed* LDL. Once again, inflammation raises its head.

In other words, this theory holds that when it comes to cholesterol we need to watch out for *oxidised LDL*, not the broader category of LDL. And two of the most common sources of oxidised LDL are smoking and car exhaust fumes:

- Multiple studies have shown that smoking increases oxidised LDL levels; statins, on the other hand, are thought to be able to reduce oxidised LDL.[32]

- Car exhaust fumes cause LDL to oxidise,[33] and have long been associated with an increased risk of heart disease. These fumes are the main culprit for many people.

What this means is that there is a significant amount we can do to reduce our oxidised LDL levels. We should stop smoking for a start, and we should not walk, exercise or live near congested traffic. A third sensible step is to take antioxidants like vitamins A, C and E that have been shown to reduce oxidised LDL levels.[34] A fourth is to use glutathione to detoxify the liver – we shall see

31 Apostolov, E. O. 'Carbamylated-oxidized LDL: Proatherosclerotic Effects on Endothelial Cells and Macrophages.' *J Atheroscler Thromb* (2013): 20: 878–92.

32 Ogawa, K. et al. 'Increase in the Oxidised Low-density Lipoprotein Level by Smoking, and the Possible Inhibitory Effect of Statin Therapy in Patients with Cardiovascular Disease: A Retrospective Study.' *BMJ Open* (2016). Available at: http://bmjopen.bmj.com/content/5/1/e005455.

33 Jacobs, L. et al. 'Traffic Air Pollution and Oxidised LDL.' *PLoS One* (2011): 6. Available at: https://www.ncbi.nlm.nih.gov/pubmed/21283820.

34 Boushehri, S. N. et al. 'Effect of Vitamin Supplementation on Serum-Oxidized Low-Density Lipoprotein Levels in Male Subjects with Cardiovascular Disease Risk Factors.' *Iran J Basic Med Sci* (2012, July–August): 15 (4): 958–64.

in the chapter on toxins that supplementing with glutathione reduces the levels of oxidised LDL[35] and also helps the liver to remove metal particles (such as cadmium) that we inhale from car exhaust fumes.

We are nearly done with this section, but before we close we need to get back to the third of Ridker's contributions that revolutionised our understanding that heart disease is primarily a problem of inflammation. By way of a reminder, his first was to show that inflammation, not blood cholesterol, is a more accurate way to determine heart-attack risk; his second was to show that statins reduce both cholesterol *and* arterial inflammation as they work to prevent heart disease. The third would answer whether cholesterol or inflammation is the root cause of heart disease.

That answer came in 2017 when, nearly two decades after his first paper on CRP was published, Ridker delivered what I consider the knockout blow to the theory that cholesterol is the root cause of heart disease. In the CANTOS study, his third major work, Ridker gave statin tablets to 10,000 heart-attack patients to optimise their heart health. He then gave half of this group an additional new anti-inflammatory medication. Although the entire group of 10,000 were on the best treatment available for heart attacks, he was able to show that those who received the extra anti-inflammatory medication had the lowest chance of getting another heart attack and the lowest chance of needing a stent, which is a procedure to clear a blocked artery.

It is worth stressing that the anti-inflammatory medication Ridker gave those patients had no effect on cholesterol; it was there merely to tackle inflammation. His study showed a marked improvement for those patients on the anti-inflammatory medication, providing the necessary proof that reducing arterial inflammation is fundamental to cutting our heart-attack risk.[36]

35 Wang, Y. et al. 'Molecular Mechanism of Glutathione-mediated Protection from Oxidised Low-density Lipoprotein Protein-induced Cell Injury in Human Macrophages: Role of Glutathione Reductase and Glutaredoxin.' *Free Radic Biol Med* (2006): 41: 775–85.
36 'Novartis Phase III CANTOS Study Demonstrates that Targeting Inflammation ACZ885 Reduces Cardiovascular Risk' (27 August 2017). Available at: https://www.novartis.com/news/media-releases/novartis-phase-iii-cantos-study-demonstrates-targeting-inflammation-acz885

Heart disease summary

- Inflammation – not cholesterol – is proving to be at the root of heart disease, as it is with other chronic illnesses. Inflammation is measured using the CRP blood test; this test should always be done when assessing heart health.

- Statin tablets have a valuable anti-inflammatory effect on the arteries. They also reduce cholesterol levels. The anti-inflammatory effects of statins are beneficial for people with a *moderate to severe* heart-attack risk. However, people with a low to mild heart-attack risk will likely find that statins' side effects outweigh their benefits; most people, therefore, should consider natural anti-inflammatory measures, including a healthy diet, exercise and stress management. We will look at diet in the next chapter, but for now it is sufficient to note that supplementing with natural anti-inflammatories such as aspirin, fish oil and alpha-lipoic acid will help our inflamed arteries.

- It is not just our arteries that can become inflamed: the LDL cholesterol that sticks to the artery walls can become oxidised and inflamed too. Stopping smoking, avoiding car fumes, and taking glutathione and antioxidant vitamins should help to prevent or reverse this process, and make our LDL cholesterol less sticky.

One of life's challenges is to be open to compelling new information that conflicts with what we 'know to be true'. That has been shown to apply particularly to the broad topic of inflammation: what causes it, how it damages us and how we can tackle it. Diet is central to the issue of rising inflammation-driven illnesses, and for that we can blame the potentially well-meaning but catastrophically misguided fat-free mantra of the 1980s. Three decades on, we know that inflammation – not cholesterol – is at the core of heart disease.

The consequence is profound: we need to rewrite fifty years of dietary advice, and we will turn to that next. In this chapter, we will look at sugar and saturated fats and how they link to inflammation; in the next chapter, we will examine nutrition more broadly.

CHEWING THE FAT

When it comes to eating macro-nutrients, we have three choices: fat, protein and carbohydrates. If we want to lose weight, we need to reduce our intake of at least one of them.

- If we reduce all three, then within a few days we will be very hungry and craving the first food we can find.
- If we cut out carbohydrates *and* fats, we will need to increase our protein intake significantly. That is not recommended, because – although the evidence is mixed – there are concerns that a high-protein diet is associated with cancer and early death.[37]
- In practice we tend to keep our protein intake constant, which is why most people trying to lose weight tend to restrict either their carbo-hydrate intake or their fat intake.

For decades, on the back of Ancel Keys' recommendations, the official advice was this: to lose weight and protect your heart, you should cut out the fat. The gospel that 'eating fat causes heart attacks' was linked to the mantra that 'you are what you eat' – if you eat fat, you will get fat and you will prob-ably have a heart attack. As a result, many of us in developed countries have spent years misguidedly eating low-fat foods.

The problem has in part been this: because our protein intake remains relatively constant, the fact that we were eating less fat means we were eating more carbohydrates. And where do we find carbohydrates? Anywhere from vegetables (very healthy), fruit (somewhat healthy), starches (bread, rice, pasta – all of which are unhealthy), and sugars, which are frankly dangerous.

Increasing our vegetable intake is the healthiest option; eating more starches or sugars causes problems, as we will shortly see. And going low-fat gets worse too, because the only way to make processed low-fat food taste tolerable is to add sugar, and plenty of it. There is already lots of sugar in most yoghurts, biscuits and breakfast cereals, as you will see by reading the label,

37 Levine, M. et al. 'Low Protein Intake is Associated with a Major Reduction in IGF-1, Cancer, and Overall Mortality in the 65 and Younger but Not Older Population.' *Cell Metabolism* (2014): 19: 407–17.

but there is far more in their low-fat cousins. That is why one catastrophic consequence of a low-fat diet has been very high sugar consumption.

Sugar and obesity

I will start by saying that you should not feel alone if you crave sugar: our bodies are hardwired for sugar and fats, and now that these two items are so easy to come by in the rich world – and increasingly in the developing world – we are consuming vastly greater amounts of them. In the 1840s, for example, the average American consumed seven kilograms of sugar each year; by the 1990s their descendants were eating nearly eight times as much.[38]

That figure has since declined by about 15 per cent (being precise is impossible due to a number of factors),[39] and it has been driven lower in part because of lower consumption of soda drinks. However, the average American still eats far more sugar than is healthy – around thirty teaspoons of added sugar or just over half a cup of sugar a day. Contrast that with the American Heart Association's recommendation of adding no more than six and nine teaspoons of sugar a day for women and men respectively,[40] and you can see the imbalance.

The rest of the world is not far behind. Indeed, as our consumption of sugar has risen, not only are more people addicted to it, but the number suffering from health woes has risen sharply. Many people know from media reports that there is a direct correlation between increased sugar consumption and rising rates of obesity: between 1980 and 2000, with sugar consumption rising fast, the incidence of obesity in the US doubled to 31 per cent of the adult population.[41] Seven years later the obesity rate had reached 38 per cent

38   Bray, G. et al. 'Dietary Sugar and Body Weight: Have We Reached a Crisis in the Epidemic of Obesity and Diabetes? Health be damned! Pour on the sugar.' *Diabetes Care* (2014): 37: 950–6.

39   See, for example: 'Just How Much Sugar Do Americans Consume? It's complicated.' Associated Press (20 September 2016).

40   See the American Heart Association: http://www.heart.org/HEARTORG/HealthyLiving/HealthyEating/Nutrition/Added-Sugars_UCM_305858_Article.jsp#.WbIi9q2Q1sM

41   Wang, Y. 'The Obesity Epidemic in the United States – Gender, Age, Socioeconomic, Racial/Ethnic, and Geographic Characteristics: A Systematic Review and Meta-Regression Analysis.' *Am J Epidemiol* (2007): 29: 6–28.

of adults, while 74 per cent of adults were classed as either overweight or obese.[42] Obesity has become a global epidemic: one in three people world-wide are overweight or obese, and obesity-related illness now kills three times as many people as malnutrition.[43]

Our eating habits have become far worse, and perhaps our biggest blind spot was failing to realise that 'low fat' means 'high sugar'. Consequently, we tend not to know how much sugar is in our favourite foods, even when that information is printed on the pack.

Half a cup of sugar a day is a lot, and in the modern world it adds up surprisingly fast: that is the amount in three cans of most soda drinks, or in three large glasses of orange or apple juice. Factor in the sugar in your breakfast cereal, bread, jam, morning biscuits, tomato sauce, pasta sauces, mayonnaise . . . I could go on. Added sugar is all around us, and if you want to know how much sugar you are eating – and I would suggest that is a very good thing to know – then you should read the packaging.

The point is that we consume a vast amount of sugar, and it is killing us. Why, though, do we love it so much? That is something we will examine more closely in the chapters on the brain, so what follows here is, so to speak, just a taster.

Sugar addicts

Our appetite for sugar is immense. Why? Because two-thirds of the surface area of your tongue is programmed to appreciate sugar. And by 'appreciate' what I really mean is 'can get addicted to'. We only need to look at the explosion of fast-food outlets throughout the world to see how our appetite for sugary foods has run rampant. In 1953, fast food accounted for 4 per cent of the money spent by US households on food away from home; by 1997, that number had risen to 34 per cent.[44] No doubt there is a convenience factor at work, but the addictiveness of sugar has surely played a role.

42   Streib, L. 'World's Fattest Countries.' *Forbes* (8 February 2007).

43   'Future Diets: The Global Rise of Obesity'. ODI (2014). See: https://www.odi.org/opinion/9329-future-diets-global-rise-obesity

44   French, S. A. et al. 'Fast-food Restaurant-use Among Women in the Pound of Prevention Study: Dietary, Behavioral and Demographic Correlates.' *Nature* (2000): 24: 1353–9.

Over the past decade, numerous studies have been published showing that sugar is overwhelmingly addictive, and why:

- Sugar's chemical structure is very similar to cocaine. In laboratory tests, rats were shown to prefer a sugar hit to a hit of cocaine.[45]
- Giving sugar to laboratory rats encouraged binge behaviour and then caused the two addiction pathways of the brain (dopamine and opiates) to surge. Stopping the sugar led to withdrawal symptoms in rats similar to those seen in drug withdrawal.[46]
- Interestingly, giving fat to rats also encouraged binge behaviour and caused dopamine brain surges. However, stopping fat consumption did not cause withdrawal symptoms.[47]
- When researchers added sugar to fat, the rats really hit their addictive stride. In bingeing sprees, they ate nearly 60 per cent of their full daily intake in the first hit of the day and rapidly put on weight.[48]

It is not hard to think of foods that combine sugar and fat – try the humble doughnut for starters. Manufacturers have spent billions finessing this potent combination as they have filled supermarket shelves with chocolate bars, biscuits and other snacks, to say nothing of the fat-and-sugar-laden ice creams, pizzas, sauces, ready meals, breakfast cereals, yoghurts – the list is practically endless. Today more than 70 per cent of food sold in supermarkets in the US has had sugar added to it.

The delicate balance of sweet and fat has been deliberately designed to make these wares difficult to resist. Even in the health-food aisle many items are packed with sugar. (For much more on the food industry and its efforts in this regard, I recommend US journalist Michael Moss' book *Salt, Sugar, Fat: How the Food Giants Hooked Us*.)

45   Ahmed, S. H. et al. 'Intense Sweetness Surpasses Cocaine Reward.' *PLoS One* (2007).
46   Hoebel, B, et al. 'Sugar and Fat-bingeing Have Notable Differences in Addictive-like Behaviour.' *J Nutr* (2009): 139: 623–8.
47   Corwin, R. L. et al. 'Limited Access to a Dietary Fat Option Affects Ingestive Behavior But Not Body Composition in Male Rats.' *Physiol Behav* (1998): 65: 545–53.
48   Hoebel, B, et al. 'Sugar and Fat-bingeing Have Notable Differences in Addictive-like Behaviour'. *J Nutr* (2009): 139: 623–8.

The point is that we are innately vulnerable to sugar and, fascinatingly, that vulnerability increases when we are tired. We will see in the chapters on the brain that, if we are in discomfort, our brain will try unceasingly to move us towards comfort. That is part of our mechanism for survival. If our ancestors were cold, tired or hungry, their brain would drive them to seek a fruit tree to get sugar and instant relief. For that reason it does not matter much if you were happy three hours ago, because if you are feeling unhappy *now* then your brain will do what it can to fix that *now*. Retailers understand that better than most, which is why the brightest and most attractive sweets are placed in the checkout aisle, which we reach when we are tired and at our most vulnerable.

Sugar is both addictive and omnipresent. What to do? Well, understanding *why* we reach out for it is the first step. When we are sleep-deprived, stressed or simply sad, our brain will look for comfort. Often that comfort is most easily found in one of sugar's many guises. Once we start on the sugar slide, our brain can quickly become addicted to it and, at that point, we will crave it regardless of whether we are happy or not.

In short, the trick to stopping sugar goes like this:

- Firstly, recognise that there is a sugar problem, and decide to do something about it.

- Secondly, do not feel guilty about it. Recognise that you likely have an issue with one or more of the Three S's – Sleep-deprivation, Stress or Sadness – and correct that. Once you have corrected the sleep, stress and sadness issues, the cravings go away on their own. (We will look at how to do that in the chapters on the brain.)

- Thirdly, throw out the sugary treats in your fridge or cupboard. (You can do this, I promise.) Then replace them with healthier treats like 70 per cent dark chocolate, berries and high-fat yoghurt (without added sugar), or coffee with cream. The next time your cravings loom, you will have plenty of healthier, non-sugary treats to satisfy them. (We will see later why I recommend certain healthy fats; for now you will have to take my word for it.)

Far from sweet

Revelations in *The New York Times*, among other media outlets, in recent years show how in the 1960s the US agricultural industry, in the form of the sugar trade group called the Sugar Research Foundation (which is today known as the Sugar Association), bribed Harvard scientists $50,000 in today's money 'to play down the link between sugar and heart disease, and promote saturated fat as the culprit instead'.[49]

The revelations first appeared in 2016 in the *Journal of the American Medical Association*, and the report's author, Professor Stanton Glantz of the University of California San Francisco, was quoted in *The New York Times* as saying that the move had allowed the sugar industry 'to derail the discussion about sugar for decades'.[50]

Another article in *The New York Times* showed that Coca-Cola donated millions of dollars 'to researchers who sought to play down the link between sugary drinks and obesity'.[51]

The food industry's efforts have not abated. In late 2016, *The New York Times* reported that a study that had just been published in a prominent medical journal and that had concluded that warnings against sugar could not be trusted was paid for by the International Life Sciences Institute, a group funded by Coca-Cola, Hershey's and Kraft, among others. Furthermore, the newspaper noted, one of the authors of the study 'is a member of the scientific advisory board of Tate & Lyle, one of the world's largest suppliers of high-fructose corn syrup'.[52]

49 Kearns, C. E. et al. 'Sugar Industry and Coronary Heart Disease Research: A Historical Analysis of Internal Industry Documents.' *JAMA* (2016): 176: 1680–5.
50 O'Connor, A. 'How the Sugar Industry Shifted Blame to Fat.' *The New York Times* (12 September 2016).
51 Kearns, C. E. et al. 'Sugar Industry and Coronary Heart Disease Research: A Historical Analysis of Internal Industry Documents.' *JAMA* (2016): 176: 1680–5.
52 O'Connor, A. 'Study Tied to Food Industry Tries to Discredit Sugar Guidelines.' *The New York Time* (19 December 2016).

A subsequent *New York Times* article has shown that, in the 1960s, the Sugar Research Foundation funded research into how sugar affected cardiovascular health 'and then buried the data when it suggested that sugar could be harmful'.[53]

When it came to the 1960s sugar corruption story, *The New York Times* noted:

'The Harvard scientists and the sugar executives with whom they collaborated are no longer alive. One of the scientists who was paid by the sugar industry was D. Mark Hegsted, who went on to become the head of nutrition at the United States Department of Agriculture, where in 1977 he helped draft the forerunner to the federal government's dietary guidelines.'

These dietary guidelines remained essentially constant for forty years advocating the benefits of a low-fat, high-carbohydrate diet and relegating saturated fats to the trash bin. Quite how many tens of thousands of lives this flagrant dishonesty has cost will never be known, yet it must rank as one of the best financial returns in history: for the paltry sum of $50,000, the sugar industry bought the world.

(Some) scientists fight back

In the world of nutrition, 2 December 2016 was a game-changer. A press release issued by the esteemed *British Medical Journal* (BMJ) stated that it would *not* retract an article that had claimed the American Dietary Guidelines (ADG) were based on 'a minuscule quantity of scientific evidence'.[54]

---

53 O'Connor, A. 'Sugar Industry Long Downplayed Potential Harms.' *The New York Times* (21 November 2017).

54 'Independent experts find no grounds for retraction of BMJ article on dietary guidelines.' *The BMJ* (2 December 2016). See press release: http://www.bmj.com/company/wp-content/uploads/2016/12/the-bmj-US-dietary-correction.pdf

The author of the article concerned was investigative journalist Nina Teicholz; it was a follow-up to her acclaimed book *The Big Fat Surprise* in which she provided extensive evidence showing that saturated fats are not bad for our health.[55] She pressed home that point in her article by accusing the ADG committee of being unscientific in its recommendation that we avoid saturated fats.

It is not hard to imagine how much pressure industry lobby groups exerted on the BMJ. The publication soon formed two independent review bodies to assess Teicholz's data. Their conclusion: Teicholz was justified in accusing the ADG committee of using weak evidence in developing the US dietary guidelines.

Oddly enough the guidelines seem healthy enough: eat plenty of vegetables, and keep sugar and alcohol to a minimum.[56] So was Teicholz being pedantic in picking a fight about whether we should or should not eat butter? Far from it.

This battle has a long and important history and, in this day of instant communications, it has gone global. In South Africa, Professor Tim Noakes, emeritus professor of sports medicine at the University of Cape Town, was brought before the Health Professions Council of South Africa (HPCSA) after a leading dietician complained that he had given unconventional advice by suggesting infants could eat a high-fat diet. After a lengthy high-profile case, Noakes was found not guilty in 2017. Bizarrely, in 2018, having lost the case, the HPCSA reopened the Noakes trial, but within a few months its effort was thrown out.

Across the water in Australia, Gary Fettke, an orthopaedic surgeon and lecturer, was less fortunate. A complaint was filed against him for advising people to eat a low-carbohydrate, high-fat diet. The Australian Health Practitioner Regulation Agency banned Fettke from giving any dietary advice to his patients; in other words, a leading surgeon

55 Teicholz, N. *The Big Fat Surprise: Why Butter, Meat and Cheese Belong in a Healthy Diet.* Simon & Schuster (2014).
56 Dietary guidelines for Americans, 2015–2020. Eighth Edition: https://health.gov/dietaryguidelines/2015/guidelines/

accustomed to amputating limbs from diabetic patients was barred from telling them to stop eating sugar. Voltaire was surely right when he said: 'It is dangerous to be right in matters on which the established authorities are wrong.'

Fettke's experience in Australia was preceded in Sweden by a case against Annika Dahlqvist, a doctor who was accused of spreading misinformation by recommending a low-carbohydrate, high-fat diet. Sensibly enough, the ruling went in Dahlqvist's favour, and she followed up on that success by writing a best-selling book on the subject. Since then, the sale of butter in Sweden has more than doubled, and the heart-attack rate has continued on a healthy downward trend[57] (although, of course, that is merely an association and does not prove anything in and of itself).

In other words, plenty of respected professionals have staked their careers on this subject, so it makes sense to look more closely at what they are so passionate about: the twin issues of why sugar is so dangerous and why saturated fats might even be good for us.

Insulin and the fat-forming pathway

The blood that moves through your body – along your arteries on its way to the extremities, and along your veins on its way back to the lungs and heart – is precisely calibrated to ensure that it contains specific amounts of oxygen and, for the purposes of what we will look at next, glucose.

This calibration process is unending: when we eat food, the protein is broken down into amino acids, the fat into fatty acids, and the carbohydrates into glucose and fructose. Logically enough, after your average meal, the amount of glucose that is then available to be carried in the bloodstream rises. But as we have seen time and again, our body needs balance, and it takes measures to ensure that our blood is not overloaded with glucose.

57 'Fewer Get Heart Attacks.' *Socialstyrelsen* (4 November 2013). See: http://www.social styrelsen.se/nyheter/2013november/farrefarhjartinfarkt

Let us take a closer look at what happens, unseen, every time we consume something:

- Carbohydrates (grains, fruits and vegetables) that are rich in fibre break down slowly into sugars; those that are low in fibre (pizza, pasta, white bread, white rice) break down into sugars much faster. The higher the fibre in the food, then, the slower is that breaking-down process, and that difference is central to modern-day diseases. In both cases, the sugars that result are comprised of glucose and fructose, and these two building blocks pass across the intestine wall and are absorbed into the bloodstream. A slow release of glucose into the blood can be used effectively throughout the body as a universal source of energy. A sudden dump of sugar, such as a fizzy drink that quickly breaks down into glucose and fructose, causes problems.

- Once glucose is in the bloodstream, the pancreas releases the hormone insulin, which pushes the glucose into the cells to be converted into energy; any excess glucose is taken by insulin for storage in fat cells. A large hit of glucose in the form of a fizzy drink or a sweet dessert requires a big release of insulin to get the glucose out of our bloodstream and locked up in fat cells. If that did not happen we would become dizzy from toxically high blood-sugar levels.

In short, some glucose is used straight away, while the rest is turned into fat. How the fat-forming process works is pretty simple: the body parcels up excess glucose with fatty acids into a compound known as a triglyceride; these sit inside the fat cells until such time as your body is short of glucose and fatty acids. At that point, the cell unwraps the triglycerides into their separate glucose and fatty acid components, allowing your body to use the glucose for energy. This process is best imagined as a bath-plug at the bottom of the fat cell: once the plug is opened, the cell unwraps the trigly-ceride, using up both the glucose and the fatty acids, which is how we start to lose our love-handles. The medical name for this bath-plug is a beta-receptor.

Here is the really important bit: if the beta-receptor, or plug, is blocked then it does not matter how hungry we feel – *we will not be able to access that stored fat for energy, and that means we will not lose weight.* What blocks the plug? Insulin. If you think about it, that is logical; after all, insulin's job is to remove glucose from the blood and store it in the fat cells, so it is hardly going to allow glucose to drain out of the bottom of the cell while packing more glucose into the top.

There is one key point to make here: what happens if the insulin cannot clear away all of the glucose? In that case, we will end up with too much glucose floating around in our arteries, in a condition known as diabetes. Why is that a problem? Because if we cannot clear glucose from our arteries, then it will cause arterial inflammation, and that brings a hugely increased risk of permanent damage to our arteries, kidneys, brain and eyes.[58] Glucose is a great energy source, but, like all fuel, excessive glucose is highly inflammatory and we need to clear it quickly from our arteries – or not eat it in the first place.

So much for the science. What this means in practice is that a diet high in carbohydrates and sugars tends to make us accumulate fat and become inflamed. In a vicious circle, fat releases inflammatory molecules, so that as our weight rises we become even more inflamed. Inflammation worsens any insulin resistance we might have, and that means insulin struggles to do its job of pushing glucose into cells. The problem compounds from there. Indeed, so dangerous are high glucose levels in our blood that the body prioritises removing it and packing it away into fat cells. The result: our pancreas generates more insulin for longer periods to process each meal. And, as the diagram shows, all that insulin in our system means we can no longer unplug the bottom of our fat cells and lose weight. By the time things reach this stage it hardly matters if we eat just a small sandwich for lunch – our excess of insulin will not allow us to lose even a small amount of weight.

58 Asmat et al. 'Diabetes mellitus and oxidative stress – a concise review.' *Saudi Pharm J* (2016): 24: 547–53.

Figure 2: Insulin unlocks the fat cell to push glucose in, and keeps the beta-receptor blocked

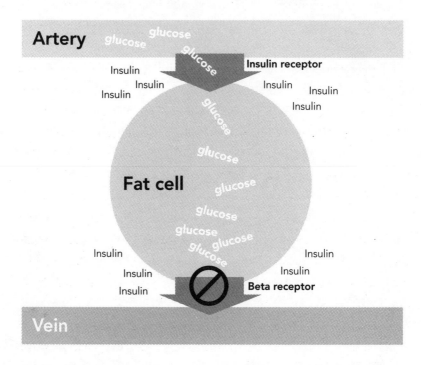

And that is why a high-carbohydrate diet can lead to fat storage, which can lead to craving more carbohydrates and which, if left unchecked, can lead to obesity and associated illnesses. We will find out later what to do about this, but for now let me tell you that the solution involves the following: avoiding all sugars and sugary carbohydrates (any time I refer to 'sugary carbohydrates' in this book, I am talking about starches, processed carbohydrates, some fruits and, of course, sugar); getting off the couch and doing some exercise; and, oddly enough, drinking a cup of coffee. Those three steps reduce insulin and unblock our beta-receptors.

Not all sugars are equal

When I think about sugar, my mind's eye shows me a bowl of bright-white sugar grains. As most people know, those grains come from cane sugar; it is also known as sucrose, and its chemical structure is 50 per cent fructose and 50 per cent glucose.

Until the 1960s, white sugar was the main form of sweetener used in food in developed countries. But with the US subsidising its farmers to grow increasing amounts of wheat and corn, corn prices eventually dropped, and processors looked to see what else they could use corn for. The result was a derivative called High Fructose Corn Syrup (HFCS), and it quickly became the go-to replacement for conventional sugar in processed foods.

HFCS had two key benefits: it was very sweet and it was cheap. Before long you could find it in countless processed products – from Coca-Cola to mayonnaise and nearly everything in between.[59] Its use was so widespread that by 1985 half of all sugar consumed in the US was in the form of HFCS. Even Lactomil, a powdered milk for infants, contained 43 per cent HFCS.

The dominance of HFCS in the US market largely stemmed from the fact that it is cheaper than cane-derived sugar. Yet since 2007 the public has grown far more aware of its harmful effects, and consumers are increasingly steering clear of HFCS-laden products.[60]

What are these harmful effects of HFCS, you might ask? The process to extract HFCS from corn (or maize, as the cereal is known in many countries) results in a product that is up to 60 per cent fructose (that is what makes it super-sweet) and 40 per cent glucose. You are probably thinking: so what? That does not seem so different from the 50:50 composition of cane sugar. That extra fructose, however, brings with it some sinister side effects.

---

59   Fields, S. 'The Fat of the Land: Do Agricultural Subsidies Foster Poor Health?' *Environ Health Perspect* (2004): 112: A820–3.
60   Lopes, M. and Prentice, C. 'U.S. Corn Syrupmakers Slash Prices to Fend Off Cheap Sugar.' Reuters (11 November 2013) .

In his excellent book – *Fat Chance: The Hidden Truth About Sugar, Obesity and Disease* – Robert Lustig, an obesity specialist and paediatric endocrinologist, spells this out, describing three basic sugars and how our bodies deal with them.

Sugar One: Glucose

This is our main source of energy. We know that glucose stimulates insulin, and we know that lots of glucose stimulates lots of insulin, which will then store the glucose as triglycerides in fat cells. Typically, 80 per cent of glucose will be used in the body for making energy or will be stored in fat cells for later energy use. The remaining 20 per cent is sent to the liver where it is stored either in the form of glycogen or as fatty triglycerides. An excess of fatty triglycerides in the liver can lead to a fatty liver, which is becoming a growing health problem.

Fatty liver

The medical world used to think that the toxin alcohol was the reason behind developing a fatty liver; we now know that is only partly true, and that sugar (and particularly fructose) is just as good at doing this.

Sugar-driven fatty liver has been given the cumbersome acronym NAFLD (non-alcoholic fatty liver disease), and up to 30 per cent of adults in developed nations suffer from this.[61] Whatever the cause, though, the result is the same: a liver that functions poorly, worsening inflammation and the chronic diseases that come with this condition. On the plus side, sugar-driven NAFLD can be reversed in weeks if we stop the sugar.[62]

---

61 Younossi, Z. M. et al. 'Global Epidemiology of Non-Alcoholic Fatty Liver Disease – Meta-Analytic Assessment of Prevalence, Incidence and Outcomes.' *Hepatology* (2016): 64: 73–84.
62 Browning, J. D. et al. 'Prevalence of Hepatic Steatosis in an Urban Population in the United States: Impact of Ethnicity.' *Hepatology* (2004): 40(6): 1387–95.

In summary – too much glucose leaves us with a high chance of insulin spikes, insulin resistance and obesity. But because not much glucose goes to the liver (just 20 per cent, typically), an excess of it brings only a minor chance of developing a fatty liver.

Sugar Two: Fructose

As you might guess from the name, fructose is found mainly in fruit and, as we saw earlier, in cereals such as corn – thus the name High-Fructose Corn Syrup (HFCS), which is made from processed corn. Fructose was originally seen as useful, particularly for athletes, because it does not cause an insulin spike and therefore allows us to keep accessing our fat stores for energy (something we will look at later). However, that overlooks three of fructose's key harmful effects:

- Firstly, fructose causes glycation, which is the sugaring of protein. Glycation is what causes hardening of the lens in the eye (cataracts) and of the kidneys (leading to kidney failure). Laboratories measure glycation using the HbA1c test; that test looks at the amount of sugaring of haemoglobin, which is the substance that transports oxygen in the bloodstream.

- Secondly, because fructose does *not* stimulate insulin, it consequently does not stimulate leptin (the fullness hormone). So if you are wondering why your children are still hungry after drinking a fructose-laden fizzy drink or fruit juice, now you know.

- Thirdly, 60 per cent of fructose goes to the liver (versus just 20 per cent of glucose) where a large proportion of it forms triglyceride fats.[63] This leaves us at a much greater risk of suffering from NAFLD (a fatty liver). By way of a comparison with the animal world, French producers force-feed corn to geese and ducks in order to make foie gras, a phrase which literally means 'fat liver'. Drinking fizzy drinks,

63 Samuel, V. T. 'Fructose-induced Lipogenesis: From Sugar to Fat to Insulin Resistance.' *Trends Endocrinol Metab* (2011): 22: 60–5.

consuming HFCS-laden foods and downing a lot of fruit juice does much the same thing.

In summary – too much fructose leaves us hungry, at risk of cataracts (and worse), and at significant risk of developing a fatty liver.

Sugar Three: Alcohol

It is even more efficient (and therefore worse for us) in terms of making fat through the liver. Eighty per cent of ethanol (an alcohol fermented from sugars) goes through the liver. This leaves us at a high risk of developing a fatty liver. It is also extremely difficult to lose weight if you continue to drink alcohol to excess.[64] A beer belly in young men and women is testament to the efficiency of this pathway. And even though some people with fatty livers might look thin, they are on the same inflamed metabolic disease pathway as most obese people.

In summary – too much alcohol (particularly beer) leaves us at high risk of a fatty liver and the ensuing inflammatory diseases. Note, too, that a fatty liver caused by the sugar in alcohol *is* a reversible condition, provided the person stops drinking alcohol and thereby eliminates that sugary intake. However, that is not the case for liver damage caused by the *toxins* in alcohol that can cause hepatitis; that damage is often irreversible.

These days the dangers of sugars are far better understood. The American Heart Association, for instance, recognises that reducing the intake of sugar could help combat obesity and heart attacks. Part of the challenge, however, is that processed sugar is so readily available. For example:

- If you have ever eaten a stick of cane sugar, you will know that it is hard work – the sugar cane stem has so much fibre that it takes five minutes to suck and chew two teaspoons of sugar, and by that time your jaw is aching from the effort. Moreover, the fibre slows the sugar absorption, which means your body does not have to deal with an overwhelming influx of sugar in the bloodstream.

64 Lustig, R. *Fat Chance: The Hidden Truth About Sugar, Obesity and Disease*. Harper Collins (2012).

- A can of Coca-Cola on the other hand, has ten teaspoons of sugar, is fibre-free and takes just minutes to drink. The result – a glucose spike causing inflammation, insulin and fatty deposits, and a fructose spike helping to develop a fatty liver.
- Or how about a theoretically healthy no-preservative, non-alcoholic can of sparkling apple juice? It contains eight teaspoons of sugar and has no fibre to slow the sugar absorption. Compare that to your average apple which contains two teaspoons of sugar. The apple has so much fibre that it is rated as having a low glycaemic load (a good thing), and is considered healthy.

The central point to bear in mind is that *all* sugars are harmful in excess, and 'excess' is precisely what the rich world has been doing for decades. Increasingly the developing world is headed the same way. But as we have seen, it is not just HFCS that is the problem – it is all sugars in excess.

And if you think this wariness over sugar is new-found, it is not. It turns out that we have known about it for decades.

Sugar and insulin resistance

The potential role of sugars in heart disease was already being studied in the 1960s. One researcher, for instance, suggested that injecting insulin into animals would stimulate blockages in the arteries.[65]

As we saw earlier, insulin is the energy storage hormone that allows us to pack away the fruits of our harvest and survive the lean winter months. But in our modern world of constant sugar harvesting, this excess of sugar and the consequent surfeit of insulin leads to insulin resistance, atherosclerosis and heart disease.

Around that time, one voice did stand up against the growing juggernaut that was the sugar-driven food industry: his name was John Yudkin, and he was for many years professor of nutrition at the University of London. In 1972, after years of research and analysis that – to him at least – showed sugar, not

---

65   Stout, R. W. 'Insulin-stimulated Lipogenesis in Arterial Tissue in Relation to Diabetes and Atheroma.' *The Lancet* (1968): 2: 7570: 702–3.

fat, was the enemy, Yudkin wrote up his thesis in simple prose and published it in a book titled *Pure, White and Deadly*. It sold well, but he was vilified by the medical profession for his efforts (not least by Keys, whose work was funded in part by the sugar industry) and was even banned from attending conferences.

Yet as the years passed, other trials looking to prove Keys' putative link between saturated fat and heart disease failed to find a connection between eating fat and obesity or between eating fat and heart disease.[66] As we saw earlier, some surmised (in the manner of Yudkin) that there was no link to be found. It is only in the past two decades that we have begun to understand that inflammation is the key element driving modern chronic illness, and that there is an unequivocal link between sugar and inflammation.[67]

As we saw earlier, when we take in sugar, insulin is released to clear the glucose from the blood and deposit it into the muscles and the liver, and particularly into the fat cells. But if our lifestyle sees us consume too much sugar, something sinister happens: both the sugar and the developing fat stores cause a low-grade inflammation to fester in the body.[68] It is this slow-burning inflammation that has been shown to trigger a very unhealthy condition called insulin resistance[69] – which is when our inflamed arteries slow down insulin from doing its job of clearing glucose out of the blood and into the cells. As a result we need more insulin to get that job done.

Insulin resistance shows up in blood tests as a rising insulin level many

66 Steinberg, D. 'Thematic Review Series: The Pathogenesis of Atherosclerosis. An Interpretive History of the Cholesterol Controversy: Part 11: The Early Evidence Linking Hypercholesterolemia to Coronary Disease in Humans.' *J Lipid Res* (2005): 46: 2: 179–90.

67 Mohanty, P. et al. 'Glucose Challenge Stimulates Reactive Oxygen Species (ROS) Generation by Leucocytes.' *J Clin Endocrinol Metab* (2000): 85 (8): 2970–3.

68 Torres-Leal, F. L. et al. 'The Role of Inflamed Adipose Tissue in Insulin Resistance.' *Cell Biochem Funct* (December 2010): Vol 28: 623–31.

69 Chen, L. et al. 'Mechanisms Linking Inflammation to Insulin Resistance.' *Int J Endocrinol* (2015): 508409: https://www.hindawi.com/journals/ije/2015/508409/

hours after we have eaten, and is associated with obesity, heart attacks and chronic illness.[70]

There are two key explanations as to why insulin resistance does such damage:

- The first explanation is that insulin resistance leads to arterial blockages and heart disease.[71] This was best described by the late Joseph Kraft in his 2008 book *Diabetes Epidemic & You*. Being a pathologist, Kraft decided to research the tissue at the site of heart attacks. His results were astounding. After performing more than 4,000 autopsies on people who had died from a heart attack, Kraft found 20 per cent of them had already been diagnosed with diabetes while the remaining 80 per cent had signs of micro-arterial diabetic change at the site of the heart attack. He called it diabetes-in-situ, and it implicates sugar, insulin and inflammation in the health of every person who has suffered a heart attack.

- Another study carried out by Kraft that links to this first explanation looked at what happens to our insulin level after we eat sugar. This is called a glucose tolerance test, and is usually done by measuring glucose levels two hours after ingesting pure glucose to see whether it has been cleared from the bloodstream. If we are healthy then it should have been cleared; if it has not been cleared then we are starting to move in the direction of insulin resistance and possibly diabetes. Kraft also looked at what happens to our insulin up to five hours after ingesting glucose (a test that doctors do not routinely do). He found that in 80 per cent of people, insulin lingers in the arteries for hours longer than it should. While a normal blood test might give someone like that a clean bill of health, Kraft's test suggests that most of us have mild insulin resistance. That is not the same as full-blown insulin resistance (which means insulin levels are still high ten hours

---

70 Semenkovich, C. F. 'Insulin Resistance and Atherosclerosis.' *J Clin Invest* (2006): 116: 1813–22.

71 Ibid.

after eating); however, it is far from ideal that such a high proportion of people had insulin lingering in their arteries between two and five hours after ingesting glucose. It indicates that many, and perhaps most, of us have glucose in our arteries much longer than we should. Kraft suggested this marked the start of diabetes and, if noticed, could be reversed before it caused trouble. The trouble it causes, of course, we already know from Kraft's first study: heart attacks, with diabetic changes visible at the site of every heart attack.

• The second explanation is one we looked at earlier: excessive insulin blocks the plugs (the beta-receptors) at the bottom of the fat cells, and prevents them from losing their fat. If someone is insulin-resistant and has excess insulin floating around their body twelve hours after they last ate, then they stand very little chance of losing fat. Fortunately there are steps they can take to reduce their insulin level and trigger the beta-receptors, including exercise, fasting and drinking a cup of coffee. All of these will see the plugs in the fat cells open, release glucose for energy and shrink their love handles.[72] However, even a mildly raised insulin level will block the beta-receptors' ability to unplug the fat cells, and – given that Kraft reckoned 80 per cent of people in his study had a mildly raised insulin level – that is a problem. Compounding this, if we are unable to access that stored glucose when we need it, we will naturally feel hungry just a few hours after we have eaten.

In summary, then, mild insulin resistance seems to be a pervasive problem, with perhaps most of us showing some signs of it. On the plus side, it is easy to measure; on the other hand, it is not routinely tested. And it is something to be aware of. This is not just about losing weight; much more seriously, as Kraft showed, it probably drove the process that resulted in the diabetic changes seen at the sites of the heart attacks of every one of his 4,000 cadavers. So although mild insulin resistance is *not* an illness, it is

72 Acheson, K. J. et al. 'Metabolic Effects of Caffeine in Humans: Lipid Oxidation or Futile Cycling.' *Am J Clin Nutr* (2004): 79: 40–6.

clearly something on which we should focus in order to optimise our health.

What can we do about it? There are several options, one of which brings us back to something we encountered in the chapter on the theories of ageing. There we saw that calorie restriction – cutting our calorie intake by about a third – is one of only two theories proven to extend healthy life. Having read this section, you will understand why: the experiments carried out on mice showed that calorie restriction decreased inflammation, reduced insulin resistance, switched on longevity genes and extended their lives.[73]

Calorie restriction is probably the best option for extending a healthy life. However, cutting out that amount of calories is a big ask, so here are some other options that mimic calorie restriction:

- High-Intensity Interval Training (HIIT): This refers specifically to short bursts of exercise. It could be as quick as a four-minute Tabata training session, where you do eight intense sets lasting twenty seconds each of, for example, star jumps or burpies, with ten seconds resting in between. It is not done for weight loss, but does greatly improve glucose metabolism and tackles insulin resistance.[74]

- Intermittent fasting: Typically this involves delaying breakfast until, say 11am, having eaten our last meal around 7pm the previous evening. That means our eating period lasts eight hours and our fasting period lasts 16, which gives a 16:8 fasting ratio. This is an easy way to mimic calorie restriction, and results in a reduction of insulin resistance and weight loss.[75]

- Ketogenic diet: This refers to a very low-carbohydrate diet (typically less than 25g of carbohydrates a day) and one that is

73 Duan, W. 'Dietary Restriction Normalizes Glucose Metabolism and Brain-Derived Neurotrophic Factor Levels, Slows Disease Progression and Increases Survival in Huntington Mutant Mice.' *Proc Natl Acad Sci USA* (4 March 2003): 100: 2911–16.

74 Cassidy, S. et al. 'High-intensity Interval Training: A Review of its Impact on Glucose Control and Cardiometabolic Health.' *Diabetologia* (2017): 60: 7–23.

75 Lee, C. 'Dietary Restriction with and without Caloric Restriction for Healthy Aging.' *Faculty Review* (2016). See: https://www.ncbi.nlm.nih.gov/pmc/articles/PMC4755412/

high in saturated fats. This forces the body to generate its energy from ketones (which are derived from fat) rather than from glucose. This not only reduces inflammation and insulin resistance; it has also been shown in animals to reverse cancer.[76] (We will look more closely at low-carbohydrate, healthy-fat diets in the next chapter.)

• The diabetic tablet Metformin: Also known as glucophage, it is used by diabetics to control the level of glucose in the blood. It works by reducing insulin resistance, and it is sometimes used as a weight-loss tablet. Metformin is interesting for our purposes because, in studies on mice, it has been shown to switch on the same longevity genes that are triggered by calorie restriction,[77] and has been found to extend the lives of a certain strain of mice.[78] That raises several questions. Can Metformin help to extend longevity in humans? And should it be used for the 80 per cent of us who have mildly raised insulin levels, or should it be given only to those people who cannot optimise their insulin level through a programme of fasting, exercise and low-carbohydrate eating? Within a few years we should be closer to answering those questions, as a study is underway to determine whether giving Metformin to healthy elderly patients will extend their healthy life.

Summary of sugar

• Sugar is inflammatory – and it does not matter whether this sugar comes in the form of glucose, fructose (including HFCS) or the sugars found in alcohol.

76 Mengmeng, L. V. et al. 'Roles of Caloric Restriction, Ketogenic Diet and Intermittent Fasting during Initiation, Progression and Metastasis of Cancer in Animal Models: A Systematic Review and Meta-Analysis.' *PLoS One* (2014): 9 (12): e115147.

77 Dhabhi, J. M. et al. 'Identification of Potential Caloric Restriction Mimetic by Microarray Profiling.' *Physiol Genomics* (2005): 23: 343–50.

78 Anisimov, V. N. et al. 'Metformin Slows Down Ageing and Extends Lifespan of Female SHR Mice.' *Cell Cycle* (2008): 1: 2769–73.

- The inflammation caused by sugar triggers insulin resistance. And what holds true for sugar is also relevant for a range of carbohydrates, including white rice, white bread, pastas and the like.
- Up to 80 per cent of us might have mild insulin resistance.
- Insulin resistance is heavily implicated in obesity, heart attacks and chronic illness.
- The following activities reduce insulin resistance and may extend a healthy life: eating a low-carbohydrate diet, intermittent fasting and doing regular high-intensity exercise.

So, with sugars and starchy carbohydrates deeply implicated in causing heart attacks and the range of other chronic illnesses, it is time to find out whether the other macronutrient – fat, and particularly saturated fat – is the evil we once thought it was.

ARE SATURATED FATS DANGEROUS?

For decades, the advice was to follow a diet loaded with fruit, grains and vegetables, and very low in fats and particularly saturated fats. The theory was based in part on an oversimplified explanation of calories: lower your intake of calories, and you will lower your weight. And because fats have more calories per gram than protein and carbohydrates, they were thought best avoided.

Calorie-counting, however, is very much a 1980s obsession. As we have seen, if we want to tackle weight loss and optimise our health then it is much more important to reduce our levels of glucose and insulin in the blood. It turns out that, for most of us, weight gain is primarily a hormone problem that revolves around insulin and sugars; it has far less to do with calories. If you are insulin-resistant – and it seems many of us are – then the excess insulin you produce after each intake of food will help to fill your fat cells with glucose and block them from emptying.

However, that is *not* to say that calories are irrelevant. It *is* true that the amount of calories we consume counts – just not in the way we used to think. For example, if we cut out starchy carbohydrates but load up on butter, nuts and full-fat yoghurt, we will reduce our insulin resistance (a good thing), but we will also find that eating so many high-calorie fats might slow down our weight loss. That is why the most effective way to lose weight is to reduce calories by minimising all sugary carbohydrates *and* fats.[79]

I am often asked how that works in practical terms, so let me tell you how I approach weight loss at my clinic. If we suddenly stop eating all sugars and fats, we will quickly become overwhelmed by cravings and return to the junk food we so love. Both sugar and fat can cause weight gain but, for the reasons described in this chapter, sugar (and its hormone-handler insulin) are *by far* the greater evil. That is why in weight-loss programmes my patients are typically advised to stop eating all sugary carbohydrates, but still to eat a reasonable amount of fats to keep the brain happy. Only once they have stopped craving sugars would I consider advising them to reduce fats temporarily in order to accelerate weight loss.

With all that said, the question still remains: is it healthy to eat butter and other saturated fats? Over the past twenty years, plenty of diets have been underpinned by just this approach. Three of the best-known in what is called the Low Carbohydrate, High Fat (LCHF) category are Atkins, Banting and Palaeolithic. When it comes to how they deal with carbohydrates, all three restrict us to less than six to nine teaspoons of sugar a day, and they limit our total carbohydrate intake (which comprises sugar, starches, fruit and vegetables) to less than 100g daily. (By comparison, government guidelines usually recommend 200–300g.)

In other words these diets would see us eat large amounts of fibrous vegetables, such as spinach and broccoli, one or two fruit portions, limited starch and virtually no added sugar. The aim is to reduce our blood glucose levels, and by extension cut inflammation and insulin resistance.

We know that reducing carbohydrates by this amount means we typically need to add fats in order to stay sated, and indeed all three diets encourage adding the saturated fats that we find in eggs, dairy and meat. However by the

---

79 Johnston, B. C. et al. 'Comparison of Weight Loss Among Named Diet Programs in Overweight and Obese Adults: A Meta-analysis.' *JAMA* (2014): 312: 923–33.

turn of this century the medical press remained largely sceptical of this type of eating.[80]

What was needed was a rigorous scientific analysis, and that did not come until 2012 when a Cochrane Library meta-analysis was published. It largely pardoned saturated animal fat. The analysis disproved our decades-long assumption that saturated fat is bad for us, and showed that eating saturated fat does *not* increase mortality from heart attacks.[81] Those findings were backed up in a 2014 meta-analysis of seventy-six studies that showed there was no evidence for the current guidelines that restrict saturated animal fats in a bid to prevent heart disease; instead it concluded that the evidence does *not* support the current guidelines that encourage us to eat polyunsaturated fats such as seeds and nuts, and that discourage us from consuming saturated fats.

What does all this mean? Simply put, most of us can confidently eat meat, dairy, eggs and coconut oil. It also means that we should use butter and avoid margarine.[82]

Now, if you are a keen follower of the American Heart Association, you might know that it does *not* agree. After assessing four studies, the AHA said in 2017 that saturated fats *could* cause heart disease, and recommended that their consumption be kept to a minimum.[83] Its announcement was controversial, and saw journalist Nina Teicholz weigh in with a sharp critique of its methodology: Teicholz accused the AHA of cherry-picking just four out of a possible ten studies that it should have used to assess heart-attack risk. She also pointed out weaknesses in the AHA's criteria, not least that it had examined soft data, such as angina, which is chest pain, rather than hard data

80   Astrup, A. et al. 'Atkins and Other Low Carbohydrate Diets: Hoax or an Effective Tool for Weight Loss?' *The Lancet* (2004): 364: 897–9.

81   Hooper, L. et al. 'Reduced or Modified Dietary Fat for Preventing Cardiovascular Disease.' *The Cochrane Library* (May 2012).

82   Chowdrey, R. et al. 'Association of Dietary, Circulating and Supplemental Fatty Acids with Coronary Risk.' *Ann Intern Med* (2014): 160: 398–406.

83   Sacks, F. M. et al. 'Dietary Fats and Cardiovascular Disease: A Presidential Advisory From the American Heart Association.' (2017): 136: http://circ.ahajournals.org/content/early/2017/06/15/CIR.0000000000000510

events, such as heart attacks, strokes and death. When Teicholz and cardiologist Eric Thorn carried out their examination of the studies, they concluded, as she wrote: 'A rigorous review of the evidence shows that when it comes to heart attacks or mortality, saturated fats are not guilty.'[84]

In other words, there is no evidence to suggest we should restrict our intake of saturated fats if we want to avoid heart disease. (If you are wondering why the AHA would behave in this way, Teicholz accuses it of sticking to outdated beliefs and says it is beholden for funding to commercial interests, such as Bayer and Proctor & Gamble.)

However, one can surely not take the word of an individual over the advice from the AHA – and we did not need to as, shortly after the AHA's announcement, the results of a much bigger study were released. The Prospective Urban Rural Epidemiological (PURE) study looked at the eating habits of 135,000 adults in eighteen countries to try to work out what is killing us: carbohydrates or fats. The PURE study showed that eating excessive carbohydrates is responsible for heart attacks and early death. Eating fats, including saturated fats, was shown to protect against heart disease and prolong healthy life.[85]

It is worth noting that the PURE research was an observational study, and therefore cannot prove cause and effect. Also, as its authors wrote, its findings '[do] not provide support for very low carbohydrate diets'. That said, its conclusions are interesting: when taken in conjunction with the two large meta-analyses, the PURE study supports the use of saturated fat in our diet. The AHA, as we have seen, is largely against it.

In light of this, my clinic encourages people to eat *healthy* saturated fats – and, given that most saturated fats come from animal sources, by 'healthy' I mean 'sourced from grass-fed animals'. When clients are trying to come off

84 Teicholz, N. (Op-Ed). 'Don't Believe the American Heart Assn. – Butter, Steak and Coconut Oil Aren't Likely to Kill You.' *Los Angeles Times* (23 July 2017). See: http://www.latimes.com/opinion/op-ed/la-oe-teicholz-saturated-fat-wont-kill-you-20170723-story.html

85 Dehghan, M. et al. 'Associations of Fats and Carbohydrate Intake with Cardiovascular Disease and Mortality in 18 Countries from Five Continents (PURE): A Prospective Cohort study.' *The Lancet* (August 2017). See: http://www.thelancet.com/journals/lancet/article/PIIS0140-6736(17)32252-3/fulltext

sugars, we typically increase their saturated fat consumption to help reduce the sugar cravings; we can do this because saturated fats are now generally seen as having a *neutral* overall effect on our health (and, as we shall see in the chapter on nutrition, they have an important positive effect in areas such as the brain and cell membranes).

Perhaps, as Teicholz suggests, it is time for health authorities to conduct a large, long-term clinical trial on the impact of saturated fats on heart disease.

Inflammation and obesity: a final word

You might wonder how serious the dangers are that sugar poses. To my mind they are so significant that sugar is one of my Three Horsemen of the Health-pocalypse. (The other two are toxins and stress, which we will deal with in subsequent chapters.)

If I were to summarise this chapter in a couple of brief sentences, it would be as follows:

- Sugar is bad.
- Saturated fat is not bad.

These days the first point is largely uncontroversial. (How things have changed in just a few decades.) Whether I am talking with dieticians, doctors or patients, there is now little defence of sugar. Indeed most people are astonished at how sugar became such a large and hidden part of our lives. Whether we grew up during the low-fat (and therefore high-hidden-sugar) decades or just because sugary fast foods were the easiest solution in a busy lifestyle, the result was the same: we ate far too much of it. I well remember how a half-litre of apple juice would count as one of my five-a-day fruit and vegetable intake (apples are fruit, after all). But when you realise that one such serving of apple juice contains nearly fourteen teaspoons of sugar, it is no surprise I was unable to shift my love handles!

Understanding sugar's multiplicity of dangers has been important in devising strategies to counter it. A number of countries are considering a sugar tax; some have already implemented one. Mexico, for example, where 70 per cent of the population is overweight or obese, and where one in six has diabetes, put in place a soda tax in January 2014. The result was a 5 per cent drop in national soda sales in the first year, and a near 10 per cent decline in the second.[86] (It is too early to tell whether this will translate into the expected reduction in obesity and chronic illness.) The UK and Ireland implemented a similar tax in 2018. Some experts want to see advertising for sugar restricted in the same way as is done for tobacco.[87]

The second point – that saturated fat is *not* bad – is still being fiercely debated. When in late 2016 Nina Teicholz concluded that the American Dietary Guidelines were based on 'a minuscule quantity of scientific evidence', we can appreciate that she was not merely trying to stir things up. Whether or not we should eat saturated fat has been a cornerstone of dietary advice for sixty years, and that in part explains the pressure that the *British Medical Journal* was under from lobby groups after it published Teicholz's article. For my part, I applaud the BMJ for focusing on the evidence, not the pressure, and for standing by her article that called for saturated fats to return to the table. In the next chapter we will look at how to apply that advice to our lives.

Key points

Obesity and chronic illness have exploded over the last fifty years along with our appetite for sugar and junk food. Sugar consumption and obesity drive inflammation, and inflammation drives chronic illness.

Heart disease is our most common chronic illness. Contrary to what we were taught, eating saturated fat does not cause heart disease. Instead, we know that sugar drives the inflammation that causes heart attacks.

- Sugar also drives insulin resistance which prevents us from losing weight. If Kraft was correct, then up to 80 per cent of us have mild insulin resistance. We can correct this by cutting out

86   Grogger, J. 'Soda Taxes and the Prices of Sodas and Other Drinks: Evidence from Mexico.' *Am J Agric Econ* (2017): 99: 481–9.

87   See, for example: http://www.bbc.com/news/health-27961475

sugar, undertaking intermittent fasting and doing high-intensity exercise.

- Sugar is addictive. If you are struggling with cravings then consider the three S's: Sleep, Stress and Sadness. Fix these and you will correct most cravings.
- Patients at my clinic who want to lose weight are advised to cut out all starchy carbohydrates, but to keep eating saturated fats. This is not only healthy eating; it also prevents sugar cravings. I would consider reducing their intake of fats only if they continued struggling to lose weight.

Chapter 4

Nutrition – Busting the Fat Myth

> I can identify the causes of obesity after listening to one stout party
> after another proclaiming the joys of bread, rice and potatoes.
>
> *Jean Anthelme Brillat-Savarin 1755–1826*

By 2014 – nearly two centuries after the death of French gastronome, lawyer and politician Jean Anthelme Brillat-Savarin, whose quote opens this chapter – almost 40 per cent of the world was overweight.

I suspect that, had Brillat-Savarin lived that long, he would not have been surprised. He understood that many of the people who were stout, as he put it, were those who ate carbohydrates to excess. He was, it seems, a man ahead of his time. Today we are still debating which is worse for us: eating fats or eating starchy carbohydrates such as bread and potatoes (and, of course, sugar)?

Before we solve that conundrum, though, let us take a closer look at what we consume and what each does to us. We can divide our nutrients into macronutrients and micronutrients. There are three groups of macronutrients, and we need to eat a lot of them: these are proteins, carbohydrates and fats. Unprocessed foods generally contain a mix of all three.

Proteins

At their basic level, proteins are comprised of small molecules called amino acids, and when we eat protein it gets broken down into these amino acids by our digestive system. We use amino acids for a range of functions, including building muscle, making white blood cells to fight infections, and constructing the machinery inside our cells.

Our body is able to make some amino acids itself, but it cannot make all of them. The latter group are called 'essential amino acids', and we have to get these from the food we eat.

We can get our protein from plants (good sources are nuts, peas, beans, hempseed and courgette, for example) and from animals (where the good sources are red meat, chicken, fish, dairy and eggs).

Carbohydrates

These are foods that are made entirely from basic sugars, such as glucose and fructose. If you were to combine those two molecules in a certain proportion then you would have table sugar, which is what we use to sweeten our teas and coffees. If you mixed them in a different combination then you would have corn syrup, which is the sweetener found in many fizzy drinks.

If you add many sugar molecules and combine them with fibre, which is indigestible and slows the rate of release of glucose into the body, then you will have what is called a complex carbohydrate. We know these better as:

- Starches, such as potatoes, rice, wheat and oats. These are made almost entirely from glucose and have some fibre. They tend to release their glucose too quickly in the body, which is why we should restrict our intake of them.
- Fruits, such as oranges, peaches, berries and apples. Fruits grow on trees (most of them, at any rate), and are full of fructose and glucose. However, they contain differing amounts of fibre and, although they contain healthy vitamins, fruit's high sugar content means it is some-times referred to as 'nature's candy'.
- Vegetables, such as carrots, broccoli, spinach, courgette, asparagus and cabbage. These grow either underground (carrots) or above the ground (cabbage). They are high in fibre and low in sugars, and this makes vegetables the healthiest category within the carbohydrate group.

Finally we have refined (or processed) carbohydrates, for which think bread, biscuits, white rice, dried fruits or candy bars to name a few. What they have in common is that humans have tampered with them, removing much of the fibre. Why does that matter? Because one of fibre's jobs is to slow down the release of the sugars from food; with no fibre to slow that release, refined carbohydrates tend to dump their sugar load into the blood, which is why we should avoid them.

An everyday example of this refining process is white bread (low in fibre) versus wholewheat bread. Lastly, and as mentioned in the previous chapter, when I refer to 'sugary carbohydrates', I am talking about these refined carbo-hydrates, along with starches, some fruits and sugar.

Fats

Our third category is fats. These are comprised of two groups of smaller mole-cules – cholesterol and fatty acids – that our body uses to build our brain and to make the cell membrane for every cell in the body. We also use fats to make hormones, our supply of vitamin D, and to create the myelin sheath that covers our nerves.

Our liver makes most of the cholesterol we need, but we can also get it from sources such as egg yolks, butter and fatty meats.

Food is the source of our essential fatty acids, which we divide into:

- Saturated fatty acids: these are called saturated because all the bonds between the fatty acids are linked. This makes them strong fats, and in this chapter we will see why that is important. Saturated fat is found predominantly in animal fat and coconut oil.
- Unsaturated fatty acids: these have one or more bonds that are incomplete, and that makes them more susceptible to heat damage. Olive oil, fish oil and seed oils such as sunflower oil are all examples of unsaturated fatty acids.

Micronutrients

The second category of nutrients is micronutrients and, as the name suggests, these are required in tiny amounts. We need them on a regular basis, and they are more commonly known as minerals and vitamins. Later in this chapter we will look at the list of my five favourite supplements.

Low-fat, low evidence?

In the chapter on inflammation we saw that the debate about carbohydrates versus fats has raged for decades. By way of a reminder, we learned how American scientist Ancel Keys seemed to have won in 1970 with his Seven Countries Study that suggested that dietary fats cause heart attacks. The loser, academically at least back then, was John Yudkin, the author of the book *Pure, White and Deadly*.

Keys' victory saw the US in 1977 embrace a low-fat approach for nutrition to prevent obesity and reduce heart attacks. Many countries followed including the UK in 1983, as well as Canada, Australia, Japan, China, Brazil, Qatar and South Africa. Finally, we saw that the problem with Keys' Seven Countries Study was that it was merely an observational study that suggested eating fat *might* be linked to obesity. It was by no means enough to hang the nutritional fortunes of the world upon.

That brings us to the present day and to a public health nutrition expert called Zoë Harcombe. For her doctorate, Harcombe reviewed the trials that led to those low-fat guidelines and concluded that they do not support them. Specifically, she showed that there is little evidence in studies – ranging from the Sydney Diet Heart Study to the Women's Health Initiative and to the Framingham Study – to suggest that a low-fat diet is beneficial to our health, and that many results showed that a low-fat diet could harm our health.[1]

In the previous chapter we encountered the argument that the cause of obesity is primarily hormone-driven rather than being an issue of consuming too many calories; in short, that it revolves around insulin and sugars, and has far less to do with calories. That said, what we eat *is* important, so in this chapter we will take a much closer look at that.

To do so requires rebalancing the three macronutrients: proteins, carbohydrates and fats. If we want to lower our intake of one of these three, then typically we have to increase how much of the other two we eat. However, given that the amount of protein we eat stays relatively constant, that means

---

1 Harcombe, Z. 'An Examination of the Randomized Controlled Trial and Epidemiological Evidence for the Introduction of Dietary Fat Recommendations in 1977 and 1983: A Systematic Review and Meta-analysis.' Columbus Publishing (2016).

a low-fat diet means eating more carbohydrates (often in the form of starch and sugars), and a low-carbohydrate diet means eating more fat.

But as we saw in the previous chapter, eating more carbohydrates means our body has to deal with more glucose, and that means it needs to pump out more insulin to take that glucose out of our bloodstream. We also know that high insulin leads to obesity, in part because it blocks the plugs at the bottom of the fat cells, and that it causes inflammation and ill-health.

All of which raises the question: what to do? It turns out that the answer lies in part in eating more healthy fats. For those worried about fat's high calorie count, we also saw in the last chapter that calorie-counting is not particularly useful, and that the high calories in healthy fats are better for us than the damaging effect of glucose (which admittedly has fewer calories per gram).

Among the most compelling studies to show that cutting out sugar, not fat, is essential to our health is the PURE study, which we saw in the last chapter, and which observed the eating habits of 135,000 people in eighteen countries. Although academics quibble about some of its methodology, its broad observations hold: a high-carbohydrate diet is associated with dying younger; eating fats generally helps us to live longer; eating polyunsaturated fats (such as seeds and fish oils) protects against heart disease; and eating saturated fats is neutral and does not cause heart disease.[2]

What the study does not go into – but which we know from other studies – is that eating processed fats increases heart-attack risk.

Brillat-Savarin – a man of influence

You can find Brillat-Savarin's wise words on obesity (and many other topics besides) in a book whose rather wonderful title in English is *The Physiology of Taste, or Meditations on Transcendental Gastronomy*. It was first published in 1825, and apparently has never been out of print.

2   Dehghan, M. et al. 'Associations of Fats and Carbohydrate Intake with Cardiovascular Disease and Mortality in 18 Countries from Five Continents (PURE): A Prospective Cohort study.' *The Lancet* (August 2017).

Fifty years after that a London physician called William Harvey suggested that one of his patients, an obese funeral director called William Banting, try out a novel diet that Harvey had encountered in France that meant he should stop eating starchy carbohydrates. It was what we would call a low-carbohydrate diet, and it worked.

Banting later wrote what was surely one of the first diet books called *Letter on Corpulence, Addressed to the Public*. More booklet than book, it was wildly successful, and what might have been the first diet craze took off. Banting's motivation, he wrote, was to help his fellows deal with a condition – obesity – that had afflicted him for thirty years:

'Of all the parasites that affect humanity, I do not know of, nor can I imagine, any more distressing than that of Obesity.'

At the start of the diet, Banting, who stood at five foot five, weighed 92kg. One year later, his weight had dropped to 71kg.

Needless to say, many in the medical profession scorned the suggestion that cutting down on carbohydrates had anything to do with the funeral director's now-svelte look; after all, popular opinion held that obesity was due to poor self-control (an opinion that remains remarkably current).

It should also be said that Banting was a fan of a good night's sleep, which – as we shall see later in this book – is at the centre of good health.

These days the undertaker whose London firm once conducted the funerals of kings, queens and princes has become a verb: the term 'to bant' means 'to eat a low-carbohydrate diet to lose weight'. And the words of Brillat-Savarin and Banting can be found in the publications of some of the world's most respected medical-nutritional writers – people like Jeff S. Volek and Stephen D. Phinney in their trailblazing *The Art and Science of Low Carbohydrate Living*, Gary Taubes' *Good Calories, Bad Calories* and Tim Noakes' *Lore of Nutrition*.

Sugar in the blind spot

I grew up at a time when most of us had a blind spot for sugar: I considered low-fat Kellogg's Special K to be a healthy breakfast option. It was 'low-fat' after all, and surely that meant 'high in health'. Had I bothered to look at the small label on the back, I might have noticed that it warned me it contained about 12g of sugar *per serving*. That compares to Coke, which comes in at 10.6g of sugar per 100ml.

I stopped eating those types of breakfast cereals many years ago, and I am glad to say that the public's knowledge of nutrition has improved immensely over the past twenty years. That does not mean that eating habits have changed sufficiently – clearly they have not or this chapter would be unnecessary – but I am encouraged by the increased interest in what we eat.

My work requires a fair amount of overseas travel, and wherever I go I entertain myself with my Yoghurt Survey. Admittedly this survey is informal and not particularly scientific, but it is useful in working out how much people in different countries know about nutrition, and how that knowledge changes over time.

Twenty years ago, most people (including me) had no idea how much sugar was in a serving (100ml) of any given yoghurt. Moreover, most people did not know that this was something worth knowing. These days I know that a good quality, full-fat yoghurt might contain 6g of sugar per serving, whereas a sugary low-fat yoghurt could contain up to 12g, which is more than a can of Coca-Cola. Interestingly, the countries where people to whom I speak are most aware of the sugar content in yoghurt – for example, the UK – are the same places where manufacturers have responded to consumer demand and offer yoghurt with a lower sugar content.

More broadly, it does not much matter these days whether I am talking to patients, other doctors or dieticians, there is widespread agreement that sugar is toxic and plays a significant role in the obesity epidemic. It may have taken a couple of hundred years, but Brillat-Savarin's advice that the way to avoid becoming stout was to avoid starchy carbohydrates such as 'bread, rice and potatoes' is more fully accepted than ever.

In the previous chapter we saw that it is essential to be aware of sugar in our diet. This chapter will focus on some of the nutritional breakthroughs the world has seen since it adopted the disastrous low-fat guidelines of the 1970s, and will work out what is relevant for us today.

The conundrum of the Blue Zones

Before we turn our attention to some of the diets and approaches seen in recent decades, consider this:

- The residents of a number of communities around the world live longer and healthier lives than the rest of us, and researchers have studied people in these so-called 'Blue Zones' to find out why. One such zone is in Okinawa, Japan; another is Ovodda on the Italian island of Sardinia.

- A newborn British girl has a life expectancy of about eighty-three (as of 2016), with a boy expected to reach seventy-nine, which on a global scale is pretty good even for a first-world country.[3] As of 2016, the UK had around two centenarians per 10,000 citizens.[4]

- On the other hand, the inhabitants of Okinawa have a life expectancy of eighty-one and the island has seven centenarians for every 10,000 citizens.[5] That is nearly four times the rate of the UK. And although the calendar might reveal an Okinawan's age to be seventy, their body often appears to be aged just fifty. What is more, many do not spend their last decade in frail-care, but are healthy until the end.

The obvious question is: why? The first place to look is their diet.

The Okinawan diet is referred to as the rainbow diet because the island's

3 Office for National Statistics. 'National Life Tables: 2014 to 2016.' Accessed at: https://www.ons.gov.uk/peoplepopulationandcommunity/birthsdeathsandmarriages/lifeexpectancies/bulletins/nationallifetablesnitedkingdom/2014to2016

4 Office for National Statistics. 'Estimates of the Very Old (including Centenarians): 2002 to 2016.' Accessed at: https://www.ons.gov.uk/peoplepopulationandcommunity/birthsdeathsandmarriages/ageing/bulletins/estimatesoftheveryoldincludingcentenarians/2002to2016#main-points

5 Willcox, B. et al. 'The Okinawa Centenarian Study.' *J Gerontol A Biol Sci Med Sci* (2006): 61: 354.

residents eat a vast array of fruits and vegetables rich in antioxidants; in addition, they consume more tofu and soya than any other population. But perhaps their most significant cultural tradition is known as *hara hachi bu*, which means: 'Eat until you are 80 per cent full.' So, whereas people in the West normally eat 1,500–2,000 calories a day, Okinawans consume on average 1,200 calories, a real-life example of the calorie-restriction theory highlighted in the chapter on the theories of ageing.

The residents of the commune of Ovodda, a farming area on the Italian island of Sardinia, live longer than the norm, but do not do it by counting calories. In fact, unlike their long-living counterparts in Okinawa, the people of Ovodda eat a lot of meat and very little tofu or soya. They do, however, enjoy the famous Mediterranean diet of olive oil, legumes, fruit, vegetables, fish and meat.

In other words, two of the world's longest-living communities have quite different approaches to nutrition, yet both work. The first group has a high-carbohydrate diet, but their overall calorie intake is low. The second group has more of a balance between the macronutrients, and their calorie intake is higher. If that seems contradictory it is worth noting that neither group eats much in the way of sugar or processed foods, which certainly helps.

But studies of the Blue Zones show there is more to their success, and not the least of these factors is lifestyle: many residents keep working into their later years (the chapters on brain health will look more closely at this); their stress level is relatively low (which we will look at later in the book too); and there is a strong sense of community.

In other words, although nutrition is important, it is not the sole factor in their success in staying younger for longer. It is simply one element in a far bigger picture of low stress, continuous brain and body activity, and community living.

Glycaemic Index (GI)

In 1981, four years after the US dietary guidelines were issued suggesting that we eat plenty of starches and fruit, David Jenkins from the University of Toronto weighed in on the dangers of sugar and introduced the world to the

Glycaemic Index. Many readers will be familiar with this, but for those who are not, the index is a measure of how quickly each food, from avocado to yoghurt, releases its sugar load into the blood. That tells us how much of a trigger that food will have on the release of insulin.

The index was initially developed to help diabetics reduce their sugar intake, and went on to influence the world of weight loss where it was used in a string of diets.

The baseline used in the Glycaemic Index is pure glucose, which is given a score of 100. Almost everything else is released more slowly into the bloodstream, and therefore has a lower number. By way of comparison, white sugar comes in at sixty-five, fruit and rolled oats measure around fifty, while many vegetables have a low GI of around thirty.

The idea is that the lower the GI score, the healthier that food is in terms of its effect on insulin release.

So how does it work in practice? By way of a simple example, we will compare a bowl of white sugar – which is comprised of two molecules, glucose and fructose – and a bowl of rolled oats, which are also comprised of glucose and fructose. Your eyes will tell you that there is an obvious difference. This lies in the length of the chain of carbohydrate: the glucose-fructose chain in oats is much longer than the glucose-fructose chain in white sugar. That is why it takes your body very little time to uncouple sugar's two molecules and dump the glucose into the blood (causing your blood glucose level to peak and trough steeply), and why it takes hours to unravel the glucose molecules from the long chain in oats. And that is why so-called long-chain carbohydrates such as oats have a lower GI score than short-chain carbohydrates. This difference, in effect, is why we should avoid short-chain carbohydrates.

The index, then, is useful, but it is not perfect. One failure is that it has a blind spot for fructose, whose GI is a paltry 19. That low GI score implies that fructose is healthy, but we saw in the previous chapter that, although it does not stimulate insulin, it does stimulate triglycerides, which are a bad fat, and leads to fatty liver, which worsens our risk of a heart attack or cancer. Fructose also pushes up our blood pressure and leaves us feeling hungry.

Glycaemic Load (GL)

Other than fructose, GI has two other blind spots: it does not take into account the portion size of the food being measured, and it ignores the effect of fibre in slowing the release of sugar from different foods.

To remedy that, a group of Harvard researchers refined the Glycaemic Index in the 1990s, developing the similarly named Glycaemic Load.

- Portion size: GL recognises how much glucose is present in a standard portion size. Why does that matter? Take a watermelon: it has a high GI score of seventy-two because it releases its glucose quickly; however, because a watermelon is 90 per cent water, its carbohydrate content is low, and that means its GL rating is low – in fact, it is just four, the same as green peas and parsnips.[6] Glycaemic Load, then, accounts for the fact that there is not a lot of sugar per kilogram in a watermelon.

- Fibre content: We know that fibre slows the release of glucose into the bloodstream, which means a much smaller insulin spike. Carrots have a GI of around thirty-nine, which is about the same as a chocolate bar. But because carrots have lots of fibre, it takes our digestive system a long time to unravel the sugar from the fibre in the carrot; the sugar from a chocolate bar, on the other hand, lands in our system within minutes. The fibre factor is one reason juicing different fruits can be problematic: although it concentrates various vitamins and minerals, it strips out the fibre, which means the sugar from the fruit is concentrated and is released quickly into the bloodstream.

Carbohydrate-counting

Many people eat a high-carbohydrate diet, by which we mean more than 200g of carbohydrates each day. However, many others choose to – or, if they are

6 You can see Harvard's comparison table for more than a hundred foods here: https://www.health.harvard.edu/diseases-and-conditions/glycemic-index-and-glycemic-load-for-100-foods

diabetic, have to – ensure that they follow a low-carbohydrate approach. What does that mean? A low-carbohydrate diet equates to less than 100g of carbo-hydrates per day.

That means you need to know what is in your food, and these days count-ing carbohydrates has become much easier since most packaged foods list their carbohydrate content, and break down their content by sugar and fats. That is useful for anyone trying to ensure a healthier lifestyle, not least parents looking to cut the amount of sugar their children consume. (Our boys are allowed the occasional sugary drink, but they must first find infor-mation on the packaging to show there is less than 10g of sugar per 100ml.)

Working that out is pretty easy: on the label in Figure 1 you can see that each serving of this product contains 25g of sugar per 80g of biscuit. This equates to 6 teaspoons of sugar per biscuit, which is a lot. When it comes to sugary drinks we should now show just as much caution. Anything under 5g of sugar per 100ml is low, 5–10g is moderate, and more than 10g per 100ml is a high sugar drink. In our family, this drink would fall just outside what is acceptable.

Figure 1: A nutrition label showing too much sugar

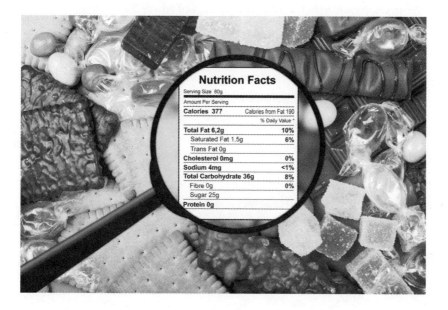

Keeping an eye on this sort of thing is also helpful when trying to follow a low-carbohydrate lifestyle. And when it comes to that, one of the most useful approaches can be found in a 2015 book called *Real Meal Revolution* that divides foods according to their total carbohydrate content. One of the co-authors, Sally-Ann Creed, refined that further in a book called *The Low-Carb, Healthy Fat Bible*. By way of a summary, her book puts foods into five categories:

- The Green list: these are foods you can eat at will. All have less than 5g of carb per 100g, and they include plants like broccoli, gem squash and peppers.
- The Gold list: these are foods you should eat with caution. Like the Green List foods, these also have less than 5g of carbohydrates per 100g, but they have a higher fat content (calories still do count). They include many dairy products such as full-fat yoghurt, cream and cheese. Someone struggling to lose weight would reduce their intake of this list of calorie-dense foods.
- The Orange list: you can eat only one item per day of this list. All of them have a carbohydrate content of between 5 and 25g per 100g. Fruits like apples and oranges feature here.
- The Red list: this is a list of high-carbohydrate foods that contain more than 25g of carbohydrates per 100g. You should avoid all of these, among them any dried fruit, sugar and chocolate.
- The Banned list: this covers seed oils, processed meats and bread which, for one health reason or another, we should not eat.

Food combining

Food combining was a popular health and weight-loss approach between the 1980s and the turn of the century. The concept is simple: protein is digested in the stomach using acid, and carbohydrates are digested in the intestine in an alkaline environment. Because of that, the idea was that we should never eat these two macronutrients at the same time because the acid and alkaline effects would cancel each other out, and that would reduce the efficiency of our digestion.

Food combining got a lot of media coverage at the time, and generated a number of spin-offs such as the acid-alkali diet. Although some of my patients like this approach, I have seen little evidence to view it as particularly useful.[7]

Protein-rich diets

In 1999, Bill Phillips launched a high-protein diet that, in my opinion, rocked the world – though not for the right reasons. As an ex-bodybuilder and owner of a protein supplement company, Phillips is very much in the world of protein. His book *Body for Life: 12 Weeks to Mental and Physical Strength* had plenty of before-and-after pictures of Joe and Jane Average becoming Joe and Jane Splendid after following his high-protein plus weight-training programme.

The logic was that all this builds muscle and, because muscle twitches all day while fat just lies there dormant, you burn more energy – even when sitting at your desk. In a triumph of marketing genius, Philips offered his red Lamborghini Diablo as a prize to whoever could shape up the best.

Since then there have been other high-protein diets including the Dukan Diet, which became well known in the UK in 2010 when Kate Middleton reportedly lost two dress-sizes on it in the run-up to her wedding to Prince William.

High-protein diets are not without risk, though: although protein is an essential nutrient, a high-protein intake is associated with stimulating insulin (which we now know is not healthy) and can result in worsening insulin resistance.[8] There is also concern that a high-protein diet, particularly in younger people, could be associated with cancer and a risk of early death.[9] In

7 Golay, A. et al. 'Similar Weight-loss with Low-energy Food Combining or Balanced Diets.' *Int J Obes* (2000): 24: 492–6.
8 Smith, G. I. et al. 'High Protein Intake During Weight-loss Therapy Eliminates the Weight-loss-induced Improvement in Insulin Action in Obese Postmenopausal Women.' *Cell Reports* (2016): 17: 849–61.
9 Levine, M. et al. 'Low Protein Intake is Associated with a Major Reduction in IGF-1, Cancer, and Overall Mortality in the 65 and Younger but Not Older Population.' *Cell Metabolism* (2014): 19: 407–17.

elderly people, on the other hand, a higher-protein diet seems to lower cancer risk and help them to live longer.

Low-carbohydrate diets

Earlier I told you that a low-carbohydrate diet involves eating less than 100g of carbohydrate a day. In fact, it can be a lot less than that depending on the diet involved. Someone on a ketogenic diet would eat just 20g of carbohy-drates a day, whereas someone on a Banting diet might eat 100g. Different eating plans suit different people, and the level of carbohydrates they should eat will often depend on the result of their insulin blood test and the level of exercise they do.

The Atkins diet, which was launched in the 1970s, remains one of the best-known low-carbohydrate diets. It was not without its shortcomings, however, including that as people progressed the diet allowed them to reintroduce many of the sugars and desserts. The diet also promoted candy bars and processed foods, which by today's standards makes it flawed.

What diets, then, *are* worth considering? Here are three examples that cover the spectrum of low-carbohydrate. Each allows different levels of carbo-hydrates, and all these days refer to 'healthy fats' and not simply 'high fats', which is a big improvement.

- Ketogenic: Our body's main energy source is glucose, which are the energy packets we derive from carbohydrates among other sources. But our body can also use ketones, which are the energy packets found in fats – thus the name 'ketogenic' – and this diet restricts our intake of carbohydrates so significantly that people enter a state known as 'ketosis' in which the liver converts fats into ketones that the brain and body can use for energy. Someone on a ketogenic diet will typically eat 20g of carbohydrates a day, the usual amount of protein and a very high amount of healthy fats. (Later in this chapter we will talk more about healthy fats.) Ketogenic diets are not new – they were originally used for epilep-tics, because using ketones to provide energy to the brain reduced the frequency of epileptic seizures.[10] Some marathon runners and extreme athletes follow a ketogenic diet to improve their body's ability to use fat for energy.[11] It has also been used to help diabetics to cut their reliance on the tablets they take and improve their blood-sugar levels.[12]

- **Banting**: Named after our old friend William Banting, this diet encourages you to eat 50–100g of carbohydrates a day, the usual amount of protein and a relatively high proportion of healthy fats. You would likely not reach ketosis eating this much carbohydrate. Fruits are very restricted; dairy is allowed.

- **Paleo**: On this diet we eat the sorts of foods that our ancestors ate in the Palaeolithic era, which ended about 10,000 years ago. As you might expect, it excludes all processed foods; it also bars dairy and – given that we were still hunter-gatherers then, not farmers – wheat. So what can you eat? Between 100–200g of carbohydrates, the usual amount of protein, and the usual amount of fats. You can also eat fruit and honey. I would not be surprised if this diet is the most familiar of the three to readers given that 'paleo' was the most-searched diet on Google in 2013.

So much for the various types of low-carbohydrate diets. How do you decide whether following such a programme is the right thing to do in the first place?

A good place to start is with the two-hour insulin glucose challenge test. Most doctors will give you a normal blood glucose test (also known as a blood sugar test), but it is essential also to measure your insulin levels. Why? Because insulin removes glucose from the blood, and the better insulin is doing its job, the better our health will be. The worse it is doing its

10   Freeman, J. M. et al. 'The Ketogenic Diet: One Decade Later.' *Pediatrics* (2007): 119: 535–43.

11   Volek, J et al. 'Metabolic Characteristics of Keto-adapted Ultra Endurance Runners.' *Metabolism* (2016): 65: 100–10.

12   Yancy, W. S. et al. 'A Low-carbohydrate, Ketogenic Diet to Treat Type-2 Diabetes.' *Nutr Metab* (2005): 2: 34.

job, the closer we are towards diabetes. Indeed, our insulin level is often the first predictor that we are on the road to developing diabetes, and it can be elevated many years before we develop it.[13]

A high insulin level means our system is not doing its job as well as we need it to and, as we saw in the previous chapter, too much insulin damages us and can lead to obesity, heart attacks and chronic illness.[14] So it is extremely important to fix this, and a low-carbohydrate diet is an excellent first step. Why? Because eating fewer carbohydrates in the first place means less glucose enters our system, and that means less pressure on our overworked pancreas to produce insulin and get it to do its job of packing away excess glucose in the fat cells.

At my clinic, we categorise the result of this blood-test as follows:

Glucose blood levels:

- Normal – below 5.5 mmol/L (millimoles per litre)
- High – anything above 5.5 mmol/L

Insulin blood levels:

- Normal – 3.9-5.5 mIU/ml
- High – anything greater than 10 mIU/ml. This is where we start to call it insulin resistance

As you can see, there is a big gap between a normal insulin level, which tops out at 5.5 mIU/ml, and a raised insulin level (anything from 10 mIU/ml upwards). So in our clinic, if someone comes in with an insulin reading in this grey zone (between 5.5-10 mIU/ml), we sit up and warn them that their insulin levels are starting to move in the wrong direction. Our approach at this early stage is for them to begin removing some of the sugary carbohydrates they are eating. Generally the person reports back that within two months their love handles have shrunk. By the time their next blood test is done, their insulin level is typically back to normal.

Our approach is supported by the work done by Joseph Kraft, the pathologist who reckoned that up to 80 per cent of us have mild insulin resistance,

13   Martin, B. C. et al. 'Role of Glucose and Insulin Resistance in the Development of Type-2 Diabetes Mellitus: Results of a 25-year Follow-up Study.' *The Lancet* (1992): 340: 925–9.
14   Semenkovich, C. F. 'Insulin Resistance and Atherosclerosis.' *J Clin Invest* (2006): 116: 1813–22.

and that glucose and insulin damage to arteries were implicated in every heart-attack case he autopsied.[15]

In other words, it is possible that *four out of five people* could benefit from a low-carbohydrate eating plan. To my surprise, I was one of them: four years ago, having noticed that my sporting performance had declined and that I was developing love handles, I decided to test my fasting blood-sugar level. To my astonishment, my insulin level was 7.0 mIU/ml, which placed me in the grey zone, and heading towards insulin resistance.

I was surprised, but on reflection I should not have been. Why? Because I was eating 250g of carbohydrates a day and, when cycling with my wife Megan most days each week, would knock back a couple of sachets of corn syrup for energy. A regular sugary treat in the evening was also not unusual.

Because I was not (yet) insulin-resistant, I did not need to consider something as drastic as a ketogenic plan, but Megan – also my coach and nutritionist – put me on 50g of carbohydrates a day. Breakfast consisted of eggs with cheese, spinach and mushrooms. Lunch and dinner were protein with salad or vegetables with butter. My cycling bottle had only water, and the day's sugary snacks were replaced with nuts. I noticed that whenever I cut back on some of the fats (the nuts, cheese and butter) I would start to crave sugar, and so I made sure to eat as many healthy fats as I needed. For the first month, I felt sluggish on my bike as my body took time to convert from its reliance on sugar for energy. But after that my energy, performance and health improved dramatically. One year later my insulin level was normal, and I graded up (carbohydrate-speaking) to a Paleo diet. Doing so provided me with three benefits:

- As someone who suffers from sinus issues, I am now less blocked up because I cut out dairy.
- Although I do not have an allergy to gluten, I do feel healthier without wheat in my diet[16].

15 Kraft, J. *Diabetes Epidemic & You.* Trafford Publishing (2008).
16 The issue of wheat and allergies is a fascinating one, and there are some good books on the topic. Two of my favourites are: *Wheat Belly* by cardiologist William Davis, and *Grain Brain* by neurologist David Perlmutter.

- The higher amount of carbohydrates available under the Paleo plan helped my high-intensity sporting performance, because I was no longer insulin-resistant.

All of that is to say that what works best for me might not work as well for you. We are all different, we all face individual challenges, and those challenges also change throughout our lives. I found that I benefited from starting on one eating programme and eventually switching to another. You might too. What is certain is that most of us should cut down on the amount of carbohydrates we consume.

Mediterranean diet

I want to close this section by looking at one of the best-known and best-studied food plans out there: the Mediterranean diet. And let me start by saying what this diet is *not*: it is not a takeaway pizza, and it is not noodles drizzled in meat sauce. Delicious though those are, they have no place in a Mediterranean diet.

Instead, this diet should contain a combination of fruits, vegetables and grains with generous portions of olive oil, fish and some meat. There are no processed foods and there are no seed oils.

That leaves a very wide spectrum of foods, and yet that is just one part of this diet. I have spoken to several chefs who follow the Mediterranean method, and the topic they all agree on is that eating is a communal event:

- Preparing the food is an enjoyable ritual that is done at home.
- Vegetables are often home-grown and are seasonal.
- People do not eat a lot of meat: one chicken could feed a family of ten. And the animals used are pasture-fed and free-range, and typically are free of added hormones.
- The meals themselves are a communal affair, drawn-out and enjoyable.

Embracing Mediterranean eating, then, combines the process of making the food with a sense of poetry, artistry and a love for life. It is a way of eating that has been shown to reduce the incidence of heart attacks, even in those who are high-risk.[17] It is a proven heart-healthy eating plan.

17 Estruch, R. et al. 'Primary Prevention of Cardiovascular Disease with a Mediterranean Diet.' *N Engl J Med* (2013): 368: 1279–90.

Local hero: Stamatis Moraitis

A friend of mine has a photograph pinned to his fridge showing an old man in mismatched, checked clothing standing in his vineyard next to an olive tree, and smiling broadly at the camera. The man was Stamatis Moraitis, and his story contains lessons we should all take to heart.

Moraitis was from the Greek island of Ikaria, a place long-famous for the longevity of its inhabitants. He ended up moving to the US in 1943 to be treated for a war injury, and decided to stay. He married and had a family. So far, so normal. But little more than two decades later, when he was in his mid-sixties, Moraitis was diagnosed with lung cancer. His doctors gave him nine months to live.

He figured that dying back in Ikaria, where his parents still lived, would be a sound financial bet as it would allow his family to keep the money that otherwise would go on medical bills. And so he and his Greek-American wife went home to Ikaria to prepare for his death.

But Moraitis did not die. In fact, he flourished. After regaining his strength, he began to take a more active role in his community. He went to church, he enjoyed the company of friends, and he tended his vegetable garden and olive trees. He got up when he wanted to, and he napped in the afternoon.

When Dan Buettner (of Blue Zones fame) met Moraitis in 2011, the returnee was still going strong at his official age of ninety-seven (although Moraitis insisted that by then he was 102). His cancer had disappeared, despite the fact he had never had any treatment for it.[18]

Even Moraitis was surprised by his recovery. And so, he told Buettner, about a decade earlier he had returned to the US to ask his doctors whether they could tell him what had happened.

18   Buettner, D. 'The Island Where People Forget to Die.' *The New York Times* (24 October 2012).

> On an island as small as Ikaria this was a well-known tale, and
> Buettner knew the answer. But he still asked Moraitis what he had
> found out.
>
> 'My doctors were all dead,' Moraitis replied.
>
> Moraitis died in 2013. When asked what he ascribed his near-
> miraculous extra decades to, he would cite three elements central to
> Ikarian life: good company, healthy food and a regular glass or two
> of wine.

Vegan and vegetarian

I am not a vegan or a vegetarian, but this chapter would not be complete without acknowledging this trend. For those who do not know the difference, a
vegan will eat only fruits, grains and vegetables, and will studiously avoid all
eggs and dairy; vegetarians, on the other hand, will eat all of the above including eggs and dairy. Neither will eat fish, or indeed any meat.

After years of feeling guilty about eating meat, Einstein reportedly became
a vegetarian and said that nothing would benefit 'health or increase chances
of survival on earth as the evolution of a vegetarian diet'.

Perhaps he did become a vegetarian, perhaps he did say that, and perhaps
he was right. In any event, a vegan lifestyle has become increasingly popular:
the number of Americans who claim to be vegan rose between 2014 and 2017
from 1 per cent to 6 per cent.[19] Even more follow a vegetarian diet.

There are plenty of reasons why people choose to shun meat, and these
include:

Ethics: with the global population now above 7 billion, the farm-to-plate
life of an animal can be cruel, and often unnecessarily so. Many people choose
not to eat meat for ethical reasons.

---

19 'Top Trends in Prepared Foods 2017: Exploring trends in meat, fish and seafood; pasta,
noodles and rice; prepared meals; savory deli food; soup; and meat substitutes.' *Report
Buyer* (2017). Accessed at: https://www.reportbuyer.com/product/4959853/top-trends-in-
prepared-foods-2017-exploring-trends-in-meat-fish-and-seafood-pasta-noodles-and-rice-
prepared-meals-savory-deli-food-soup-and-meat-substitutes.html

Hormone toxins: research suggests that toxins, also called 'obesogens', are linked to the world's obesity crisis.[20] The concern with meat is that hormones are often used to make animals grow faster in order to get them ready for slaughter sooner, and that these hormones affect us too.

Health: others are concerned that eating meat is simply dangerous. A World Health Organization study has shown, for instance, a link between processed meat and a higher incidence of colorectal cancer (although the WHO did note that the risk was small).[21] There are also concerns that eating too much red meat could cause colon cancer, although the evidence is mixed. Lastly, studies suggest that people who follow a vegetarian diet live longer.[22]

In other words, there are some understandable reasons why people choose not to eat meat. That said, when it comes to the argument about toxins, matters are less clear-cut. Why? Because ditching meat means eating more vegetables, and that could simply see us swap one set of toxins for another: the pesticides and herbicides used on plants are unequivocally bad for our health, and to avoid that risk would require going organic.

And there seem to be other factors that account for vegetarians and vegans living longer. After all, vegetarians not only tend to eat healthily, they are also more likely to exercise, to drink less alcohol and to avoid smoking. In other words, the reason they live longer could be more nuanced than simply their diet. Indeed, studies seem to bear that out: when researchers in Australia looked at vegetarians and meat-eaters who made similarly healthy lifestyle choices, it turned out that both groups live equally healthy, long lives.[23]

That tells me that there is no reason to avoid going vegetarian, but there are three important issues that people who follow that road need to be aware of:

20   Holtcamp, W. 'Obesogens: an environmental link to obesity.' *Environ Health Perspect* (2012): 120: a62–a68.

21   'IARC Monographs evaluate consumption of red meat and processed meat.' WHO Internat. Agency for Research on Cancer (2015). Accessed at: http://www.iarc.fr/en/media-centre/pr/2015/pdfs/pr240_E.pdf

22   Orlich, M. J. et al. 'Vegetarian Dietary Patterns and Mortality in Adventist Health Study 2.' *JAMA* (2013): 173: 1230–8.

23   '45 and Up Study.' Saxinstitute. Accessed at: https://www.saxinstitute.org.au/our-work/45-up-study/

Sugar: because both vegans and vegetarians do not eat meat, they could end up eating an excess of starchy carbohydrates; the risk is that this can lead to insulin resistance.

Vitamins: it is difficult for vegans and vegetarians to ingest enough of the vital, fat-soluble vitamin D and vitamin A in their diet. Levels of vitamin D, for instance, are thought to be 74 per cent lower in vegetarians than in people who eat meat.[24] Vegetarians and vegans therefore need to ensure they supplement for these, and for vitamin B12 too, as their diet can lack them.

Fish oil: EPA and DHA, both of which are found in fish oil, are essential fatty acids. Given that they are from fish, vegans and vegetarians will not take these supplements, and instead use flaxseed oil. However, the conversion rate to EPA and DHA from flaxseed oil is poor, which is why vegans generally have a 50 per cent lower level of these protective oils than people who eat fish do.[25] For vegans and vegetarians, algae is a better source of these essential fatty acids than flaxseed oil.

The decision to eat meat or not is, of course, a personal one. Carnivores should avoid eating processed meat, and instead use meat that is grass-fed and organic, and that has no added hormones. Vegetarians and vegans should avoid eating excessive starch, should supplement with vitamins A, D and B12, and should take algae oil instead of flaxseed oil to ensure they get enough of the essential fatty acids that they need.

The four pillars of nutrition

No matter what eating plan works best for you, there are four pillars of nutrition that we cannot compromise if we want to be healthy, and we will spend the rest of this chapter on them.

24 Craig, W. J. 'Nutritional concerns and health effects of vegetarian diets.' *Nutr Clin Pract* (2010): 25: 613–20. Accessed at: https://www.ncbi.nlm.nih.gov/pubmed/21139125

25 Rosell, M. S. et al. 'Long-chain n–3 polyunsaturated fatty acids in plasma in British meat-eating, vegetarian, and vegan men.' *Am J Clin Nutr* (2005): 82: 327–34. Accessed at: https://academic.oup.com/ajcn/article/82/2/327/4862944

In summary they are:

- Pillar 1 – Cut out sugars.
- Pillar 2 – Eat healthy fats.
- Pillar 3 – Ensure your gut is healthy.
- Pillar 4 – Choose the right supplements.

Pillar 1 – Cut out sugar

By now we have spent a large portion of this and the previous chapter building the case against sugar and starches. These days it is near impossible to find anyone – outside those involved in making money out of sugar – who will defend it as healthy. In that way, the case against sugar is a lot like that against tobacco a couple of decades ago.

More people then ever understand that they must be much more careful of their sugar consumption. Why? Because we know that sugar causes inflammation, and sets off a hormonal cascade that leads to a fatty liver, obesity, diabetes, heart disease and cancer.

However, there is no single optimal eating plan for everyone. We know the people of Okinawa do well on their diet, as do the Sardinians (as do the residents of Ikaria, like Stamatis Moraitis, whom we met on page 125). But their diets are dissimilar, with different macronutrients. And yet, both live long, healthy lives.

What we can say is that you might thrive on the low-calorie eating (*hara hachi bu*) favoured by the Okinawans. Or your body might prefer the low-stress community eating of Sardinia, with plenty of olive oil, vegetables and wine. What is likely true is that many, and perhaps most, of us have a mildly raised insulin level, as Joseph Kraft found with 80 per cent of the thousands of bodies he studied; for that reason people with higher-than-healthy insulin levels would benefit from a low-carbohydrate approach to correct that problem.

In any event it is clear that Brillat-Savarin was correct in his observation that starch should not play much of a part in our diet. Sugar, as we now know, should play pretty much no role at all.

Pillar 2 – Eat healthy fats

Fats and fatty acids

Fatty acids, like everything else in the universe, are comprised of atoms – in this case a chain of hydrogen and carbon atoms that is topped by a second cluster of atoms called a carboxyl group. The chain of hydrogen and carbon is what gives us the 'fatty' part of the phrase; the carboxyl top makes it an 'acid'. Thus the term fatty acid.

Figure 2: Fatty acids – the building blocks of fat – are a chain of hydrogen and carbon atoms topped by a carboxyl group

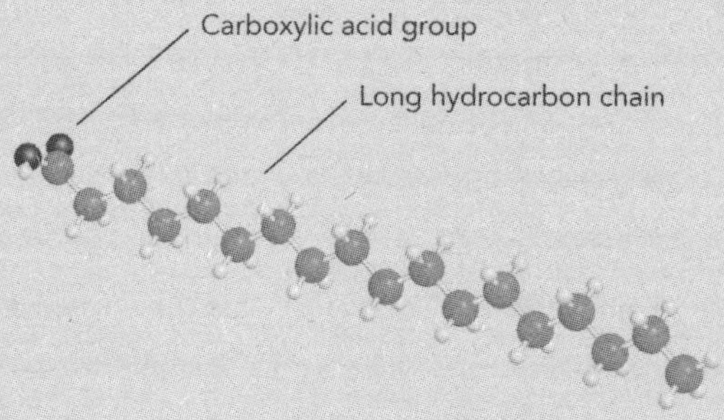

Carboxylic acid group

Long hydrocarbon chain

Two things determine which of the dozens of fatty acids we are talking about: firstly, how the hydrogen and carbon atoms *connect* on that chain; and secondly, the *length* of that chain. It is these characteristics at the molecular level that determine how good or bad different fatty acids are for us.

Fats are simply what you get when a number of fatty acids combine. In other words, fatty acids are the building blocks of fats. And it is the types of fatty acids that the fat is comprised of that give the fat its characteristics – whether it is saturated or unsaturated.

Saturated fats are normally solid at room temperature, and come mainly from animal fat, dairy and tropical plants such as coconuts. Until recently saturated fats were considered bad for our health, but many experts are starting to refine that position. These types of fats are called 'saturated' because the fatty acids of which they are comprised have two hydrogen atoms attached to every carbon atom all the way along the fatty acid chain – thus the chain is 'saturated' with hydrogen atoms, which means there is no room on that chain for any more hydrogen atoms. Palmitic acid and stearic acid, both of which are widely found in food, are two examples of fatty acids that give us saturated fats.

Unsaturated fats come mainly from fish and plants, including olives, nuts and seeds, and are considered to be healthy. They are 'unsaturated' because instead of every carbon atom on the chain being connected with two hydrogen atoms, two or more of the carbon atoms are instead connected to each other. If an unsaturated fatty acid has just one of these carbon-carbon bonds, like oleic acid, then it is called 'monounsaturated' ('mono' meaning 'one'); if there is more than one such bond, as with linoleic acid, then it is known as 'polyunsaturated' ('poly' from the Greek word for 'many'). Unsaturated fats are normally liquid at room temperature.

It is important to know that heat corrupts fats, and can turn even the healthiest fat toxic.

Only a few years back, people talked about a 'low-carb, high-fat' diet. Sensibly, the term 'high fat' has these days been replaced by the term 'healthy fats', and many more people understand the benefits that healthy fats convey. (Another term, which you will often see in eating plans that involve healthy fats, is 'real food'. It means many things to many people; I view it as food cooked from scratch, with nothing packaged or processed.)

But what exactly do we mean by healthy fats? It is perhaps easier to start by talking about one very *unhealthy* fat: trans fats. Some animal products such as milk and meat naturally contain trans fats, but only in tiny amounts. Most of the trans fats in our modern diet are the result of an industrial process known as hydrogenation, in which hydrogen atoms are forced through the oil breaking the carbon-carbon bonds (see the box on fatty acids) and forcing them to bind with the hydrogen. The result is a partially hydrogenated vegetable oil, which – as it is now saturated – is solid at room temperature.

Why do this? Because it makes the fat last longer, and hydrogenated and partially hydrogenated fats have some useful properties when it comes to manufacturing processed foods, such as margarine, biscuits, cakes, microwave popcorn and many others. The problem is that hydrogenation hugely increases the amount of trans fats, and those are toxic: they damage our cells, resulting, for instance, in a higher risk of strokes and heart attacks.[26] Denmark banned all trans fats in 2004, and a follow-up study in 2016 found that the number of heart attacks had dropped significantly.[27] From a health perspective, margarine belongs in the dustbin of yesterday along with other disasters such as bloodletting or using mercury to cure ailments.

Now that we have put hydrogenated fats and trans fats in their place, it is time to look at the rest of this group to see how our body uses fats and oils. Earlier in this chapter we saw that there are two types of fats – cholesterol and fatty acids – so let us see what our body does with these. For this thought experiment we will dream up a virtual meal of olives, fish, sunflower seeds and butter. All of these contain fatty acids and some contain cholesterol, but in both cases the body needs to break them down into these smaller components. How does that happen? Meet your gall bladder: it releases bile salts, which are made from recycled cholesterol, and these head to the small intestine to separate the fat into fatty acids and cholesterol. After that they will be absorbed.

Cholesterol

In our virtual meal, cholesterol is mainly present in the butter, but there is also some in the fish (and in any animal product we eat). Most of the cholesterol in our body, though, comes not from the food we eat, but is manufactured by our liver. This remarkable organ is the ultimate cholesterol regulator: if we do not eat enough cholesterol then the liver will make more; if we eat a lot of cholesterol, then it will make less. Why is that important?

26 Hirata, Y. et al. 'Trans-fatty acids promote pro-inflammatory signaling and cell death by stimulating the apoptosis signal-regulating kinase 1 (ASK1)-p38 pathway.' *J Biol Chem* (2017). Accessed at: http://www.jbc.org/content/early/2017/03/29/jbc.M116.771519.abstract
27 Restrepo, B. J. et al. 'Denmark's policy on artificial trans fats and cardiovascular disease.' *Am J Prev Med* (2016): 50: 59–76.

Because carrying out that function requires our liver being healthy; the less healthy our liver – due to, say, non-alcoholic fatty liver disease from consuming too much sugar – the worse our internal cholesterol control.[28] So even if cholesterol were bad for us (and it is not), when it comes to how much cholesterol is in our blood it is our liver's health that counts far more than the amount of cholesterol we eat.

Fatty acids

Saturated fatty acids: butter is the main source in our virtual meal. As the box on page 130 explains, 'saturated' simply means there is no room on the fatty acid chain for any more atoms, and that makes its bonds strong and hard to damage. This is why saturated fats such as coconut oil and butter are far healthier options for frying food than the likes of sunflower oil or canola oil.

Unsaturated fatty acids: in our virtual meal these are found predominantly in the olives, the fish and the sunflower seeds, and are further divided into:

- *Monounsaturated fatty acids*, which are found in the olives. These fatty acids have *one* double bond or weakness in each chain. This makes them quite good for cooking, but that single (mono) weakness leaves this oil less stable to heat than the saturated fatty acids found in coconut oil.

- *Polyunsaturated fatty acids*, which are in the fish oil and sunflower seeds. These fatty acids have *multiple* bonds in each chain. More bonds means these fatty acids have a higher chance of weakening; heat, for instance, can quickly turn them rancid and toxic – which is why we should not fry with sunflower oil, because the heat damages the oil. But heat can also damage the fish oil tablets that many of us take, which is why it is important to be suspicious if fish oil supplements have developed a fishy smell or are cloudy. It is also why your fish oil tablets should only have been through a 'cold-pressed' extraction process. Similarly, any seed oil (such as sunflower oil or canola

28 Simonen, P. et al. 'Cholesterol synthesis is increased and absorption decreased in non-alcoholic fatty liver disease independent of obesity.' *J Hepatol* (2011): 54: 153–9.

oil) can go rancid if the oil is extracted using heat, so if you are using sunflower oil on your salad, then make sure it is from a cold-pressed source. And do not fry food with sunflower oil or canola oil, as the heat turns the oil toxic.

The fatty acids and cholesterol we have listed here are essential nutrients. (Trans fat, of course, is not.) Now that we have broken down our delicious virtual meal into its constituent parts, it is time to follow the route these take through the body and see what they do that is so important.

Once the bile salts have helped our intestinal wall to absorb the cholesterol and fatty acids, they are processed and then sent out to the body in chylomicrons, which we can think of as boats. These transport the cholesterol and essential fatty acids to wherever they are needed in the body.

We will start with cholesterol, which has some important jobs. It is used to make:

- Cell membranes: logically enough, these surround every cell in the body; membranes also surround the individual machinery, such as the mitochondria, within the cells. Cholesterol acts as the strongman of these membranes, supporting their other components.
- Hormones: the hormones produced by our adrenal cortex (which is part of our adrenal glands that sit above our kidneys) are made from cholesterol. Among these are cortisol, testosterone, oestrogen, progesterone and DHEA (examined in the upcoming chapters). Without cholesterol, we cannot make these hormones.
- Vitamin D3: sunlight converts cholesterol under the skin into the hormone cholecalciferol, which most of us call vitamin D3. It has about 300 functions in the body ranging from boosting the immune system to protecting against skin cancer, and supporting the liver and thyroid gland.
- Myelin sheath: the axons (or arms) of your nerves are insulated with a myelin sheath, which allows them to pass messages along their length faster. Multiple Sclerosis is a disease where the body's immune system destroys these myelin sheaths.

Fatty acids have two main functions:

- Formation of cell membranes: fatty acids are used to build cell membranes, and they keep the walls flexible so that nutrients can get in and toxins can be removed. You can think of them as being a bit like those 1970s string curtains that stopped people seeing into the kitchen. Once the walls get stiff, which is often an effect of unhealthy fats, then cells become sickly and die.

- Managing inflammation: fatty acids provide the building block for the body to make a group of fats known as prostaglandins that our body uses when it needs to heal damage. Some prostaglandins encourage inflammation; others reduce it. Inflammation is not necessarily bad – for example, it is essential for healing injuries; without inflammation we could not form a scar to heal a cut on our skin, and we would be unable to strengthen our muscles after exercise. But as we saw in the previous chapter, excessive inflammation can harm us and cause a range of ills including asthma, arthritis, heart attacks and cancer.

The final point I want to make is to explain the different *omega* fatty acids. We can find omega fatty acids, which have important effects on inflammation, in the sunflower seeds and the fish. Sunflower seeds are a source of omega-6, while fish is a source of omega-3. Our body needs both of these omegas, but our modern diet tends to be overly heavy in omega-6, because corn (also known as maize) has a high omega-6 content and is used in everything from cattle feed and chicken feed to corn syrup in fizzy drinks, and many other places besides.

The result is that our omega-6 levels are too high, and that is a problem because omega-6 fatty acids have a tendency to be converted into something called arachidonic acid, which gets turned into *pro-inflammatory* prostaglandins. On the other hand, omega-3 fatty acids – which we find in oily fish – convert only into *anti-inflammatory* prostaglandins.

Because we cannot convert omega-6 fatty acids to omega-3, we must instead balance our intake of fish oils and our intake of plant oils. The solution is part diet and part exercise:

- Eat more fish and less corn and corn-related foods. So choose butter and meat sourced from pasture-fed cows rather than corn-fed, for example, because grass is full of omega-3.

- Exercise, because this damages our muscles, and rebuilding them requires arachidonic acid. In other words, every time you exercise you burn off arachidonic acid. Bodybuilders know this, because they punish their muscles so much that they need to *supplement* with arachidonic acid simply to continue building more muscle. (Incidentally, anti-inflammatories such as aspirin and ibuprofen stop inflammation by switching off the formation of arachidonic acid, which is why when ibuprofen was given to bodybuilders after a work-out, it impeded their muscle rebuilding.[29]) Daily exercise uses up excess arachidonic acid and reduces inflammation.

Laboratory testing

As pathology laboratories improve, we can test areas that we once only dreamed of assessing – including our levels of omega-3 and omega-6 fatty acids. That allows us to work out exactly which of these essential fatty acids we are deficient in.

If your local laboratory cannot perform these tests, then the following will provide a good balance of omega-3 and omega-6 fatty acids:

- Fish oil capsules (lots of omega-3) that contain 1,000mg of EPA and DHA. What are these useful for? EPA helps with pain and inflammation. DHA is good for the head and specifically brain health.
- Evening primrose oil contains an essential omega-6 oil that we are often deficient in called gamma-linolenic acid (GLA). Although most omega-6 oils tend to turn into arachidonic acid, which is inflammatory, GLA is unusual in that it is anti-inflammatory. Among its uses are as a treatment for breast pain in women.
- Flaxseed oil is one source of the omega-3 fatty acid called alpha-linolenic acid (ALA). ALA is a good source of omega-3 for

29 Trappe, T. A. et al. 'Effect of ibuprofen and acetaminophen on postexercise muscle protein synthesis.' *Am J Physiol Endocrinol Metab* (2002): 282: E551–6.

vegans, but there is some concern that for many people it does not convert well into the active EPA and DHA that we find in fish oil. However, ALA has a number of benefits, and if you are vegan it is probably the best source of omega-3 that you will get.

Pillar 3 – Love your intestines

Most of what we eat and drink enters our body via our intestines, so it makes sense to keep these in tip-top order. That is not always easy, as many of my patients know.

For example, take Sarah (not her real name). When she came to see me she was thirty-two and had been struggling with low energy for a year. Her lifestyle was not out of the ordinary: she worked hard, partied once a week, and most nights got six hours of sleep. When asked, she said she regularly had some bloating and stomach cramps, as well as acne and mild thrush.

The way to measure the health of your intestines is with a stool test, and after getting Sarah's results back we sat down and discussed what we had found. To do that, though, required telling Sarah how the gut works.

It is comprised of three key zones: the stomach, the small intestine and the large intestine. The stomach secretes acid to break down protein and kill off any incoming bugs. The small intestine breaks down the carbohydrates and fats, and is also where the good bacteria and yeasts that we call flora live. This layer of organisms provides additional protection against bugs, and in that way prevents the symptoms associated with mild intestinal infections, including bloating, nausea and diarrhoea. (Incidentally, the effect these organisms have extends far beyond the gut. They seem to protect our skin from the bacteria that cause acne and rosacea, and their anti-inflammatory effect seems to guard our brain against a worsening of anxiety and depression.)[30]

Finally we have the large intestine. Its main function is to convert food into faeces, and in that process it extracts any minerals and water from what has

---

30 Bowe. W. et al. 'Acne vulgaris, probiotics and the gut-brain-skin axis – back to the future.' *Gut Pathogens* (2011): 3: 1.

passed through the small intestine before expelling what is left from the body. The large intestine has a completely different set of bacteria – called E. coli – that help to break down food, make a vital product called vitamin K, and play a big role in protecting us from dangerous strains of E. coli.

In other words, all three zones have factors that protect us from bacterial infections: stomach acid, the flora in the small intestine, and E. coli in the large intestine. This army of helpers is vast, with our gut containing ten times as many helpful bacteria as there are cells in our body.[31] This microbiome, to give it its proper name, contributes hugely to our health.

And yet, although many people know their intestinal flora is essential to good health, most do not understand how important stomach acid is. Consider, for a minute, scavenger animals or even man's best friend, the dog. All have much stronger stomach acid than we do, and that is likely because it protects them from bacterial infections when eating the rotting flesh of dead animals or, like Fido, when snuffling through the refuse.

As we get older, however, we produce less stomach acid, and that leaves us more susceptible to gut infections from the food we eat.[32] It also means we are more vulnerable to overgrowth of our *own* bacteria – something called Small Intestinal Bacterial Overgrowth, or SIBO, which is what happens when the numbers of our friendly flora rise too high, and which causes bloating, fatigue and abdominal cramps. In part, that happens because there is less stomach acid to cull the flora, and it turns out that many people with Irritable Bowel Syndrome, which is characterised by bloating and abdominal cramps, have SIBO.[33] The solution is to use antibiotics or herbs to pare back the numbers of our good flora, and consider taking before mealtimes Betaine HCL (hydrochloride), an acid that tops up our dwindling stomach acid levels.

31 Holzapfel, W. H. et al. 'Overview of gut flora and probiotics.' *Int J Food Microbiol* (1998): 41: 85–101.
32 Beasley, D. E. et al. 'The evolution of stomach acidity and it's relevance to the human microbiome.' *PLoS One* (2015): 10: e0134116.
33 Dukowicz, A. C. et al. 'Small Intestinal Bacterial Overgrowth.' *Gastroenterol Hepatol* (2007): 3: 112–22.

In other words, rather like Baby Bear's porridge that was neither too hot nor too cold, our body requires a delicate balance between these trillions of bacteria. We do not want too many of them, and we do not want too few. The balance needs to be just right.

All of which allows me to explain what Sarah's results meant to her and to many of the rest of us too. Firstly, Sarah's stool sample showed she had a very low count of small intestinal flora and an overgrowth of the candida yeast. That was why she had repeated bouts of thrush, which left her susceptible to inflammation and more significant bacterial infections.

Secondly, her large intestine had far too many bad E. coli bacteria. It was also inflamed and had a low antibody count, which meant her immune system was too tired to fight those unhealthy E. coli. This combination of excessive unhealthy E. coli and inflammation caused the bloating, cramps and poor energy.

Knowing this, I could easily devise her treatment. The first step was to boost her system, which was tired. That meant toning down on the weekly parties, and making sure she slept eight hours a night in order to rebuild her immune system. Next I introduced her to the Four Rs:

- Remove: that meant cutting out any foods that might be upsetting her. In Sarah's case that was alcohol, but it could just as easily have been an allergy to wheat or a minor intolerance that left her intestines susceptible to damage. Because alcohol destroys the intestinal flora, stopping drinking allowed her flora to flourish and improved this line of her gut's defence system.

- Repair: our gut repairs itself every four days, and central to that process is an amino acid called glutamine. Also helpful are ginger and quercetin, which is found in peppers, tomatoes, berries and broccoli, and both of which have powerful anti-inflammatory properties. A US company called Metagenics (with which I have no affiliation) makes an excellent repair product called UltraInflamX that contains these and other ingredients.

- Restore: taking probiotics helps to restore the flora in the small intestine. Probiotics generally contain lactobacillus and biffidobacterium bacteria, and these form the backbone of our small intestinal flora.

This flora needs food to eat and this comes in the form of pre-biotics. Fermented foods like kimchi or sauerkraut do the job, providing our flora with the food it needs to thrive. Taking E. coli helps to build up levels in the large intestine. Synexa (with which I also have no affiliation) is an international firm that produces healthy E. coli for us to take each day.

- Replace: finally, as Sarah's stomach acid was probably deficient, which left the entire gut susceptible to bacterial infections, we also needed to replace those levels. This is easily done using a hydrochloric acid tablet that is taken before eating. This is typically a temporary measure in someone Sarah's age, but in a seventy-year-old it might need to be taken permanently. Unhealthy, processed foods should be ditched in favour of portions of kefir or sauerkraut.

Pillar 4 – Choose your supplements

We are bombarded from all sides by adverts for countless supplements that promise essential benefits, so I am never surprised when a patient turns up dragging a sack of pills behind them. As we saw in the chapter on the theories of ageing, taking too many vitamin supplements runs the risk of turning off our internal antioxidant system, so we need to be careful about that. However, it is also likely that many people *are* deficient in certain nutrients, and that means taking some supplements is probably useful.

A sack of pills, though, is not the answer. As a rule I focus on a maximum of five supplements, and in this section I will tell you what those top five are. First, though, I want to hand out some medals to three contenders that did not make the list, though each came close.

The first of our three also-rans? Probiotics. Why did I omit them? Because although we have seen how important our gut flora is and how easy it is to upset the microbiome with alcohol, antibiotics and stress, I do not think we should take probiotics every day. Instead, probiotics are probably better taken on an occasional basis. What we *should* do is help our flora by enjoying a daily dollop of foods that our probiotic flora like to eat. As we saw above, this type of indigestible carbohydrate is termed 'pre-biotic', and it includes sauerkraut, which is fermented cabbage, kefir, which is a strain of fermented milk, and kimchi, which is a mix of fermented vegetables.

Our second contender is alpha-lipoic acid. This is an intra-cellular antioxidant, which means it works inside the cell (and there are not many antioxidants that do this). In that way it protects our DNA from damage. We will see in the chapter on anabolic versus catabolic hormones that alpha-lipoic acid protects us from glycation, which causes cataracts, skin hardening and kidney damage. It also has an important role in helping insulin to do its job, and in that way lowers our insulin resistance.

The third wannabe is vitamin A, which is essential for maintaining good vision, is a powerful immune-booster, and – as we shall see in the chapter on the skin – stimulates new cells and is therefore often used in creams to strengthen our skin. Lastly, vitamin A is important during gene transcription, the process in which cells divide and our DNA shares its messages to make proteins and new cells.

Enough of feeling sorry for the three that did not make my top five. It is time to meet the winners, and here they are from fifth place to first.

5. *Multivitamins*

I am all for eating nutrient-dense foods, and in an ideal world we would not need supplements. In practice, however, I believe many of us do not get enough minerals and nutrients from what we eat, and some recent research backs that up. A 2010 study in the US suggested that 20 per cent of the population was on a diet at any one time, and that made them nutrient-deficient.[34] And a 2017 study on more than 10,000 people showed that many who were not taking vitamin supplements were deficient in numerous vitamins, and that when they started taking supplements their vitamin levels improved.

These studies suggest that many of us are at significant risk of being vitamin- and mineral-deficient. The solution is a high-quality multivitamin taken twice a week. Another Metagenics product that fits this bill is PhytoMulti;

---

34 Calton, J. 'Prevalence of micronutrient deficiency in popular diet plans.' *J Int Soc Sport Nutr* (2010): 7: 24.

Solgar's VM-2000 is another. If you cannot find either of those then my rule of thumb is to check the label of your multivitamin and see what type of 'folate' it contains; if the answer is 'folic acid', then do not bother with it because half of the population has a genetic mutation or some other issue that means they cannot absorb folic acid. If, on the other hand, the label tells you that it contains a natural folate such as 5-MTHFR then the rest of the multivitamin is very likely to be good quality.

4. Coenzyme Q10

This supplement is essential for energy inside the cell, and that means it is essential for our energy. Your body's cells have an energy engine-room called a ribosome, and that organelle uses what are called mitochondria to make energy. Central to that manufacturing process is, you guessed it, coenzyme Q10.

Interestingly, though, our bodies 'forget' how to make coenzyme Q10 from around the age of thirty-five. That is also the age when we no longer make as many mitochondria. What this means is that if you are over thirty-five and are chronically tired, and you have checked that you are not anaemic and that your adrenals are healthy, then the chances are that you will benefit from taking coenzyme Q10 tablets to boost your cellular energy supply.

The good news is that the benefits to taking coenzyme Q10 do not end there, because this is one of our few intracellular antioxidants, and that means it protects the DNA in our cells from becoming damaged. Coenzyme Q10 also has a big effect on the brain's dopamine system, and for that reason is used in the natural treatment of attention deficit disorder.

All of that, and coenzyme Q10 made it only to number four on my list. Imagine how powerful the next three items must be.

3. Vitamin D3

These days we are able to measure our vitamin D level, which is why we know many – and perhaps most – of us are deficient in it. (We will learn why that is the case in the chapter on the skin.)

There are a number of good reasons why vitamin D3 takes the bronze medal, not least because it pulls calcium into the bones, which keeps them strong.

However, if we are deficient in vitamin D3 (and in vitamin K2) then we will not be able to get that calcium into our bones in the first place, and that not only increases the chance of them becoming brittle; it also means we accelerate the calcification of our arteries, muscles and brains – and that really is bad news.

Vitamin D3 also helps our liver's detoxification pathways (as we will see in the next chapter) and assists our body to make thyroid hormone. In addition to that, vitamin D3 boosts our immune system against all-comers, including the common cold, and has proved useful in the fight against cancer. Finally, it is involved in making dopamine, the hormone that helps us to focus and stops cravings and addictions.

2. Fish oil

This is the number one supplement for many people, and while it is superb it only takes silver. As the saying goes, second place is no disgrace, and fish oil gets to the podium because of its high levels of the active omega-3 fatty acids EPA and DHA.

These are two key aspects of any fish oil supplement, so make sure that at least 500mg of your 1,000mg tablets are comprised of EPA and DHA. (Cheaper tablets often top out at just 180mg.) These omega-3s help to reduce inflammation in our body, and that is important because our arteries, brain, joints, intestines and lungs all tend to inflame, and that leads to disease. Although fish oils have repeatedly been shown to be important in reducing inflammation, a 2018 review by the Cochrane Library pointed out that they have not been shown to reduce deaths.

Our bodies have to battle inflammation on a number of fronts, not least from our diet, with so many processed foods chock full of sugars and the like, and that also makes a regular dose of anti-inflammatory fish oil vital. Lastly, fat is a key component of our brain tissue, and fish oil helps to keep it strong and functioning well; it also keeps our cell membranes supple, which means nutrients can pass into the cells and toxins can pass out.

One final note about fish oil: buy cold-pressed fish oil (because heat damages it), keep it in a cool, dry place, and make sure that it is reputably certified as being mercury-free.

1. Glutathione

The gold medal position goes to this relatively unknown supplement, so let me tell you why it is so special. Firstly, glutathione is the brain's universal antioxidant; in that way it stops inflammation in the brain, makes us feel calmer, stops damage to the brain, and reduces the chance of Alzheimer's disease.[35]

Glutathione is also used to stabilise the brain and help people with schizophrenia and bipolar disorders.[36] It reduces the production of mucous in the lungs and the sinuses, and is used in all manner of treatments from cystic fibrosis to post-nasal drip.[37] It is also a vital antioxidant in our body as a whole, and helps to keep our arteries clear of blockages.

Lastly, and possibly most importantly, glutathione oversees the removal of mercury and other toxins via the liver. Without glutathione we accumulate these toxins, and that leaves us susceptible to heavy metal poisoning. We will look more closely at this subject in the chapter on toxins.

As we age, we deplete our glutathione stores and need to pay more attention to replacing them. If we drink alcohol or are inhaling the smog of city air, our glutathione stores will decline.

I am strongly convinced that the most beneficial way to take glutathione is by having a monthly glutathione drip, but there are other options. Companies such as Xymogen make tablets and powders of stable glutathione, or you can take tablets of a substance called N-acetylcysteine, which is what we call a precursor for glutathione – that means it converts into glutathione in your body.[38]

35   Rose, S. et al. 'Evidence of oxidative damage and inflammation associated with low glutathione redox status in the autism brain.' *Transl Psychiatry* (2012): 2: e134.
36   Dean, O. M. et al. 'A role for glutathione in the pathophysiology of bipolar disorder and schizophrenia? Animal models and relevance to clinical practice.' *Curr Med Chem* (2009): 16: 2965–76.
37   Bishop, C. 'A pilot study of the effect of inhaled buffered reduced glutathione on the clinical status of patients with cystic fibrosis.' *Chest* (2005): 127: 308–17.
38   Pizzorno, J. et al. 'Glutathione.' *Integr Med* (2014): 13: 8–12.

NUTRITION: A FINAL WORD

After reading this chapter, you no doubt have a good grasp on how diets have evolved over the past century or so, and a much better insight into which diets are flawed, and why, and which might be helpful, and why.

As we have seen, there is no one 'right' diet, and it is clear that different eating plans provide different benefits. But whatever approach we choose, we must be more mindful about how much sugar and starch we eat.

Indeed our increasing sugar consumption has very likely driven the global obesity epidemic, although there is still some debate as to whether this is due to the 'excessive calories' found in sugar or to the fact that sugar triggers insulin. My work tells me both factors are important, but ultimately it is very difficult for obese people to lose weight until their raised insulin levels have normalised.

People who are insulin-resistant (which means an insulin level greater than 10mIU/ml) will likely benefit from following a very low-carbohydrate diet, such as the ketogenic diet, for a period of time. However, if someone wants to reduce their starchy carbohydrate intake and has an intolerance to gluten or suffers from sinus issues, then the wheat-free and dairy-free approach of a Paleo diet might be better.

Someone with a normal insulin level, who feels healthy, might do best sticking to a Mediterranean diet; it has a more balanced array of the three macronutrients, and focuses on a relaxed, community aspect of eating.

Sugar, processed foods and fast foods are central to the obesity epidemic, and healthy nutrition is central to ensuring optimal health. If we do not take in the right nutrients, then we are not giving our body a chance of attaining good health. And so whichever plan you decide to follow – from vegan to ketogenic to any other – all of them them insist on eating healthy, unprocessed food. All have their good points, and all have a couple of weak points. There is no perfect eating plan, so the best advice I can give is that you choose the one that works best for you.

Better nutrition is an essential part of what is known as preventative medicine, which we can regard as taking steps now to improve our health, rather than waiting until things go wrong. And on that note, it is worth closing with a quote from one of South Africa's most famous sons, the late Dr Christiaan Barnard, who performed the world's first successful heart transplant in 1967: 'I have saved the lives of 150 people through heart transplants,' he once said. 'If I had focused on preventative medicine earlier, I would have saved 150 million people.'[39]

Key points

The mainstream eating plans we have looked at agree on the following pillars of nutrition:

- Cut out sugars and limit your intake of starches.
- Eat healthy fats (olives, seeds, nuts).
- Saturated fats, such as those found in butter and eggs, have health benefits and are no longer regarded as unhealthy.
- Avoid seed oils (sunflower oil, canola oil and others) unless they have been cold-pressed. Why? Because the heating process used for extraction generally damages the oil, which then gets further damaged when we cook with it. Never use processed fats like margarine.
- Optimise your gut health. That means eating some sauerkraut, kefir or kimchi, and intermittently using probiotics. And remember the Four Rs: remove, repair, restore, replace.
- Choose the right supplements. My favourites are a good multivitamin, coenzyme Q10, vitamin D3, high-quality fish oils and glutathione.

---

39 Noakes, T. and Sboros, M. *Lore of Nutrition: Challenging conventional dietary beliefs.* Penguin Random House (2017), p. 22.

Chapter 5

Toxins – The Fate of the Mad Hatter

Giving up smoking is easy. I've done it hundreds of times.

Attributed to Mark Twain

'A proper pea-souper.' That is what Londoners called the Great Smog of December 1952, although in truth most ignored it. After all, they had experienced many of these winter windless, coal-fire and factory-driven smogs. Only later, once the statistics came out showing that this pea-souper had caused 12,000 deaths, did the authorities make changes.[1] The Clean Air Act of 1956 sought to deal with this decades-long health problem.

These days it is not London, but New Delhi, Tehran, Beijing and Ulaanbaatar vying for the unenviable title of 'most polluted' capital. However, they are not the only places that poison their residents on a daily basis, and this avalanche of air pollution is responsible for one in every eight deaths worldwide according to the WHO. Small wonder the UN's main health body rates air pollution as 'the world's largest single environmental health risk', and says cutting air pollution could save millions of lives each year.[2]

---

1 Bell, M. et al. 'A Retrospective Assessment of the London Smog Episode of 1952: the Role of Influenza and Pollution.' *Environ Health Perspect* 112.1 (2004): 6–8.
2 'Seven million premature deaths annually linked to air pollution.' World Health Organization press release (2014): http://www.who.int/mediacentre/news/releases/2014/air-pollution/en/

There are three big medical factors – which I call 'The Three Horsemen of the Health-pocalypse' – which cause many of us to live shorter and unhappier lives than our parents. They are:

- Sugar
- Toxins
- Stress

We looked at the dangers of sugar in the chapters on inflammation and nutrition, and we will tackle stress – one of my favourite topics – in the chapter on adrenal strain. For now, we will take a long look at the Second Horseman: toxins.

THE INVISIBLE THREAT

With toxins a potentially massive threat to our health, we should start by defining what we are talking about: a toxin is simply something that damages the body. It could be an obvious toxin like alcohol that the body needs to clear in order to feel normal again. Or it could be largely invisible, like the car exhaust we inhale while going about our daily lives or the fumes that leach from certain cleaning products or carpets.

Fortunately your body has an amazing detoxification system and does a great job in removing unwanted, dangerous substances, typically via the liver. As we age, however, a tired, overloaded liver will not clear toxins as efficiently as it once did – rather like the way an old or dirty fuel filter in your car means it no longer runs as well. Your liver is little different: a struggling liver can leave you feeling tired and depressed, susceptible to developing allergies and infections, looking pale and even running the risk of developing serious health issues, such as a heart attack and cancer, and lead to early death. So, it is well worth looking after it; you get just one liver, and most of us need it to last a good eighty or so years.

That is no easy feat given that, as you will discover in this chapter, we live in a sea of toxins. In the past, though, *proving* that certain toxins were a factor in illness was about as straightforward as identifying who killed JFK. That said, the evidence against toxins is impossible to ignore:

- According to the WHO, toxins have been shown to be responsible for the increase in cardiovascular diseases[3] (CVDs), the world's number-one killer for the last sixty years and the cause of three in ten deaths.
- In many countries, cancer is now the second-biggest killer. A presidential cancer panel concluded in its 2010 report to then-President Barack Obama that 'the true burden of environmentally induced cancers has been grossly underestimated'.[4]

What is taking so long?

The problem is that it often requires lengthy studies to prove that a substance is toxic to our health. That is because, for governments to take it seriously, the toxin generally needs to be shown to be, say, cancer-forming. For example, it took over 100 years to prove that mercury amalgam fillings were dangerous – and the evidence is still not universally accepted. Other toxins – like some of the herbicides used in agriculture – have taken fifty years to prove their toxicity.

The reason it takes so long to prove the toxicity of even substances that seem obviously dangerous is simple: if I can prove that being exposed to a toxin increases the chance of getting a certain illness, that merely shows *correlation*. It is interesting and it might be important, but it does not prove *causation* – that Toxin A *caused* Illness B. For a toxin to be banned, we generally need to show causation, and that takes a lot more work.

In other words, it is often not a good idea to wait for government guidance; each of us should be vigilant about the possible damage different toxins can cause. Whether in the air, food or water, or in the items we use each day, toxins are ever-present, and I am convinced that many more will eventually be shown to be among the key causes behind disease and ill-health.

The good news is that by end of this chapter you will know how to

---

3 Azevedo, B. F. et al. 'Toxic Effects of Mercury on the Cardiovascular and Central Nervous Systems.' *J Biomed Biotechnol* (2012): doi: 10.1155/2012/949048.

4 'Cancer and Toxic Chemicals.' Physicians for Social Responsibility (2010). Found at: http://www.psr.org/environment-and-health/environmental-health-policy-institute/responses/environmental-and-occupational-toxicants-and-cancer.html

recognise and therefore choose to avoid different toxins; consider the different supplements that have been shown to enhance liver health; and understand how to remove heavy metals, like mercury, which might already have accumulated in your system.

With that said, let us look at a few common categories of toxins, including heavy metals, pesticides and endocrine disruptors.

1. Heavy metals

We have been exposed to some heavy metals for centuries, but it is only in recent times that legislation is starting to protect us from them. For the sake of brevity, we will look only at lead, cadmium and mercury; there are, however, many more.

- Lead was added to petrol in the early 1920s by a man called Thomas Midgley. In the air, lead is so toxic that Midgley became known as the man who 'had more impact on the atmosphere than any other single organism in Earth's history'[5]. (His other invention was CFCs, also now banned, and used for decades in refrigeration and aerosol canisters; CFCs harm the ozone layer.) Lead can damage almost every organ in the body, and is particularly injurious to the brain. In high doses, lead will make us mad, but even low doses affect intelligence and stunt children's IQ development. Since the 1970s governments have gradually banned lead in petrol and paint; as a result, blood-lead levels have dropped 80 per cent.[6] A 1990 report concluded that lead in petrol was the environmental mistake of the twentieth century.[7]

- Cadmium is found in cigarettes and some foodstuffs. In the 1990s it was proven to be a carcinogen, meaning that it causes cancer

5 McNeill, J. R. *Something New Under the Sun: An Environmental History of the Twentieth-Century World* New York: Norton, xxvi, 421 pp (2001).
6 'Blood Lead Levels Keep Dropping; New Guidelines Recommended for Those Most Vulnerable.' CDC (1997). Found at: https://www.cdc.gov/media/pressrel/lead.htm
7 Shy, C. M. 'Lead in Petrol: The Mistake of the XXth Century.' *World Health Stat Q* (1990): 43: 168–76.

(particularly lung cancer). As a result, its industrial use has been limited.[8]

- Mercury: who could forget characters such as the Cheshire Cat, the White Rabbit and the Mad Hatter in Lewis Carroll's *Alice in Wonderland?* The Mad Hatter's name is no coincidence. In medieval times, hatters did go insane, and that was due to their use of the liquid metal mercury, then known as quicksilver, to cure the felt of the hats they made. We now know mercury has severe effects on the nervous system. Today our main exposure to mercury is eating fish: it accumulates in algae and then passes up the food chain to predator fish such as tuna before ending up on our plate. The result is that predator fish can accumulate significant amounts of mercury before we eat them, as was shown in a massive US population study called the NHANES survey (National Health and Nutrition Examination Survey): people who ate a lot of fish had a much higher mercury level than the rest of the population.[9]

The Minamata poisoner

The reality of mercury poisoning was cruelly exposed in 1956 by the people of Minamata, a small city on the west coast of Japan's Kyushu Island. For years the Chisso Corporation, which manufactured chemicals, released waste products – including methyl-mercury – from its factory into the bay. Over time, the shellfish in the bay absorbed the mercury and, given that shellfish were a dietary staple for many residents, so did many local people. Mercury levels were so high that thousands of people were poisoned. The worst-affected suffered paralysis, coma and death. Mercury poisoning is still known as Minamata Disease.

8 Waalkes, M. P. 'Cadmium Carcinogenesis in Review.' *J Inorg Biochem* (2000): 79: 241–4.
9 Xue, J. 'Methyl-Mercury Exposure from Fish Consumption in Vulnerable Racial/Ethnic Populations: Probabilistic SHEDS-Dietary Model Analyses Using 1999–2006 NHANES and 1990–2002 TDS Data.' *Sci Total Environ* (2012): 373–9.

2. Pesticides and herbicides

In our enthusiasm to protect our plants we often use chemicals that are highly toxic, and these comprise our second broad category of toxins. The first mass-produced pesticide (a substance devised to kill insects) could be considered to be DDT, which stands for dichloro-diphenyl-trichloroethane. Developed in the 1940s, DDT killed more than just mosquitoes – it was toxic to humans and animals alike, and was described by the then-leading environmentalist Rachel Carson as being 'as crude a weapon as the caveman's club'.[10] By 1972 it was banned in the US.

Since DDT, three other agricultural chemicals have grabbed our attention:

- Organophosphates: when I worked in casualty in South Africa, I regularly saw children from farms rushed in, foaming at the mouth and rolling their eyes in a state of delirium – after swallowing an organophosphate pesticide. Organophosphates have been called 'junior-strength nerve agents' and, if they are inhaled, swallowed or come into contact with the skin, can easily kill.[11] Organophosphates are associated with cancer, but are not proven to cause it; as a result, they are banned for residential use (you cannot buy them at a nursery, for instance). As horrific as it was to see their effect on children, organophosphates remain approved for agriculture and are widely used.

- Neonicotinoids: these seemed to have a much safer profile than organophosphates until researchers noticed that they not only killed pests, they also wiped out bee colonies. The bee crisis has been in the news for years with nicotinoid pesticides blamed for the decimation of populations in Europe, the US, Australia and beyond, and in that way hurting nature's ability to pollinate our plants.[12] Neonicotinoids are now being linked in the UK (currently this is correlative, not

---

10 Carson, R. *Silent Spring.* Houghton Mifflin (1962).
11 'Organophosphates: A Common But Deadly Pesticide.' *National Geographic* (2013).
12 'Neonicotinoids, Bee Disorders and the Sustainability of Pollinator Services.' *Current Opinion in Environmental Sustainability* (2013): 5 (4): 293–305.

causative) to plummeting bird populations in areas that show high pesticide levels.[13]

- Glyphosate: this is the latest of the agricultural chemicals to hit the news and can be found in many herbicides, including Monsanto's Roundup. We will see later what a slow process it has been to prove glyphosate's probable toxicity.

3. Endocrine disruptors

Our third category of toxins comprises chemical compounds that are toxic in the sense that they interfere with the endocrine (hormone) system by mimicking the female hormone oestrogen. These are associated with early puberty in girls, breast- and fat-formation in boys, infertility in men and, potentially, cancer in everyone. They are not damaging enough to warrant banning and so we remain very exposed to them.

This broad group of chemicals, all of which mimic oestrogen, includes:

- Parabens, a group of preservatives widely used in cosmetics and creams.
- Phthalates, dioxins and Bisphenol A (BPA), found in plastics.
- Atrazine, a weedkiller that is banned in the EU but that is widely used in the US, Australia and other countries.

Although oestrogenisation (increasing oestrogen levels) is a significant problem in the world, these chemicals remain a part of our daily existence. You will find them in plastic bottles, microwaved foods, meals-in-a-bag, and in beauty and hygiene products including shampoos, shower gels and moisturisers.

4. Electronic fog

There are two types of electromagnetic radiation, otherwise known as electronic fog. The first is regarded as damaging, while the second – although all around us – is not yet recognised as problematic, and will likely take years to prove its harm. This fog is so prevalent, and the industries driving it so powerful, that it is worth mentioning.

---

13 Goulson, D. 'Ecology: Pesticides linked to bird declines.' *Nature* 511 (2014): 295–6.

The two types are:

- Ionised radiation: this has so much energy that it knocks electrons out of atoms and is therefore considered to be damaging to humans. We find this sort of radiation in X-rays (low risk), medical radiation for cancer (higher risk) and nuclear explosions (very high risk). Once exposed, we have a raised life-time risk of developing cancer.[14] A WHO report in 2005, for example, reckoned that the Chernobyl nuclear reactor disaster in 1986 (the largest in history) would eventually kill 4,000 people through radiation exposure.[15]

- Non-ionised radiation: this does *not* have the energy to knock out atoms and so is *not* considered damaging to humans. This includes EMF radiation from mobile phones, Wi-Fi, Bluetooth and microwaves. As a result, the official advice in many countries is that having a mobile phone tower near your house will not harm your health. However, research shows that although mobile phones do not knock electrons out of atoms, they do open up electronic channels leaving cells susceptible to oxidative damage.[16] In 2011, the WHO classified the radio-frequency electromagnetic fields emitted by wireless devices like mobile phones as 'possibly carcinogenic' for a specific brain cancer called a glioma. However, a lot more work needs to be done to determine these effects.[17]

14   Gilbert, E. S. 'Ionising Radiation and Cancer Risks: What We Have Learned from Epidemiology?' *Int J Radiat Biol* (2009): 85: 467–82.

15   'Chernobyl: The True Scale of the Accident.' WHO (2005). Found at: http://www.who.int/mediacentre/news/releases/2005/pr38/en/

16   Pall, M. L. 'Scientific Evidence Contradicts Findings and Assumptions of Canadian Safety Panel 6: Microwaves Act Through Voltage-gated Calcium Channel Activation to Induce Biological Impacts at Non-thermal Levels, Supporting a Paradigm Shift for Microwave/Lower Frequency Electromagnetic Field Action.' *Rev Environ Health* (2015): 30: 99–116.

17   'IARC Classifies Radio-frequency Electromagnetic Fields As Possibly Carcinogenic to Humans.' *World Health Organization* (May 2011). Found at: http://www.iarc.fr/en/mediacentre/pr/2011/pdfs/pr208_E.pdf

An hour in our toxic fog

The list of dangerous and suspect toxins that surround us is long. Some years back I decided to spend the day writing down every toxin I encountered, but I quickly gave up; there were simply too many. Here is what I jotted down in that first hour.

From the moment I climb out of bed and breathe, I inhale the volatile organic compounds (VOCs) in paint, carpets and my memory-foam pillow. VOCs are believed to be cancer-causing (or, in medical-speak, carcinogenic), and they certainly worsen my asthma. (You will find carpets containing VOCs in cheap hotels – look for that plastic smell when you enter the room and, the following morning, mild swelling around the eyes.)

The paint on the walls of my apartment was applied before 1992 so I can expect a mild dose of lead in the air, which will eventually settle in my brain and other organs and probably cause damage. Opening the cupboard, I inhale some fresh mould spores from the damp bottom corner, which will worsen my allergies and put an added strain on my immune system. In the bathroom, having showered and shaved (more chemicals), I wash my face and apply face cream (with paraben preservatives, which have an oestrogenic effect) and sunblock cream containing titanium dioxide (a metal, and the ingredient that blocks the sun's damaging rays).

After getting dressed, I open my laptop to check my emails, and am surrounded by that pervasive electronic fog – which, given that my apartment has Wi-Fi, is omnipresent regardless. My mobile phone rings; being right-handed, I clamp it to my right ear (possible increased risk of brain tumour, damage to memory and mood) and then walk down the corridor (the varnished wooden floor has more VOCs) to the kitchen. My drink of tap water contains high levels of chlorine (which will irritate my bowel and my prostate) and probably some mercury and/ or oestrogen depending on my local water table. But I am grateful because the water quality could be far more dangerous: many people in countries like India and Cambodia have high levels of arsenic in their water and no way of avoiding it.

Time for breakfast: I whisk some eggs (non-organic and therefore loaded with oestrogen) and put them in the microwave in a plastic container, which

– as the plastic heats up – releases Bisphenol A (BPA) and dioxins that have (you guessed it) more oestrogenic effects. I pour some orange juice from the carton that has leached phthalates (more oestrogenic toxins) into the juice in the weeks that it took to get from the factory to my fridge.

I will leave it there with me standing at my kitchen counter waiting for my scrambled eggs to cook. There is little need to tell you about the toxins I inhale from the cleaning products used at home or from the car fumes as I commute to work or the mercury that I swallow from the salmon I buy at my favourite sushi shop. By now you get the point: toxins are everywhere and, as far as I am concerned, they contribute to most illnesses and are one of the most significant health problems of modern living.

It sounds hopeless, but it turns out that there is a lot we can do to limit our exposure to this strange soup of toxins:

- Fit VOC-free carpets that have a high wool-content (read the label).
- Use low-toxin paint (it is usually labelled low-VOC).
- Use eco-friendly pillow fillers; for example, those made from kapok, wool or down.
- Check your beauty products to make sure they do not contain paraben preservatives; sadly, the majority do.
- Switch off Wi-Fi at night, use a hands-free set when talking on a mobile phone, avoid Bluetooth headphones, and try not to live close to a mobile-phone mast, if possible.
- Use a high-quality filter on your drinking-water tap.
- Buy fresh, organic fruit, eggs, dairy products, vegetables and meat. And avoid processed and packaged food.

And while these might seem like small details, cumulatively they can make a big difference to your toxic load.

THE SERIAL OFFENDERS

At the start of this chapter we saw how London's Great Smog compelled a change in legislation to protect people's health. Yet although air quality in the

UK has improved in many ways, it has deteriorated badly in much of the rest of the world.

A report in 2017, for instance, linked pollution to 9 million premature deaths worldwide. Almost all were in low- and middle-income countries, where air pollution accounts for up to a quarter of deaths; air pollution also kills tens of thousands in developed nations each year, and poor air quality is linked to heart attacks and lung cancer.

As the study's lead author, epidemiologist Professor Philip Landrigan, pointed out: 'Pollution is much more than an environmental challenge – it is a profound and pervasive threat that affects many aspects of human health and well-being[18] . . . In the most severely affected countries, pollution-related disease is responsible for more than one death in four.'

Meanwhile, a vast study funded by the Bill & Melinda Gates Foundation, and also published in 2017, reckoned that indoor and outdoor air pollution killed around 6.4 million people in 2015, and that Qatar, Saudi Arabia and Egypt were the worst countries for air pollution.[19] Reducing exposure, the authors concluded, would bring 'potential for substantial health benefits'.

And do not think you are sitting pretty just because you live in the UK or the US. In Scotland and in colder climes in North America, farmers reportedly use a technique called 'desiccation' to treat their wheat crop. This involves spraying the crop with glyphosate, which softens the wheat stalks ahead of harvesting and in those cold places helps to protect the combine harvesters.[20] The combine harvesters are grateful, but we, the general public, get exposed to an increased dosage of herbicide when eating our bread, pasta or cereal.

18   Landrigan, P. J. et al. 'The Lancet Commission on Pollution and Health.' *The Lancet* (Oct 2017). Found at: http://www.thelancet.com/journals/lancet/article/PIIS0140-6736(17)32345-0 /abstract

19   Cohen, A. J. et al. 'Estimates and 25-year Trends of the Global Burden of Disease Attributable to Ambient Air Pollution: An Analysis of Data from the Global Burden of Diseases Study 2015.' *The Lancet* (2017). Found at: http://dx.doi.org/10.1016/S0140-6736 (17)30505-6.

20   Benbrook, C. M. 'Trends in glyphosate herbicide use in the United States and globally.' *Environ Sci Eur* (2016): 28: 3.

As the Gates Foundation report suggests, reducing our exposure to toxins would help our health, but it requires governments to act. And experience shows that legislation does work, as we can see with the example of our old enemy lead: this heavy metal was used in piping that funnelled water around Victorian London, for instance, poisoning generations. It took decades before researchers could prove that increases in Parkinson's disease, heart attacks and Alzheimer's were at least in part as a direct result of lead poisoning.[21]

These days, as we saw earlier, the dangers of lead are well documented, and we shake our heads at the Victorians' foolishness. However, I suspect generations to come will be astonished at how we surround ourselves with different toxins – and far more of them, given the advances in the chemicals industry, than the Victorians ever encountered.

Change can happen, but the difficulty remains in *proving* that a substance is toxic, and then getting governments to ban it. The following three examples illustrate this: one has been successful, one partially so, and one remains a work-in-progress.

The success story: tobacco

The dangers of smoking are widely known: it has been proven to precipitate emphysema, heart disease, strokes and cancers. Despite that, more than a billion people light up every day, most of them in poor- and middle-income countries. One in seven of the global population consume tobacco, and it kills 6 million people a year.[22]

Even after the US surgeon general's famous report in 1964, it took years to rein in cigarette advertising. By the 1990s, the major tobacco companies had fended off hundreds of lawsuits that claimed they had withheld information

21 Wu, J. et al. 'Alzheimer's Disease (AD)-Like Pathology in Aged Monkeys after Infantile Exposure to Environmental Metal Lead (Pb): Evidence for a Developmental Origin and Environmental Link for AD.' *J Neurosci* (2008): 28: 3–9.

22 'Tobacco control can save billions of dollars and millions of lives.' World Health Organization Media Centre (2017). Found at: http://www.who.int/mediacentre/news/releases/2017/tobacco-control-lives/en/

from the public about the dangers of smoking. Their decades-long show of brazenness ended around that time when a number of states sued Big Tobacco for the medical costs incurred in treating sick and dying smokers.[23] As one attorney-general put it at the time: 'You caused the health crisis; you pay for it.'

Today residents of the developed world are no longer subjected to aspirational adverts of beautiful people, white linen, seaplanes and exotic locations, and Big Tobacco has been forced to confine its most egregious marketing practices to developing nations.

The fact is that banning tobacco advertising works, as the UK showed: in the carefree days of the 1970s more than half of Britain's adult population smoked; by 2004 that number had halved and two years later, after the government introduced a ban on smoking in public areas, it dipped further to 23 per cent. Although cigarette manufacturers are fortunate that humans are creatures of habit, years of warnings, restrictions and higher taxes have curbed demand: in 2014, the proportion of British adults who smoke had dropped below 20 per cent.[24] Proof, as if it were required, that the war against toxins is worth fighting.

The partial success story: amalgam fillings

Until about 200 years ago, our dentally challenged ancestors would have had a couple of options when dealing with a rotten tooth: have it pulled out, which was cheap and painful, or have the hole filled with liquid gold, which was expensive and painful. The idea of combining mercury with an alloy of silver, tin and copper must have seemed the perfect solution: amalgam, still commonly known as 'silver fillings', is pliable, cheap, durable and painless. Little wonder that it caught on across Europe, the US and the world.

23 'The Master Settlement Agreement: An Overview.' The Public Health Law Center (2015). Found at: http://publichealthlawcenter.org/sites/default/files/resources/tclc-fs-msa-overview-2015.pdf
24 West, R. and Fidler, J. 'Smoking and Smoking Cessation in England 2010: Findings from the Smoking Toolkit Study.' University College London (2011).

Unfortunately, silver fillings are about 50 per cent mercury and, in 1843, the US dental association banned them due to health concerns.[25] However, that proved an unpopular decision, and a few years later the pro-amalgam lobby won and silver fillings were back on the dental menu. It was another century before scientists finally proved that amalgam is one of our greatest sources of mercury poisoning. As you might expect, it took a vast amount of research to persuade governments of the dangers.

The Scandinavian countries reacted quickly: in 2008, Norway became the first to ban amalgam fillings; later that year Denmark and Sweden followed suit.

Matters have moved much more slowly in the European Union. In 2008, the EU said there was not enough evidence to ban amalgam fillings and reiterated that position in 2015.[26] The following year, after much debate, the EU provisionally agreed that, from 2018, amalgam fillings would not be permitted for use in pregnant and breastfeeding women or in children under fifteen years of age.[27] Most nations, however, still allow the use of amalgam fillings. The tide may be turning but it took 150 years to begin to prove the toxicity of amalgam fillings, and longer still to get governments to act.

The work-in-progress: glyphosate

The latest herbicide that, according to some research, has been shown to damage our health is glyphosate, which we met earlier in this chapter. Glyphosate is the key ingredient in Monsanto's multi-billion-dollar product Roundup, whose herbicidal properties were discovered by one of the company's scientists in 1970.

25 For the history of amalgam fillings see, for instance, Rathore, M. et al: 'The Dental Amalgam Toxicity Fear: A Myth or Actuality.' *Toxicol Int* (2012): 19 (2): 81–8.

26 'The Safety of Dental Amalgam and Alternative Dental Restoration Materials for Patients and Users.' Scientific Committee on Emerging and Newly Identified Health Risks (SCENIHR) (2015). Found at: https://ec.europa.eu/health/scientific_committees/ emerging/docs/scenihr_o_046.pdf

27 'EU Agrees Dental Amalgam Ban in Children, Pregnant and Breastfeeding Women.' World Alliance for Mercury-Free Dentistry press release (8 December 2016). Found at: http://www.eeb.org/index.cfm/library/eu-agrees-dental-amalgam-ban-in-children-pregnant-and-breastfeeding-women/

In many ways, Roundup is the perfect weed-killer: it targets a weed's amino acids and destroys them, causing the plant's death. In the 1990s, Monsanto built on Roundup's success by developing genetically engineered soybean, maize and cotton variants (and, later, alfalfa and sugar beets) that were resistant to Roundup, and which they christened 'Roundup Ready'. The advantage for farmers was that they could spray their crops with Roundup, which would kill the weeds and leave the harvest unharmed.

Roundup is cheap and effective, and – according to the company – safe for humans when used as directed. Too good to be true? Some think so: concern about Roundup's effect on human health has been growing for decades, and has accelerated in recent years.

In 2012, a study in the *Food and Chemical Toxicology* journal concluded that Roundup and Roundup Ready maize caused cancer in laboratory rats,[28] although the conclusions described in the article were later described as 'unreliable'.[29]

In 2015, the International Agency for Research on Cancer (IARC), a branch of the World Health Organization, concluded that glyphosate is 'probably carcinogenic to humans', that 'there is sufficient evidence of carcinogenicity in experimental animals', and that it 'caused DNA and chromosomal damage in human cells'.[30]

In contrast to the IARC report, the European Food Safety Authority said in late 2015 that, after assessing the literature, Roundup was unlikely to cause cancer in humans.[31]

And in 2016, the WHO and the Food and Agriculture Organization (FAO) concluded (in contrast to the WHO's IARC assessment of the previous year)

28 Séralini, G.-E. et al. 'Long term toxicity of a Roundup herbicide and a Roundup-tolerant genetically modified maize.' *Food Chem Toxicol*, 50 (2012): 50: 4221–31.

29 Wallace Hayes, A. 'Editor in Chief of Food and Chemical Toxicology answers questions on retraction.' *Food Chem Toxicol* (2014): 65: 394–5.

30 'Evaluation of Five Organophosphate Insecticides and Herbicides.' *IARC Monographs*, Volume 12 (2015). Found at: https://www.iarc.fr/en/media-centre/iarcnews/pdf/MonographVolume112.pdf

31 'Conclusion on the Peer Review of the Pesticide Risk Assessment of the Active Substance Glyphosate.' European Food Safety Authority. *EFSA Journal* (2015): 13(11): 4302: DOI: 10.2903/j.efsa.2015.4302

that 'glyphosate is unlikely to pose a carcinogenic risk to humans from exposure through the diet'.[32] In other words, the UN bodies felt that the amounts we consume on a daily basis are probably not risky.

What to make of this contradictory research? I prefer to err on the side of caution. For their part, different countries have come to different conclusions. By 2016, four decades after Roundup was launched, many cities in Canada, the US and Europe had banned glyphosate from use in public places; Sri Lanka outlawed glyphosate in 2014; in early 2017, Malta banned it entirely. In many cases the actions against Roundup mean farmers are still free to use the herbicide, but parks, golf courses and plant nurseries either cannot use or sell glyphosate herbicides or are encouraged not to do so.

Summary

The point of these three examples is that it can take a very long time indeed to prove that a substance is so toxic that it needs to be banned. It takes longer still for governments to act. Which means it falls to us to act. To that end there are three things you can do:

- The first, and most obvious, step: be vigilant and avoid potential toxins.
- The second step is to optimise your liver to ensure that your detoxification system is working smoothly; next we will look at how to keep your liver in peak condition.
- And the third is to *consider* removing heavy metal toxins that have already accumulated in your body, with which we will close out this chapter.

Optimise your liver

Earlier I told you that your liver is your key detoxification organ, and that the better its condition, the better it will function. How well it does that depends

---

32 'Joint FAO/WHO Meeting on Pesticide Residues: Summary Report.' WHO (16 May 2016). Found at: http://www.who.int/foodsafety/jmprsummary2016.pdf

on factors such as age, genetics, diet and your toxin load, and there are differ-ent ways we can see how well it is operating.

The standard way to measure its function is by using a blood test called a Liver Function Test (LFT). However, the LFT is designed to help diagnose severe illnesses such as hepatitis, and *not* to detect the mild wear and tear of your average forty-year-old.

That means we need a different approach to determine the extent of the more common 'gentle deterioration' that most livers experience. It is a subtler way to look at how the liver works, and there are three good ways to do this: seeing how well the liver metabolises testosterone; testing for Non-Alcoholic Fatty Liver Disease, or NAFLD; and genetic testing.

Testosterone metabolism

For this, I am going to bring in a relatively healthy forty-year-old male subject (we will call him Stan) and, for now, will move away from processing environ-mental toxins such as lead and mercury and look instead at how his liver performs one of its most important tasks: removing one of the steroid hormones called testosterone.

Once a man produces testosterone, his body needs to remove it quite quickly, and it does this via the liver. If this process does not happen effectively in men then it can have a toxic effect. (Because women have a naturally high oestrogen level it does not help to look at how a woman's liver changes testosterone into oestrogen, because that level would be overshadowed by her normally high oestrogen level.)

We start life with healthy liver pathways, but as our liver accumulates damage over the years these pathways become less effective. Yet, because we still need to get rid of our hormones, the ageing liver does its best pushing them down its slowing pathways.

And so it is with Stan: as testosterone enters his liver to be metabolised, it enters one (or both) of two pathways. Simply put, Pathway 1 uses an enzyme to convert the testosterone into oestrogen, which is then removed by the liver from the body. Pathway 2 uses an enzyme to convert the testosterone into something called DiHydroTestosterone, or DHT; that DHT is then removed by the liver from the body.

These two pathways are rather like plumbing pipes that wash testosterone through the liver, which processes it before removing the metabolised oestrogen or DHT (or both) from the body. But as Stan ages, these pathways no longer work as well as they once did and, as a result, his liver's ability to do its job of removing DHT and oestrogen worsens,[33] and Stan's levels of DHT and oestrogen start to rise. This degeneration in how these pathways process testosterone is a key reason why men at twenty – who typically have healthy livers – look lean, muscular and have a full head of hair, while the same men at forty are fatter, balder or both.

Figure 1: The pathway of testosterone metabolism, which typically becomes less efficient as men age

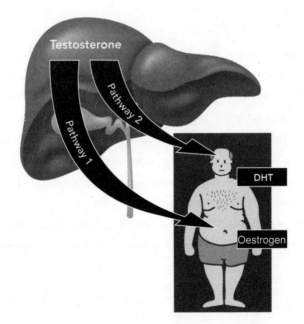

Figure 1 shows how that process plays out in Stan: although his testosterone still travels along one or both pathways, its progress is slower and less efficient. This slowing-up means Stan starts to accumulate oestrogen or DHT

33 Krieg, M. et al. 'Effect of Aging on Endogenous Level of 5-alpha-Dihydrotestosterone, Testosterone, Estradiol and Estrone in Epithelium and Stroma of Normal and Hyperplastic Human Prostate.' *J Clin Endocrinol Metab* (1993): 77 (2): 375–81.

(or both), and we can see the result. As Pathway 1 slows, this version of Stan accumulates oestrogen and as a result, tends to develop a beer belly. As Pathway 2 slows, the other version of Stan accumulates DHT, and as a result his hair starts falling out and he goes bald. (Genetic reasons can also play a part in baldness, of course.) If *both* pathways are affected Stan suffers the double hit of getting a beer belly and going bald.

If Stan were a patient of mine, I would advise the following. First, a simple blood or urine test would show his DHT and oestrogen levels, and that would tell me how well his liver was metabolising testosterone and which pathway his body favoured.

In Stan's case, I might find that his oestrogen levels are several times higher than they ought to be for a man of his age. Indeed, this is something I see regularly: male patients in their forties with a normal Liver Function Test (LFT) result, but whose oestrogen levels are climbing dangerously. Typically, I would correct this with oestrogen-lowering tablets and liver-support supplements: these not only help to detoxify this vital organ; they also improve our chances of ageing healthily – as many studies have shown:

- A raised oestrogen level doubles the risk that a man will die from a heart attack, stroke or prostate cancer.[34]
- Unsurprisingly, lowering his oestrogen level cuts his risk of cardiovascular events and of prostate cancer.[35]
- Reducing[36] high levels of DHT lowers the risk of enlargement of the prostate[37] and of male-pattern[38] balding. We can use progesterone

34   Jankowska, E. A. et al. 'Circulating Estradiol and Mortality in Men with Systolic Chronic Heart Failure.' *JAMA* (2009): 301 (18): 1892–901.

35   Abbott, R. D. et al. 'Serum Estradiol and Risk of Stroke in Elderly Men.' *Neurology* (2007): 68 (8): 563–8.

36   Klaiber, E. L. et al. 'Serum Estrogen Levels in Men with Acute Myocardial Infarction.' *Am J Med* (1982): 73 (6):872–81.

37   Krieg, M. et al. 'Effect of Aging on Endogenous Level of 5-alpha-Dihydrotestosterone, Testosterone, Estradiol and Estrone in Epithelium and Stroma of Normal and Hyperplastic Human Prostate.' *J Clin Endocrinol Metab* (1993): 77 (2): 375–81.

38   Mauvais-Jarvis, P. et al. 'Inhibition of Testosterone Conversion to Dihydrotestosterone in Men Treated Percutaneously by Progesterone.' *J Clin Endocrinol Metab* (1974): 38 (1): 142–7.

to help the DHT pathway work more efficiently,[39] or we can block it completely using certain drugs.

Stan's experience, then, shows not only how we can test for mild weaknesses in the liver; it also illustrates why it is not sufficient to carry out the standard LFT and simply assume that the liver is functioning well. It makes much more sense to check the liver's health by testing for elevated oestrogen and DHT levels.

Non-Alcoholic Fatty Liver Disease

The second way to assess the more subtle dysfunction that can afflict our liver is to test for Non-Alcoholic Fatty Liver Disease, or NAFLD. This is a very common condition that, simply put, means the liver is not functioning properly. And once again, just as we saw in Stan's case, the LFT blood test might be normal even though the liver is not.

So, what exactly is NAFLD and what causes it? This condition describes a liver that is fatty and damaged but which, on the positive side and provided the right steps are taken, has a 90 per cent chance of returning to normal.[40] And it is important that action is taken, because if left to fester, NAFLD can lead to various cancers.[41] It is generally caused by eating too many sugary carbohydrates, and the reason *those* lead to NAFLD is because the resultant insulin surges mean fat is stored in the liver to the point that it damages it.[42]

The crunch question is whether NAFLD weakens the liver's ability to detoxify. Unfortunately the answer is yes, and that is because NAFLD 'causes inflammation, scarring and impedes the liver's ability to process steroid

---

39   Ibid.

40   Browning, J. D. et al. 'Prevalence of Hepatic Steatosis in an Urban Population in the United States: Impact of Ethnicity.' *Hepatology* (2004): 40(6): 1387–95.

41   Sanna, C. et al. 'Non-Alcoholic Fatty Liver Disease and Extra-hepatic Cancers.' *Int J Mol Sci* (2016): 17: 717.

42   Nseir, W. et al. 'Relationship Between Non-Alcoholic Fatty Liver Disease and Breast Cancer.' *Isr Med Assoc J* (2017): 19: 242–5.

Paschos, P. and Paletas, K. 'Non-Alcoholic Fatty Liver Disease and Metabolic Syndrome.' *Hippokratia* (2009): 13 (1): 9–19

hormones'.[43] The other bad news is that NAFLD is common. Why? Because, as we saw in the chapter on inflammation and obesity, the world has become obsessed with eating sugary carbohydrates; it is thought that 20–30 per cent of people in developed nations have NAFLD.[44]

To illustrate NAFLD, let me introduce Felicity. She is thirty-nine, eats a low-fat diet, does Pilates twice a week and does not drink much alcohol. Despite this, she is developing a bigger belly that she cannot shift. Felicity's standard liver blood test results (the LFT) are normal, but the clue here is in her cholesterol: she has a high triglyceride level. Why would that be? Felicity is on a low-fat diet, but she is eating more sugary starches and drinking more fruit juice; some of this excess sugar is being stored as triglyceride fat in the liver. The result is a fatty liver that does not function as well as it should. Indeed, the blood triglyceride level[45] is the first marker that will indicate NAFLD; insulin resistance and belly fat quickly follow.

If a fatty liver is left untreated it can result in a significant heart-attack risk.[46] The good news is that NAFLD is easily treated: if Felicity cuts out the fruit juice and sugary starches her liver will return to normal within weeks, and her belly fat will start to melt away in a matter of months.

Genetic testing

This is the third way to find how well your liver is functioning. Gene testing is a simple process: you rub the inside of your cheek with a swab and send it off to a laboratory. The cells are analysed and, some days or weeks later, the result shows which of your liver pathways are weak and therefore in need of support.

43   Browning, J. D. et al. 'Prevalence of Hepatic Steatosis in an Urban Population in the United States: Impact of Ethnicity.' *Hepatology* (2004): 40(6): 1387–95..

44   Younossi, Z. M. et al. 'Global Epidemiology of Non-Alcoholic Fatty Liver Disease – Meta-Analytic Assessment of Prevalence, Incidence and Outcomes.' *Hepatology* (2016): 64: 73–84.

45   Zhang, Q. Q. et al. 'Non-Alcoholic Fatty Liver Disease: Dyslipidaemia, Risk for Cardiovascular Complications and Treatment Strategy.' *J Clin Transl Hepatol* (2015): 3: 78–84.

46   Ballestri, S. et al. 'Risk of Cardiovascular, Cardiac and Arrhythmic Complications in Patients with Non-Alcoholic Fatty Liver Disease.' *World J Gastroenterol* (2014): 20(7): 1724–45.

That brings up the question: how best to support these weak liver pathways? To explain that, we need to learn a little more about the main liver pathways, and that means knowing how the detoxification process works.

DETOXIFYING THE LIVER

Toxins are processed through the liver in two phases. For our purposes, we can compare it to taking out the rubbish at home:

- Phase 1 – someone takes the rubbish bag outside, which leaves the house looking cleaner.
- Phase 2 – the garbage truck removes the rubbish before it starts to fester.

In the same way, detoxifying the liver uses a two-step process.

Figure 2: The liver's detoxification pathway

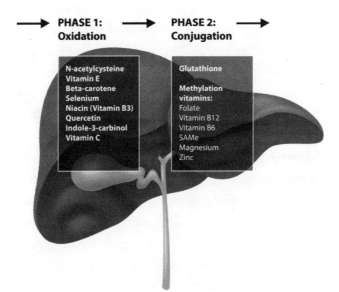

Figure 2 shows how the different pathways in Phase 1 (the Oxidation Phase) require various vitamins to support them; it also shows how the two main pathways in Phase 2 (the Conjugation Phase) require various supplements to support them. Both phases also require enzymes in order to function properly.

Phase 1 – the Oxidation Phase requires vitamins A (seen here as beta-carotene), B3, C and E as well as nutrients such as selenium and indole-3-carbinol (the latter is found in cruciferous vegetables such as broccoli and cauliflower) to function smoothly. It uses these vitamins and nutrients to process the particular toxin into a different state.

Phase 2 – the Conjugation Phase removes the products that the first phase has converted the toxins into. To do that, it needs a master antioxidant called glutathione to strip out metals like mercury, and it needs the methylation pathway (requiring folate and the B vitamins) to remove many other toxins from the body.

Sticking with our home analogy, if we were to take the rubbish out of the house and leave it festering, the smell would soon be overwhelming. That is why we need to complete Phase 2 and take the rubbish to the dump. If we went on a detoxification programme that saw us eat only carrots for a few days, then the vitamins in the carrots would help to accelerate the toxins through Phase 1 but, after a day or two, we would suffer from overwhelming feelings of fatigue and headaches. Why? Because the toxins would have hit a bottleneck at Phase 2. Headaches are not a 'healing crisis', as some people call them, but an accumulation of toxins at the end of Phase 1. And that is *not* a healthy state. The solution is to add glutathione, vitamin B12 and others to pull the toxins through Phase 2 and out of our system. In other words, effective detoxification means coordinating the vitamins and minerals used in both Phase 1 *and* in Phase 2.

This is where the genetic test comes in: it is useful in showing which of these Phase 1 and Phase 2 enzymes we are deficient in. Once we know that, we can supplement for them. For example, many people are deficient in the enzyme that converts folic acid into active folate – which is essential to Phase 2 and helps with the removal of mercury, lead and alcohol. Someone with this genetic defect should take an active folate supplement (see box on page 170), not a folic acid supplement, or their Phase 2 cycle will not function properly. (Indeed, giving folic acid to someone with that genetic deficiency can increase their cancer risk.)[47]

47   Bailey, R. et al. 'Unmetabolized Serum Folic Acid and Its Relation to Folic Acid Intake from Diet and Supplements in a Nationally Representative Sample of Adults Aged >or= 60y in the United States.' *Am J Clin Nutr* (2010): 92: 383–9.

L-5-MTHF and glutathione

If your gene test shows you are deficient in the enzyme that converts folic acid to folate, then you ought to avoid vitamin tablets that contain folic acid. Why? Because you cannot convert that folic acid into active folate, and that could be harmful. Instead, you should make sure you eat more foods that contain active folate (whose full name is L-5-methyltetrahydrofolate, or L-5-MTHF), such as spinach, broccoli, asparagus and Brussels sprouts, or take a multivitamin that contains active folate.

A genetic test can highlight any number of deficiencies, advantages or quirks in the body. For example, it might tell you that you have a mutation in the gene that prevents glutathione from doing its job. And what job is that, you ask? The very important one of removing heavy metals such as mercury. Someone who has a problem with this gene might accumulate mercury much faster than the next person[48] or, if you are like me, be less able to rid the body of mercury. After I learned that this was a problem for me, I supplemented with glutathione, as we will see in the next section.

To recap: we know that a good result on the standard liver test (the LFT) is no guarantee that our liver is functioning at its best. And typically I will advise patients to look at the following three areas in order to get a better idea of how healthy their liver is:

- A raised oestrogen level in a man is a sign that his liver is processing testosterone poorly. Improving his liver pathways and removing oestrogen will help.
- A raised triglyceride level and some belly fat indicates a fatty liver and an increased heart-attack risk in both men and women. Cutting out sugar and sugary carbohydrates goes a long way to reversing this.

48 Andreoli, V. and Sprovieri, F. 'Genetic Aspects of Susceptibility to Mercury Toxicity: An Overview.' *Int J Environ Res Public Health* (2017): 14: 93.

- Gene-testing shows where along the liver's processing pathways we are weak, and therefore how we should support the liver. Doing this improves liver functioning and health.

REMOVING HEAVY METALS

Finally, I want to talk about whether or not we should remove toxins from the body. Although some people reckon doing this is nonsense and a waste of money, and while it is true that some detoxification products are worthless, detoxifying *is* a powerful and important health tool, and one that we should be aware of.

One method, as we have seen, is to improve how well the liver's pathways function. Another, known as chelation, is used in particular to rid the body of heavy metals, and is something my clinic has used for years. This is a robust technique that involves giving the patient a particular substance (called a chelator) as a tablet or in a drip. This substance attaches to a particular toxin and removes it from the body.

One such substance is DMSA (which stands for dimercaptosuccinic acid). It is given in tablet form, and is very successful in attaching to mercury, lead and arsenic, and then washing these out of the body.[49] There is a problem though, because DMSA also attaches to minerals such as magnesium and calcium; losing these can harm bone strength and cause fatigue. The solution is to supplement with minerals at the same time, and monitor their levels.

Another chelator is EDTA (which stands for ethylenediaminetetraacetic acid). EDTA is used in industrial processes to dissolve limescale, and in medicine to remove mercury from the body. (There are gentler ways to do this, including by using alpha-lipoic acid, chlorella and active charcoal.)

Something to bear in mind is that chelation might put strain on your immune system. There are no good studies to support this, but anecdotally many practitioners are wary of being too robust with chelation because of the

---

49 Rush, T. et al. 'Effects of Chelation on Mercury, Iron & Lead Neurotoxicity.' *Neurotoxicology* (2009): 47–51.

pressure the adrenal gland might suffer. We will cover the adrenal gland and its immune system hormones in the next two chapters, but for now understand that if you are susceptible to coughs and colds then you might be well advised to improve your immune system before starting on a liver detoxification programme.

Finally, using chelation to remove metals and other toxins is helpful inasmuch as it prevents that toxin from damaging the body further. However, it might not undo the damage already done, and in some cases that damage can be permanent.

Supporting the liver

Chelation, in which chelators like DMSA and EDTA attach themselves to heavy metals, pull them out of the cells and wash them out of the body, is not the only way to remove these toxins from the body. And chelators have the distinct disadvantage of leaching minerals from the body, which means the patient can quickly become mineral-deficient.

There is another way, as Figure 3 shows. On the left of this simplified diagram you can see how mercury, lead, dioxins (which are often the by-products of industrial processes) and PCBs are helped through Phase 1 of the detoxification process by an enzyme called Cyp1b1.

What comes next is Phase 2, part of what we call the glutathione reaction that rids the body of many chemical and metal toxins including mercury.[50] Glutathione is not the only antioxidant in this process but it is central to it, and if the liver does not have enough glutathione then mercury and other toxins will accumulate and damage our cells. Studies have shown that, in the laboratory at least, adding glutathione to a cell helps to remove mercury toxicity.[51]

50 Dutczak, W. J. and Ballatori, N. 'Transport of the Glutathione-Methylercury Complex Across Liver Canalicular Membranes on Reduced Glutathione Carriers.' *J Biol Chem* (1994): 269: 9746–51.
51 Kaur, P. et al. 'Glutathione Modulation Influences Methylmercury-induced Neurotoxicity in Primary Cell Cultures of Neurons and Astrocytes.' *NeuroToxicology* (2006): 27(4): 492–500.

Patricia Kane was one of the first health practitioners to show the benefit of using glutathione drips to remove mercury from the body;[52] in my clinic, I have seen many patients reduce their blood levels of mercury through the use of glutathione drips. We also add other vitamins from the methylation pathway and from Phase 1 to enhance the entire liver detoxification process.

Figure 3: The methylation cycle and the glutathione reaction – two of the liver's detoxification pathways

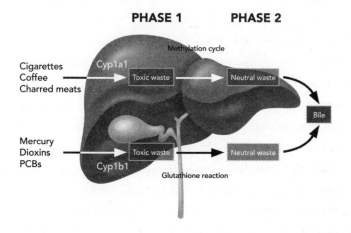

Of course, the body needs to get rid of numerous other toxins too, including hormones and those found in alcohol and countless other substances. It does this every minute of the day, and it is in the liver that we get a sense of just how remarkable the body is. By taking the appropriate supplements to support both Phase 1 and Phase 2 liver detoxification, we can expect our liver to work far more efficiently than it currently does, and we can avoid the headaches of that old carrot-and-vitamin detoxification programme.

For the sake of completion, Figure 3 also illustrates a second pathway called the methylation cycle: this shows how the liver processes toxins such as those found in coffee, burned meat and cigarettes. This is also a two-stage process,

---

52 Kane, P. et al. *The Detoxx Book: Detoxification of Biotoxins in Chronic Neurotoxic Syndromes* (2009).

with its Phase 1 stage helped by an enzyme called Cyp1a1. Interestingly, someone with a defective Cyp1a1 gene cannot make an effective version of this enzyme, and that means they will struggle to remove these toxins. Typically, a person with that deficiency would, for instance, feel wired for hours after drinking coffee.

TOXINS: A FINAL WORD

Toxins put a massive – and largely under-recognised – stress on the body, and we are flooded by them on a daily basis. Cancers, nerve damage, hormone damage and cardiovascular disease are all strongly associated with toxin exposure, while metal toxicity leaves us fatigued, with allergies, foggy thinking, depression, genetic mutations and countless other disruptions large and small. Indeed, one study concluded that just 5–10 per cent of all cancers are caused by genetics,[53] with the rest due to environmental factors.

Whatever the precise figures, I have no doubt that the toxins we are exposed to have a significant role to play in causing them, and they are something to which we are all exposed. With the massive burden of death and disease associated with toxins, much more can and must be done in many areas including the use of herbicides and pesticides, with products such as amalgam fillings and plastics, and with industrial pollution.

The world is becoming a worryingly polluted place, and the level of toxins is a disturbing health risk that costs us all, both in terms of health and money. We have seen how hard it is to prove that products like amalgam fillings are toxic and how long it takes for governments to legislate. Indeed, there are so many toxins around us that we tend to put up with them until they are proven to be toxic; it makes more sense to avoid them long before that. For example, until electromagnetic radiation from Wi-Fi and mobile phones is proven *not* to be damaging, it would be sensible to limit your exposure to it.

53   Anand, P. et al. 'Cancer is a Preventable Disease that Requires Major Lifestyle Changes.' *Pharm Res* (2008): 25: 2097–116.

If avoiding toxins is a sensible first step to ensuring optimal health, then clearing the existing toxic burden from our body is generally a wise second step, and boosting our detoxification system is an obvious third. Given that our liver is our key detoxification organ, and given that it needs to last us around eighty years, it goes without saying that looking after it is paramount to healthy ageing. We can help ourselves by working out how well our liver works: by testing our genes, our triglyceride level and the levels of certain hormones.

It is a sobering thought that nearly every patient tested at my clinic has exhibited toxic levels of some or other heavy metal. And so, although we *can* surely survive in the modern world, we need to take toxins seriously if we want to thrive. That means helping our liver by avoiding potential toxins and supplementing with drips or tablets to get rid of those that are already in our system. I would go so far as to say that the air in most of our cities is more polluted than we can safely cope with, and that at the very least we should support our liver with glutathione drips to stay on top of the toxic load.

This topic is certainly not all doom and gloom, and there are various factors that are pointing us in the right direction: social media today highlights potential toxins far faster than any medium has done in the past; increased public awareness means governments will be forced to act more quickly on suspected toxins; and in the UK, a full ban on the use of microbeads – tiny plastic particles that can enter the marine foodchain – in cosmetics and personal care products came into effect in 2018. We are making progress, but we do need to make more.

Key points
- We are surrounded by multiple toxins and cannot avoid them all of the time. It can take years before science proves certain substances are toxic; even longer before governments legislate. That is why knowledge counts – if we know what toxins to avoid, or if we suspect that certain substances are toxic, then we should avoid them.

- The better we look after our liver the better it will perform. There are three ways to assess if our liver is working well: measuring oestrogen and DHT levels in men assesses how well the liver is processing hormones like testosterone; an increase in triglyceride levels and expanding waist circumferences in men and women suggests a fatty liver – cutting out sugary carbohydrates usually reverses this toxic state; and gene tests can show where our liver pathways are weak, and suggest healthy supplements to support them.

- There are two ways to remove heavy metal toxins once they have accumulated: using chelation, which is effective but which leaches valuable minerals from the body; and enhancing our glutathione liver detoxification system, which is done with glutathione and vitamin drips.

- Looking after the liver is essential, not only because this organ processes toxins but also because it removes hormones, and its ability to do both fades with age. It is my opinion that we are so overwhelmed with toxins in our modern world that, even if we are vigilant in avoiding toxins, we should be assisting our liver with drips or supplements.

- Over the next few chapters we will look at our hormones, and methods to rebalance their levels in a fatigued body. None of that is sustainable unless our liver is healthy.

- The hatters of old surely knew that working with mercury was causing them terrible problems, yet they had little choice in those times. Today we know far better what is toxic, what is likely to be toxic, and how to avoid or remove toxins. We can and must be better than the hatters of old.

Chapter 6

Anabolic versus Catabolic Hormones – Building Up, Breaking Down

> Those who don't find time for exercise will one
> day need to find time for illness.
>
> *Plato, aged eighty-three, around 500 BCE*

We spend the first twenty years of our lives becoming stronger, faster and brighter. This is nature at its best: building us up in a process known as 'anabolism', from the Greek word meaning 'ascent', and which refers to the building of bones, muscle mass and the like. By the age of twenty we are fertile, energised, mentally sharp, physically strong and, for most of us, about as sexy as we are ever going to be.

After that – well, you know what happens: the slow slide sets in, the decline as nature intended it. By thirty few of us are as fast as we were (the world's best sprinters tend to peak in their twenties). Equally dismally, we are no longer as mentally acute as we were (the best mathematicians typically have their biggest breakthroughs in their twenties).[1] After that it gets worse. By the time we reach our late thirties, grey hairs start to appear, our bodies are stuck with stubborn flab, men often start balding and women struggle with cellulite. And how is it that our ability to drink what we thought were heroic amounts of alcohol in our twenties seems to have gone the way of our once-perfect skin?

In short, our bodies are starting to break down. It is as frustrating and infuriating as it is apparently unavoidable. But why are our bodies unable to

---

1 Singh, S. *Fermat's Last Theorem*. Fourth Estate (1997).

continue being as phenomenal as they were when we were in our early twenties? What is going on?

The short answer is what scientists call 'catabolism', from the Greek for 'throwing down': our bodies have started to crumble (if it helps, think catastrophe for catabolism) and, just as nature planned it, we are quietly being removed to make way for the next generation. It is the natural order.

Nobody likes bad news but I would encourage you to retain hope. As you will see, all is not lost. Because you, me and everyone around us are remarkable beings, and in the following pages I will prove that to you. Start with this: on average your body replaces nearly 300 billion cells every day. By way of putting that figure into perspective, 300 billion pieces of paper stacked on top of each other would make a pile reaching halfway to the moon.

Now consider that each of your cells has a cellular brain in the form of DNA. This DNA 'brain' talks to the information messengers known as mRNA, which in turn take those messages to the ribosomes inside the cell; those ribosomes manufacture the structures the cell needs to build and divide, an unceasing process of maintaining our bodies.

Given that each human adult has an estimated 37 trillion cells, this frenetic activity of protein-building in every one of your cells every day of your life, around the clock, makes the Herculean effort needed to organise the Olympic Games look like a picnic.[2] The sheer extent of the activity going on inside us is astonishing. For instance:

- The next time you cut your finger, notice how it heals completely in less than a week.
- Your body has twenty-two metres of intestine, and you replace all of it every four days throughout your life.
- When a bacterium enters your body, the white blood cells – the macrophages – identify it as an enemy and try to destroy it by swallowing it. What is astonishing is that the macrophages somehow know not to eat our own body elements, only foreign bodies. Should the

2   Bianconi, E., et al. 'An estimation of the number of cells in the human body.' *Ann Hum Biol*, November–December 2013, Vol. 40, No. 6: Pp 463–71.

bacterium manage to slip past the macrophages, the chemicals released during that tussle will kick-start the next line of defence: our Beta-cells, which attack and destroy the bacterium and print out warning antibodies that will recognise this specific danger for the rest of your life. Every time a bacterium like this enters our body, the specific anti-bodies recognise it and set off the alarm, calling in the body's defences.

In this way, our body acquires immunity to that bacterial infection.

The list goes on: your brain tells your body to produce hormones at the precise time they are needed, and in precise amounts; those hormones travel to the specific cells they are designed for and tell the DNA what to do. The consequence of this hormonal instruction is that your cells build their protein blocks, function exactly as they are meant to, replicate and eventually die – all in a manner more reliable than the finest clock.

That precision and reliability, however, does not mean the process is flawless. Every so often, unavoidably, in a body of 37 trillion cells and countless messages, something goes wrong. In most instances the consequences are insignificant. The cell's brain (the nucleus) follows the recipe to make a new cell in a process known as cellular transcription but occasionally this recipe flops. When that happens, the body makes a damaged cell and, over time, we will notice that damage as grey hair, wrinkles, depleting energy or a fading memory.

The ageing world

In the end, as the wags tell us, there are only two certainties in life: death and taxes. I am no expert on the second but I can tell you something about the first. If we look at life expectancy in the US, for example, the statistics show that, over the past century or so, people lived two years longer per decade. Or to put it another way, average life expectancy for men and women in the 1930s was fifty-nine but, as the world's richest country got richer, advances such as vaccinations, heating, lower levels of pollution, the wide availability of antibi-otics, and improved sanitation all contrived to bump up that number. By 2010, the average American could expect to live to seventy-eight.[3]

3 The Centers for Disease Control and Prevention's National Center for Health Statistics. Life Expectancy by Age, National Vital Statistics Reports (2011). http://www.cdc.gov/nchs

Figure 1: Life expectancy in the US (and elsewhere) has risen steadily over the past century

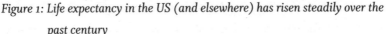

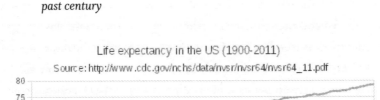

Fantastic though these improvements are, they will not get you and me as far as we would like. As we saw in the chapter on the theories of ageing, the goal of this book is to optimise our Healthspan, the number of years that we are healthy; it is not to try to stay alive for as long as possible at all costs. Yet it is interesting to consider what *is* possible. If we assume our genetic life potential is 120 years then – assuming the same rate of improvement of two years per decade – it will take a further two centuries before US society reaches its potential age. That is not going to help you or me.

Ageing – and combating it – has been a concern of mankind since the ancient Greeks and likely long before them. After all, the Fountain of Youth is the subject of many a fable. The Old Testament prophet Moses, who lived around the time of the ancient Greeks and reputedly reached the grand age of 120, also pondered the ageing process and had this to say: 'The length of our days is seventy years – or eighty if we have the strength.' That is not too different from today, so perhaps things have not changed that much in three millennia? If so, what is to blame? The negative consequences of industrialisation? Mankind's propensity to go to war? The stresses of life in general?

Indeed, is it unrealistic to think that we can extend our lives much beyond eighty? Or, given the modern epidemic of obesity, the flood of toxins to which we are exposed and the stresses of modern life, is it even possible our lives could shorten? It is true that, as life expectancy in many countries soared, it stuttered in the US and then, between 2014 and 2016, declined. Among the likely reasons: nearly 60 per cent of calories consumed by Americans come from ultra-processed foods;[4] and half of that country's population is either diabetic or pre-diabetic.[5] We should not take it for granted that each generation will live longer than the last.

Furthermore, if we want a good Healthspan then the chapter on toxins shows how important it is to recognise and avoid toxic substances. And the chapter on inflammation shows how important it is to understand the damaging effects of sugar and junk food.

For my part, I am convinced we can reach our genetic potential of 120 years, so the average lifespan of seventy-eight means we are well short of what is possible. Closing that gap, though, requires more than relying on antibiotics and cutting air pollution. We will dig into what is needed in the next few chapters; first we need to start by working out how to optimise our anabolic processes and reducing those that are catabolic. The good news is that this is eminently doable.

MEET YOUR ANABOLIC AND CATABOLIC PLAYERS

Earlier I told you that our bodies become more catabolic through our adult life – breaking down more than they build up as we age. Let us say, theoretically, that we could turn that on its head: if we could reverse this natural decline, we could postpone being removed from the playing field and, instead of our bodies breaking down in middle-age, they could rebuild themselves. Logically,

---

4   Steele, E. M. et al. 'Ultra-Processed Foods and Added Sugars in the US Diet: Evidence from a Nationally Representative Cross-Sectional Study.' *BMJ Open* (2016): Accessed at: http://dx.doi.org/10.1136/bmjopen-2015-009892

5   Menke, A. et al. 'Prevalence of and Trends in Diabetes Among Adults in the United States, 1988–2012.' *JAMA* (2015): 314 (10): 1021–9. Reference: doi:10.1001/jama.2015.10029

then, if we want to ensure that we are healthier today than we were yesterday, we would need to make sure that our body's 37 trillion cells manufacture better building blocks today than they did yesterday. And we would also have to do that tomorrow and the next day and the next.

It might sound fantastical but it is possible. As we saw earlier, the magicians that oversee the anabolic (building up) process each day are our anabolic hormones, and for the purposes of this discussion these are growth hormone, testosterone, oestrogen and DHEA. (Thyroid hormone is also a building-up hormone but is only partially anabolic. Insulin is another anabolic hormone but anything beyond a very low blood level is associated with inflammation and an early death. For the purposes of this chapter we will ignore both.)

Our anabolic hormones tend to peak around the age of twenty, which is why we look so good at that age.[6] We are not only at our most attractive; we are also at our most fertile, giving us the best chance of passing on our genes.

In the chapter on the theories of ageing, we saw that hormonal decline is believed to cause us to age, so with that in mind let us take a closer look at these hormones:

- Growth hormone (GH) causes our growth spurt as teenagers. Some adults inject it to stay lean and mean but there are good reasons to worry that too much GH can accelerate ageing. We will read more about GH in the next section.

- Testosterone has various health benefits from reducing arterial plaque to improving brain functioning. And while testosterone replacement does strengthen bones, skin and muscle, the jury is out as to whether it shortens or lengthens our lifespan. We will read more about testosterone in the chapter on men's health.

- Oestrogen replacement strengthens bones, skin and soft tissue. Hormone replacement therapy (HRT) during menopause has

6 Orentreich, N. et al. 'Age Changes and Sex Differences in Serum Dehydroepiandrosterone Sulfate Concentrations Throughout Adulthood.' *J Clin Endocrinol Metab* (1984): 59: 551–5.

endured much criticism over the last twenty years, but we have learned that if it is done correctly then undergoing HRT is healthier for women than not taking hormones.[7] We will learn much more about HRT's potential benefits in the chapter on women's health.

• DHEA is probably the least-known of the anabolic hormones, yet has the greatest potential for keeping us anabolic as we age. In young people, DHEA builds muscle and boosts energy. In the elderly, it has the additional task of being converted into testosterone and oestrogen as required by the body, and that outcome allows those anabolic hormones to rebuild bone, muscle and skin. Low DHEA in older men is a predictor of an early death.[8] We will go into this subject in greater detail in this chapter.

At the opposite spectrum are the breaking-down effects of our catabolic hormones (cortisol, adrenalin and glucagon, among others). At some point in our adult life the anabolic hormones take a back seat and the catabolic hormones dominate. Of these, cortisol is the most important, and excessive levels of it have important consequences: raised sugar levels, increased abdominal fat, muscle-wasting, thinning skin, wrinkles, weakened bones and lowered immunity. If you want to picture the physical effect of excess cortisol you could do worse than imagine a worn-out taxi driver: an older, stressed man with a fat belly and matchstick legs.

Cortisol is produced by your adrenal glands, and in the next chapter – which is about stress – we will see what happens when stress burns us out and depletes our cortisol store. You might think from what I have said about cortisol's catabolic effects that this would be a good thing. It is not. Healthy living is about the search for balance and, when it comes to cortisol deficiency, a lack of it is even more devastating than an excess.

7 Sarrel, P. M. et al. 'The mortality toll of oestrogen avoidance: an analysis of excessive deaths among hysterectomized women aged 50 to 59 years.' *Am J Public Health* (2013): 103: 1583–8.
8 Mazat, L. et al. 'Prospective measurements of dehyrdoepiandrostenone sulphate in a cohort of elderly subjects: relationship to gender, subjective health, smoking habits, and 10-year mortality.' *Proc Natl Acad Sci USA* (2001): 98: 8145–50.

That discussion, however, must wait. For now our focus is how the process of ageing is intimately connected to our hormones, and how, as we age, we accumulate more catabolic than anabolic hormones. What we know so far is that:

- Hormones are central to the ageing process. Anabolic hormones build us up while catabolic hormones break us down. The hope is that, if we can stay more anabolic than catabolic as we age, our bodies should not break down.

- DHEA has intriguing possibilities not least because a healthy DHEA level in older people is associated with living longer.

- As we age, DHEA is our primary anabolic hormone and cortisol is our primary catabolic hormone. One possible way to optimise our health could be to reduce excessive cortisol and boost flagging DHEA.

Jump around

If you are like most people in their thirties, forties and beyond, then you have probably noticed that you feel more tired, less enthusiastic and some-what worn down. Life is not like it was when you were twenty, a time of seemingly boundless energy and that truly alive feeling. Now the years seem to zip past, and the zing of those youthful days seems more absent than present. As the old phrase has it: 'My "get-up-and-go" got up and went.'

Unsurprisingly the issue of middle-age fatigue has caught the attention of some fine medical minds, and in this chapter we will benefit from their wisdom. In short, though, as Stephen Cherniske puts it in his book *The Metabolic Plan*: 'You are not tired because of a caffeine deficiency.'

But if it is not a lack of coffee, then what is it? Metabolically speaking we become tired – and here I do not mean sleepy, but lethargic in that middle-aged, burned out way – through inactivity.

So here is the bad news: the less we do, the less energy we have, and that is largely due to the brain. When we go for a run, for instance, the muscles send a message to the brain, and that stimulates BDNF (brain-derived neurotrophic factor) to make more neurons.[9] The end result is that the brain sends messages back that enhance the muscle. Lots of parts of your body win. But if we sit on the couch it all goes the wrong way.

The same argument was put another way in a 2016 study in which scientists found that the reason elderly people have weak muscles is mainly because they have fewer nerves connecting those muscles to the brain. For example, the quadriceps (thigh) muscle has 70,000 nerves connecting it to the spine, but sedentary elderly people can lose up to 40,000 of those nerves, and that means their thigh muscle gets considerably weaker.[10] It seems to me as though the older we get, the more we need to move in order to ensure the brain keeps sending messages to rebuild nerve and muscle.

It gets more interesting still: one reason high-intensity interval training (HIIT) is so popular is that it packs intense exercise into a ten-minute slot. But perhaps more significantly, HIIT has been shown to increase new mitochondrial formation inside our cells.[11] Why is that important? Because mitochondria are the cellular engines that make our energy that gives us our zip, but as we age we tend to lose them – and that is one reason we feel more sluggish in our fifties and sixties. HIIT exercise becomes important as we age, because it stimulates new mitochondria and improves our daily energy.

In addition, excess stress tends to burn out hormones like DHEA and, as we run out of DHEA, our brain can become depressed and we slump into inactivity.[12] With inactivity, the brain no longer gets the message to rebuild the muscles, and the body defaults to storing food as fat in order to get us through the presumed upcoming winter.

9   Zoladz, J. A. et al. 'The effect of physical activity on the brain derived neurotrophic factor: from animal to human studies.' *J Physiol Pharmacol* (2010): 61: 533–41.

10   Piasecki, M. et al. 'Age-related neuromuscular changes affecting human *vastus lateralis*.' *J Physiol* (2016): 594: 4525–36.

11   Little, J. P. et al. 'A practical model of low-volume high-intensity interval training induces mitochondrial biogenesis in human skeletal muscle: potential mechanisms.' *J Physiol* (2010): 588: 1011–22.

12   Souza-Teodoro, L. H. et al. 'Higher serum dehydroepiandrosterone sulfate protects against the onset of depression in the elderly: Findings from the English Longitudinal Study of Ageing (ELSA).' *Psychoneuroendocrinology* (2016): 64: 40–6.

The result of this double whammy of burning out our hormones with stress in our thirties is that we enter our middle-age years a little depressed, overweight, inactive and feeling too worn out to do much about it.

Now here is the good news: the more years you spend doing daily exercise, the longer your body will send messages to the brain telling it to turn some of the food that you eat into muscle and the rest into usable energy. Exercise is crucial to a Younger for Longer life. *Whatever you can do to keep your body exercising throughout your life should have a profound positive effect on your health and longevity.*

Jack LaLanne: king of the road

For my money the king of the active approach was an American called Jack LaLanne, who thought nothing of doing 900 push-ups a day – when he was in his eighties. I consider that I am in pretty good shape for someone in his fifties but I cannot manage more than 100, and that is on a good day.

LaLanne was famous in the US for most of his long life. In the 1940s he was promoting weight training with a high-protein, low-carbohydrate diet, and in the 1950s he had a long-running TV show that promoted his approach to health. He was a consistent voice against the high-carbohydrate philosophy that dominated thinking between 1970 and 2010. He was also a man who believed in showing by example:

- In 1957, at the age of forty-three, he swam across San Francisco's Golden Gate Strait while towing a cabin cruiser that weighed just over one ton.
- In 1984, aged seventy, LaLanne swam one mile towing seventy rowing boats, one of which was filled with passengers.

He celebrated his ninetieth birthday in 2004 by hosting a marathon 24-hour TV special of the original *Jack LaLanne Show*. He died in 2011 at the age of ninety-six after showing the world that his way of healthy living had allowed him to live a life of vitality long after most of his peers had died.

The way he did it was simple enough: he ate and exercised with a focus on maintaining anabolic muscle mass. The result was that for his entire adult life his body told his brain that it was active and needed the food he ate to be converted into usable energy and sustainable muscle. Even in his nineties he had an astonishing physique, far closer to Arnold Schwarzenegger's than you would believe possible for an aged pensioner.

Predicting longevity

Jack LaLanne's approach (see box above) on its own, of course, does not necessarily prove anything. He was just one person, no doubt he had good genes and, the sceptics might mutter, perhaps he was just lucky. Well perhaps he was, although I do not believe that accounts for it. I am a firm believer in scientific studies, and it turns out that there are quite a few to back up LaLanne's approach.

When it comes to predicting longevity in older people, a number of metabolic factors are important. In the chapter on the theories of ageing we saw that exercise, non-smoking and good health are common characteristics of people who reach 100. As important as these are, once you are elderly there are three predictors that will keep you healthy.

- *Predictor 1: Muscle mass* – I said at the beginning of this book that I am very wary of single-study results but the findings of this Italian study of eighty-four people aged between ninety and 106 are fascinating: researchers found that, in this group, muscle mass was the most important longevity factor.[13] Dwindling muscle mass in an elderly person indicates increasing frailty and vulnerability. That said, muscle mass is not solely determined by the amount of time

13 Ravaglia, G. et al. 'Determinants of Functional Status in Healthy Italian Nonagenarians and Centenarians: A Comprehensive Functional Assessment by the Instruments of Geriatric Practice.' *J Am Geriatr Soc* (1997): 45: 10: 1196–202.

spent in the gym or doing other exercise – as we saw earlier, muscle development is controlled by our anabolic hormones, and it is the *levels* of these hormones that count. The exhortations of sports brands to 'Just Do It' will not add up to much unless our bodies have the underlying anabolic hormones to get us off the couch in the first place.

- *Predictor 2: DHEA* – we have seen that several anabolic hormones are concerned with building us up and, among those, DHEA is proving to be the best predictor of longevity. The Italian study about muscle mass in the very elderly also found there was a greater risk of death when DHEA levels started to decline.[14] Interestingly, DHEA was for many years a bit of a medical conundrum – an odd adrenal hormone that seemingly had no portfolio. We now know that DHEA helps with about 150 different metabolic functions: it contributes to keeping your immune system in peak condition, lowers cholesterol, protects you from heart attacks, strokes and cancer, maintains your sex drive, and helps with both mood and memory. We will look more closely at DHEA shortly.

- *Predictor 3: Living in a community* – there is an African proverb that says, 'It takes a village to raise a child,' which if nothing else is a testament to the power of community. These days, though, many of us tend to live less in communities and more behind high walls. A New York study of 119 centenarians found that elderly people who live in a community setting generally have very good mental health, and we know that a healthy, happy brain contributes significantly to a healthy body.[15] In his book *The Blue Zones*, Dan Buettner looked at six factors for living longer lives: one of the most important is belonging to a community.[16] As we will see in the chapter on brain health, our

---

14   Ibid.

15   Jopp, D. S. et al. 'Physical, Cognitive, Social and Mental Health in Near-Centenarians and Centenarians Living in New York City: Findings from the Fordham Centenarian Study.' *BMC Geriatr* (2016): 16: 1.

16   Buettner, D. *The Blue Zones: Lessons for Living Longer from the People Who've Lived the Longest*. National Geographic (2010).

brain shrinks when we live in isolation but thrives when we are surrounded by family, friends and pets.

Three factors

There are a further three factors that I consider key for maintaining health and body mass in the aged. They are not predictors, as they cannot easily be measured, but they are important:

Amino acids

These are the building blocks that make proteins, and include what are called branch chain amino acids (BCAAs), which are amino acids that we cannot make ourselves, and that means we need to eat them.[17] The king of amino acids is glutamine, which we get from red meat and which helps to build our muscles, bones, skin and hormones. Glutamine's most important work, potentially, as we age is to rebuild our intestine allowing us to absorb nutrients properly and maintain our body mass. Glutamine levels in ageing rats have been shown to decrease as they age but, if glutamine is added to the diet, the rat's intestine rebuilds and the body mass of the ageing rodent is restored.[18]

Glutathione

This is one of our most important nutrients. It is not a BCAA and, although its name sounds similar to glutamine, the two are quite different. You might recall meeting glutathione in the chapter on toxins, and you probably remember that it took the gold medal in my list of top supplements.

Glutathione controls the most important detoxification pathway in the liver and, without enough of it, our bodies accumulate heavy metals like lead and mercury. Glutathione also crosses the blood-brain barrier where it works

---

17 The three main BCAAs are valine, leucine and iso-leucine, and they are found in meat, fish, dairy and eggs, as well as in beans, lentils and nuts – to name a few sources.
18 Maynial-Denis, D. 'Glutamine Metabolism in Advanced Ageing.' *Nutr Rev* (2016): 74: 225–36.

as the brain's primary antioxidant reducing inflammation there and, in so doing, likely helping to counter depression, bipolar disorders and dementia. (We will look further at brain inflammation in the chapters on brain health.) A lack of glutathione in the lungs worsens asthma;[19] in the arteries it leads to inflammation and blockages.

The bad news is that glutathione levels decline with age. The good news is that glutathione levels automatically increase with exercise.[20] Turning that on its head, a significant side-effect for people who do *not* exercise daily is that they fail to replenish their glutathione levels each day, and this increases their chances of damage from raised toxin levels, as well as the possibility of developing dementia, heart attacks and lung damage.

Glutathione can be taken as an oral supplement, but the body absorbs it better if taken as a drip.

Detoxification

If there is one element that can make us look older than our years, it is an unhealthy liver detoxification system. Twenty-year-olds look fantastically healthy because they have high hormone levels and a healthy liver to remove those spent hormones when needed. But as we age, a weakening liver means oestrogen is not removed effectively in women, for instance, which contributes to cellulite formation. Men who have a weak liver cannot remove testosterone effectively, which leads to baldness and prostate problems, among other ailments. We have to be careful giving ageing people anything stronger than low-dose hormones, because their liver might not cope with anything more powerful, which is why maintaining a healthy liver is essential to healthy ageing.

19   Kloek, J. et al. 'Glutathione Prevents the Early Asthmatic Reaction and Airway Hyperresponsiveness in Guinea Pigs.' *J Physiol Pharmacol* (2010): 61: 67–72.
20   Jeevanandam, M. et al. 'Altered Plasma Cytokines and Total Glutathione Levels in Parenterally Fed Critically Ill Trauma Patients with Adjuvant Recombinant Human Growth Hormone (rhGH) Therapy.' *Crit Care Med* (2000): 28: 2: 324–9.

Longevity and gene-testing

In looking at how to predict longevity I have stayed away from genetic testing because, apart from obvious genes like the BRCA1 gene (which significantly increases the risk of breast cancer in women who carry it), most of the gene tests we do are for *low-penetrance* genes. What we mean by that phrase is that individually these genes have a very low impact on our health. In fact, studies have shown that our genes account for just 25 per cent of the variance of our lifespan – 75 per cent is determined by how we live.[21]

For example, smoking tobacco turns on hundreds of bad genes whereas exercising turns on hundreds of good genes. In other words, how we live our life does affect our genes, and the term for that is epigenetics. For most people, how they live their life is far more important than the cards they were dealt at birth.

Gene testing is at its most useful showing us which good habits we should focus on to remove the effects of bad genes. The advice in this book will cover most of the good habits needed to neutralise our bad genes.

THE RISE (AND FALL) OF GROWTH HORMONE

Growth hormone, or GH, is produced by your brain's pituitary gland and is regarded by many as the mother hormone that influences all others. As its name suggests, GH makes us grow when we are young, and adults who inject themselves with it feel healthier, stronger and more energised. For that reason it is often perceived as the ultimate youthful hormone.

Our GH levels decline as we age, and it is thought this contributes to our

21 Christensen, K. et al. 'The Quest for Genetic Determinants of Human Longevity: Challenges and Insights.' *Nat Rev Genet* (2006): 7: 436–48.

bodies weakening. For that reason, researchers wondered whether injecting with GH could reverse that process, and indeed a seminal 1990 study of twenty-one elderly men showed that those who were injected with GH for six months had stronger bones, improved muscles and less body fat than those who were not injected.[22] As a result, thousands of elderly people were given GH injections to boost their fading vitality.

The studies that followed generally agreed that such injections delivered positive *anabolic* effects to bone, muscle and fat. However, a review of the literature in 2007 suggested that GH injections could *not* be recommended because there were too many side effects, including swelling and painful joints.[23] That drew a rebuttal from a group of anti-ageing physicians called the A4M who said that their review of the literature suggested most people benefited greatly from GH injections, and that the dosage could be lowered for those people experiencing side effects.[24]

In my opinion, both the review and the rebuttal missed the point. The concern ought not to be whether GH causes or does not cause swollen joints in some people; it should be to determine whether GH makes patients look and feel better for a period before causing premature death or whether it can help them to stay healthier for longer. Or to put it another way, does GH make us shine like a comet for a while, but burn us out sooner than we should?

Concerns about growth hormones

Concerns about GH are not new: among the first to worry about its long-term effects were researchers carrying out a 2004 study on mice. These laboratory rodents get examined from every angle, and the researchers

22 Rudman, D. et al. 'Effects of Human Growth Hormone in Men over 60 Years Old.' *N Engl J Med* (1990): 323: 1–6.

23 Liu, H. et al. 'Systematic Review: The Safety and Efficacy of Growth Hormone in the Healthy Elderly.' *Ann Intern Med* (2007): 146: 104–5.

24 'Analysis of Faulty Data Yields Inaccurate Results: Thousands Benefit from Growth Hormone Replacement Therapy for Aging-Related Disorders – Proven, Real-World Track Record of Benefits of Adult Growth.' *Worldhealth.net* (15 January 2007), A4M in the Media. http://www.worldhealth.net/news/analysis_of_faulty_data_yields_inaccurat/

noticed that some with low GH levels looked small, fat and unhealthy and yet lived 25–60 per cent longer than other mice.[25]

Why was that? One suggestion was that mice with low GH levels have a low body temperature, and that is a factor that has been shown to extend life, as we saw in the chapter on the theories of ageing.[26] Another suggestion, derived from a study on fruit flies, was that GH stimulates insulin, which switches off some of our longevity genes.[27]

We have seen this association of high GH and dying younger in other animals: large-breed horses and dogs have higher GH than smaller breeds, and they typically die younger.[28] The pattern is that high GH in animals is associated with growing larger but dying sooner. But is that the case for humans? A good place to start is with people with dwarfism, as that is a condition caused by insufficient GH. Here is what researchers found:

- A small study of eleven people with dwarfism caused by low GH showed that they all died much younger (on average aged fifty-one) than their siblings, who did not have dwarfism and who lived on average to seventy-eight.[29] This suggests that a higher level of GH is necessary for a longer, healthier life.

- In contrast, a 2011 study showed that people from North Ecuador with dwarfism and with growth hormone deficiencies live longer than average and tend to be free of cancer and heart attacks.[30] This suggests that a *lack* of GH helps us to live healthier and longer.

25 Brown-Borg, H. M. et al. 'Life Extension in the Dwarf Mouse.' *Curr Top Dev Biol* (2004): 63: 189–225.

26 Bartke, A. et al. 'Does growth hormone prevent or accelerate aging?' *Exp Gerontol* (1998): 33: 675–87.

27 Clancy, D. J. et al. 'Extension of life-span by loss of CHICO, a Drosophila insulin receptor substrate protein.' *Science* (2001): 292: 104–6.

28 Patronek, G. J. et al. 'Comparative Longevity of Pet Dogs and Humans: Implications for Gerontology Research.' *J Gerontol A Biol Sci Med Sci* (1997): 52A: B171–8.

29 Besson, A. et al. 'Reduced Longevity in Untreated Patients with Isolated Growth Hormone Deficiency.' *J Clin Endocrinol Metab* (2003): 88: 80: 3664–7.

30 Guevara-Aguirre, J. et al. 'Growth Hormone Receptor Deficiency is Associated with a Major Reduction in Pro-aging Signaling, Cancer and Diabetes in Humans.' *Sci Transl Med* (2011): 3 (70): 70.

- The theory that low GH is healthier was further supported by studies showing that GH deficiency in humans could protect from cancer[31] and heart attacks.[32] Another study of nearly 200 New Yorkers aged ninety-plus showed that women with low GH levels had a better life expectancy than their peers with high GH. It also showed that men and women who had survived cancer had a much better life expectancy if they had low GH levels.[33]

- We know that gigantism – a condition in which high GH levels cause large bones – shortens lifespan in humans by causing heart attacks and diabetes. But when people with gigantism had their GH levels lowered, their life expectancy improved to match that of the general population.[34]

- And finally, an elegant study from 2003 showed that both low GH levels *and* high GH levels in humans are detrimental to cardiac function.[35] Injecting GH into 'normal' patients who had suffered cardiac damage *did* benefit their hearts. However, people with acromegaly, a condition caused by a constant overproduction of GH, are known to suffer heart damage from high GH levels. This study's conclusion was that GH replacement has a part to play in rebuilding a damaged heart (or damaged bones and muscles) but that, when it is given in excessive amounts for prolonged periods, it is unhealthy.

So what does this tell us? Most of these studies are of people with naturally low GH levels, and they suggest that low GH protects against early death.

31   Shevah, O., Laron, Z. 'Patients with Congenital Deficiency of IGF-I Seem Protected from the Development of Malignancies: A Preliminary Report.' *Growth Horm IGF Res* (2007): 17: 54–7.

32   Shechter, M. et al. 'Obese Adults with Primary Growth Hormone Resistance (Laron Syndrome) have Normal Endothelial Function.' *Growth Horm IGF Res* (2007): 17: 165–70.

33   Milman, S. et al. 'Low Insulin-Like Growth Factor 1 Level Predicts Survival in Humans with Exceptional Longevity.' *Aging Cell* (12 March 2014). http://onlinelibrary.wiley.com/doi/10.1111/acel.12213/full

34   Orme, S. M. et al. 'Mortality and Cancer Incidence in Acromegaly: A Retrospective Cohort Study.' *J Clin Endocrinol Metab* (1998): 83: 2730–4.

35   Sacca, L. et al. 'Growth Hormone, Acromegaly and Heart Failure: An Intricate Triangulation.' *Clin Endocrinol* (2003): 59: 660–71.

What happens, though, if we inject GH into elderly people who have low GH in order to help boost their anabolism? We saw earlier that this will make them look and feel better. But does it shorten their lives? To answer that, scientists experimented on mice. In one study they found the mice lived shorter lives;[36] in another, that they lived longer.[37] And as there are no reliable large studies of GH supplementation for elderly humans, that is where matters currently stand: we cannot say whether *supplementing* with GH is a good idea.

We also know that GH reduces the wear and tear of cartilage in our joints, and in this and other catabolic conditions such as osteoporosis and broken bones (and even with heart attacks) it might well have a short-term place.[38] Many elderly people are immobilised by osteoporosis and broken bones, and using GH to help rebuild them over a six-month period might help. However, there is currently too much doubt over GH to recommend long-term injections for the elderly in the hope that it will improve anabolism and longevity.

Maintaining GH levels naturally

That said, there is nothing wrong with *maintaining* our GH levels naturally as we age. Healthy GH levels will keep our joints, bones and ligaments strong, and allow us to be active well into our eighties and nineties.

The following help to stimulate GH naturally:

- Supplementing daily with glutamine, an amino acid that makes GH.
- Daily exercise, particularly lifting weights or doing squats.[39]

---

36 Vergara, M. et al. 'Hormone-Treated Snell Dwarf Mice Regain Fertility But Remain Long Lived and Disease Resistant.' *J Gerontol A Biol Sci Med Sci* (2004): 59: 1244–50.

37 Panici, J. et al. 'Early Life Growth Hormone Treatment Shortens Longevity and Decreases Cellular Stress Resistance in Long-lived Mutant Mice.' *FASEB J* (2010): 24: 5073–9.

38 Chrisman, O. D. 'The Effect of Growth Hormone on Established Cartilage Lesions. A Presidential Address to the Association of Bone and Joint Surgeons, 1974.' *Clin Orthop Relat Res* (1975): 107: 232–8.

39 Eto, B. et al. 'Glutamate-Arginine Salts and Hormonal Responses to Exercise.' *Arch Physiol Biochem* (1995): 103: 160–4.

- Lowering the intake of glucose, because glucose affects the production of growth hormone and DHEA.[40]
- Intermittent fasting.[41]
- Cutting out alcohol, because alcohol blocks the production of GH.[42]
- Sleeping well, because deep sleep stimulates the production of GH, whereas sleeplessness and stress reduce our GH levels.[43]

The adrenal glands

Your adrenal glands are small: each is about the size of an acorn and they weigh just a few grams, yet their importance far exceeds their modest size. Each sits above a kidney, and it is no great stretch to consider the adrenal glands as your body's 'brain outside its brain'.

Figure 2: The adrenal glands, which sit on top of the kidneys, and which can be thought of as your body's brain outside its brain

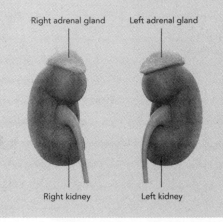

Right adrenal gland   Left adrenal gland

Right kidney   Left kidney

40   Manglik, S. et al. 'Serum Insulin but not Leptin is Associated with Spontaneous and Growth Hormone (GH)-releasing Hormone Stimulated GH Secretion in Volunteers with and without Weight-loss.' *Metabolism* (1998): 47: 1127–33.

41   Denti, L. et al. 'Effects of Aging on Dehydroepiandrosterone Sulfate in Relation to Fasting Insulin Levels and Body Composition Assessed by Bioimpedance Analysis.' *Metabolism* (1997): 1246–51.

42   Xu, X. et al. 'Ethanol Suppresses Growth Hormone-Mediated Cellular Responses in Liver Slices.' *Alcoholism: Clin Exp Res* (1995): 19: 1246–51.

43   Van Cauter, E. et al. 'Age-related Changes in Slow Wave Sleep and REM Sleep and Relationship with Growth Hormone and Cortisol Levels in Healthy Men.' *JAMA* (2000): 284: 861–8.

Testosterone and oestrogen are related to DHEA in that all three are made from cholesterol, which is why they are known as steroid hormones; and although they are produced in different parts of the body, in many ways they begin life in the two adrenal glands.

In fact, the significance of the adrenal glands and the steroid hormones they produce makes this subject far too large for one chapter, which is why the next chapter will look solely at what happens to our adrenals and our health under the stress of our fast-paced modern lifestyle. The two chapters after that will examine testosterone and oestrogen respectively.

THE ROLE OF DHEA

Having looked at GH, it is time now to turn to DHEA, the other key anabolic hormone that this chapter will cover. DHEA, which is made in the adrenal glands and in the brain, was once thought to be a bit of a medical oddity, but some researchers reckon it could be our most important hormone in terms of anabolism, or rebuilding us. It has been studied intensively over the past thirty years and, as we saw earlier, one important result is that a deficiency of DHEA in older people is a strong predictor of mortality. We also know that lower DHEA levels and higher cortisol levels as we age are associated with increased catabolism, a worsened immune system and an increase in arterial blockages.[44]

Not surprisingly, some researchers have theorised that low DHEA is a contributing risk factor to early death. However, although a deficiency in DHEA is *associated* with dying early, it has never been shown to *cause* early mortality; in addition, replacing DHEA has also *not* been shown to make us live longer. That said, supplementing with DHEA has been shown to improve various aspects of our health, including our brain, our risk of having a heart attack or stroke, and our immune system, and we will look at each of those aspects now.

44   Valenti, G. 'Neuroendocrine Hypothesis of Ageing: The Role of Corticoadrenal Steroids.' *J Endocrinol Invest* (2004): 27: 62–3.

DHEA and the brain

The chapter on the brain will go into much more detail on this, but for now it is worth noting two points: firstly, our body's overall health is dependent upon good brain health; secondly, a deficiency of DHEA harms the brain, which is why supplementing with DHEA can improve brain function.

There is plenty of evidence to show a connection between DHEA and depression. For example, we know low levels of DHEA are associated with dysthymia, or 'the blues', in ageing adults, and studies have shown that boosting DHEA in men and women results in an improved feeling of well-being.[45] Another study found that people suffering major depression who supplemented with DHEA significantly improved their mood.[46] And DHEA also improves libido in ageing men.[47] A study of hundreds of post-menopausal women found low DHEA levels were associated with depression.[48]

Finally, a deficiency of DHEA is associated with worsening Alzheimer's disease and brain degeneration, and studies have shown that Alzheimer's patients have only half as much DHEA as non-sufferers of the same age.[49] However, although replacing DHEA does help memory,[50] it has *not* been shown to improve Alzheimer's.

45 Morales, A. J. 'Effects of Replacement Dose of Dehydroepiandrosterone in Men and Women of Advancing Age.' *J Clin Endocrinol Metab* (1994): 1360–7.
Bloch, M. et al. 'Dehydroepiandrosterone Treatment of Midlife Dysthymia.' *Biol Psychiatry* (1999): 45: 1533–41.
46 Wolkowitz, O. M. et al. 'Double-blind Treatment of Major Depression with Dehydroepiandrosterone.' *Am J Psychiatry* (1999): 156 (4): 646–9.
Schmidt, P. et al. 'Dehydroepiandrosterone Monotherapy in Midlife-Onset Major and Minor Depression.' *Arch Gen Psychiatry* (2005): 62: 154–62.
47 Reiter, W. J. et al. 'DHEA in the Treatment of Erectile Dysfunction. A Prospective, Double-blind, Randomized, Placebo Controlled Study.' *Urology* (1999): 53: 590–4.
48 Barrett-Connor, E. et al. 'Endogenous Levels of Dehydroepiandrosterone Sulfate, But Not Other Sex Hormones, are Associated with Depressed Mood in Older Women: the Rancho Bernardo Study.' *J Am Geriatr Soc* (1999): 47: 685–91.
49 Bastianetto, S. et al. 'Dehydroepiandrosterone (DHEA) Protects Hippocampal Cells from Oxidative Stress-induced Damage.' *Mol Brain Res* (1999): 66: 35–41.
50 Alhaj, H. A. et al. 'Effects of DHEA Administration on Episodic Memory, Cortisol and Mood in Healthy Young Men: A Double-blind, Placebo-controlled Study.' *Psychopharmacology* (2006): 188: 541–51.

DHEA and CVD risk

Heart attacks and strokes (cardiovascular diseases, or CVDs) are the leading cause of mortality worldwide[51] and account for one in three deaths, according to a huge 2017 study that examined every country on earth over the past twenty-five years, and whose lead author described CVDs as 'an alarming threat to global health'.

The publication in which the study's findings appeared said what will seem obvious to readers of this book: 'The . . . paradox is that medicine remains very expensive, yet we don't put efforts into promoting health at younger ages, which could be a cost-effective method to preventing the onset of the disease. Instead, we continue to only invest in treating advanced manifestations of cardiovascular disease.'

How does this relate to DHEA? Many studies have shown a link between DHEA deficiency and our risk of suffering a heart attack or a stroke:

- A study of more than 1,700 middle-aged and elderly men with type-2 diabetes who showed low DHEA levels were independently associated with a worsening heart-attack risk.[52]
- Low DHEA levels are associated with worsened arterial blockages in men[53] (although not in women).[54]
- Low DHEA is associated with high LDL cholesterol levels (so-called 'bad cholesterol') and low protective HDL cholesterol levels ('good

51 Roth, G. et al: 'Global and National Cardiovascular Disease Prevalence, Mortality, and Disability-Adjusted Life-Years for 10 Causes, 1990 to 2015.' *J Am Coll Cardiol* (May 2017).

52 Feldman, H. et al. 'Low Dehydroepiandrosterone Sulfate and Heart Disease in Middle-Aged Men: Cross-Sectional Results from the Massachusetts Male Aging Study.' *AEP* (1998): 8217–28.

53 Fukui, M. et al. 'Serum Dehydroepiandrosterone Sulfate Concentration and Carotid Atherosclerosis in Men with Type-2 Diabetes.' *Atherosclerosis* (2005): 181: 339–44.

54 Yoshida, S. et al. 'Dehydroepiandrosterone Sulfate is Inversely Associated with Sex-Dependent Diverse Carotid Atherosclerosis Regardless of Endothelial Function.' *Atherosclerosis* (2010): 212: 310–15.

cholesterol').[55] Supplementing with DHEA reduces bad LDL cholesterol levels.[56]

- In a study of more than 32,000 women, low DHEA was associated with a greater risk of having a stroke.[57]

DHEA and immunity

Researchers have shown that low DHEA has a negative effect on the immune system, and that supplementing with DHEA improves it. For example, elderly people with low DHEA responded worse to the influenza vaccine,[58] while elderly men who supplemented with DHEA significantly boosted their immune system.[59]

DHEA summary

In elderly people, low DHEA is associated with worsening catabolism and an increased risk of death. Supplementing with DHEA improves key factors such as mood, cholesterol levels and the immune system, but it has not been shown to make us live longer. That said, it makes sense to keep DHEA at an optimal level throughout our life, and to pay particular heed to it as we reach old age.

Long before that, though, we need to reduce the stress that damages us in the first place, and we must make sure that our DHEA level stays healthy.

55 Okamoto, K. 'Relationship Between Dehydroepiandrosterone Sulfate and Serum Lipid Levels in Japanese Men.' *J Epidemiol* (1996): 6: 63–7.

56 Nestler, J. et al. 'Dehydroepiandrosterone Reduces Serum Low Density Lipoprotein Levels and Body Fat but Does not Alter Insulin Sensitivity in Normal Men.' *J Clin Endocrinol Metab* (1988): 66: 57–61.

57 Jimenez, M. et al. 'Low Dehydroepiandrosterone Sulphate is Associated with Increased Risk of Ischemic Stroke Among Women.' *Stroke* (2013): 44: https://www.ncbi.nlm.nih.gov/pmc/articles/PMC3811081/

58 Fulop, T. et al. 'Relationship Between the Response to Influenza Vaccination and the Nutritional Status in Institutionalized Elderly Subjects.' *J Gerontol Biol Sci* (1999): 54: M59–64.

59 Khorram, O. et al. 'Activation of Immune Function by Dehydroepiandrosterone (DHEA) in Age-advanced Men.' *J Gerontol A Biol Sci Med Sci* (1997): 52 (1): M1–7.

We can boost our DHEA with moderate exercise – but note the use of the word 'moderate'. Moderate exercise helps the body to rebuild itself, but excessive exercise will exhaust our DHEA supply and eventually drop our DHEA level.

Our lives are not short of stress, and there are plenty of good reasons to control it. Increased stress at work is associated with a shorter life,[60] and we know too much stress damages our brain, our hormones, our arteries and our DNA.[61] Excessive stress is probably the main reason our DHEA levels decline as we age.

To summarise, then, boosting low DHEA will benefit our health, but will *not* reverse the damage that excessive stress has caused – which is the reason why supplementing with DHEA improves our health but does *not* help us to live longer. Achieving that means avoiding excessive stress in the first place or finding something that can reverse stress's negative effects; we will find out more about that in the chapters on adrenal health and the brain.

WORKING OUT YOUR ANABOLIC-CATABOLIC BALANCE

Before I treat someone for a presumed hormonal imbalance I need to know the levels of their anabolic and catabolic hormones. This is easily done: we simply draw blood and send it to a laboratory that measures their DHEA to cortisol level. Why this combination? Because as we move into catabolism due to ageing or ill-health, our DHEA (anabolic hormone) level drops and our cortisol (catabolic hormone) level rises. Knowing the proportion of each tells me what I need to know about rebalancing them, something that is particularly important in middle-age.

60   Goh, J. et al. 'Exposure To Harmful Workplace Practices Could Account For Inequality In Life Spans Across Different Demographic Groups.' *Health Affairs* (2015): 34: 1761–8.
61   Hara, M. R. et al. 'A Stress Response Pathway Regulates DNA Damage Through β 2-Adrenoreceptors and β-Arrestin-1.' *Nature* (2011): 477: 349–53.

By way of an example, let me introduce you to Mike (not his real name). In his twenties, Mike had been so fit and healthy that he had competed in triathlons. But by the time he came to see me in his forties he was living a high-stress, executive life with time mostly for work and a little left over to spend with his wife and children.

Mike had hit the midlife blues, and was concerned about his growing belly and his thinning legs. His blood results showed his DHEA level was way down and his cortisol level was too high. The solution in his case was to supplement with DHEA – that gave him the energy boost he needed to start exercising again, the incentive to eat healthily, and the lift to ensure he spent more quality time with his family.

Six months later, Mike was a changed man: his cortisol levels were lower, his DHEA was higher, and life had become fun again. In short, Mike's adrenals were once again working well, and that meant he could stop supplementing with DHEA.

What does Mike's story tell us? Firstly, that excess stress was largely to blame for his predicament. Indeed, the insidious effect of stress is one of the most common reasons for this imbalance, because initially it causes the levels of *both* DHEA and cortisol to rise. If the stress goes on for months or years then one or both of these hormones starts to wilt. Commonly it is DHEA that drops first, which leaves the person with an imbalance of too much cortisol and too little DHEA. That means the body has more catabolic than anabolic hormones, and this causes it to move to a breakdown state – the skin wrinkles, the muscles get thinner and fat starts to spread.

We can get a good idea of our health simply by seeing whether we are ageing prematurely in our forties, and the DHEA-cortisol test is a simple, cheap and useful measure of how catabolic we are. If our cortisol is high then we know this is contributing to increased catabolism. If it shows DHEA is low then that person is not sending enough anabolic building messages to their body, which also contributes to decline. It is a double whammy. The solution is to support DHEA, reduce stress (because stress makes the body produce more cortisol) and improve liver function – partly because a healthy liver lowers the level of excess evening cortisol. Indeed, a recent study showed that correcting the DHEA-cortisol imbalance in ageing people restored their immunity and reduced all-cause mortality.[62]

Before closing, it is worth making clear that cortisol – although it seems the villain of the piece – is not only a good hormone, it is *essential*. Far worse than excess cortisol is zero cortisol, because without it we would die in hours. Like so much else in life, we need balance. Improving DHEA is only half the battle; we also need to counter stresses, and the earlier we do that, the better. Only then can we expect to enjoy that Younger for Longer life.

CATABOLISM

So much for trying to keep anabolism, or the building-up process, going as we age. The other side of the coin is to try to avoid catabolism – or even to reverse it.

Peter Medawar, the 1960s Nobel Laureate, put it this way: as we age, the damage in our body accumulates at a faster rate. It is not that different from owning an old car: if it already has a problem with the brakes, the headlights and the starter motor, then at any time those problems could play up and, as every year goes by, there is a good chance that a new problem will be added to the list.

The question is, what causes this accumulation of damage? There are two key aspects:

- Free radical damage, which is the harm done by free radicals as they knock around in our cells;
- Glycation, which is the damage done when sugar molecules attach to fat or protein, and which has been linked to an array of age-related diseases.

If we could block these *and* if we could maximise anabolism, then we would be well on our way to slowing the ageing process and living our best possible life. But *can* we block them? Let us start by looking at the first of these.

62   Phillips, A. et al. 'Cortisol, DHEA Sulphate, Their Ratio and All-cause and Cause-specific Mortality in the Vietnam Experience Study.' *Eur J Endocrinol* (2010): 163: 285–92.

Free radical damage

Earlier in the book we encountered a number of theories of ageing, some more plausible than others. Among the most important is the theory that we age because, as our cells go about their business of making and storing energy, the free radicals generated during that process damage them. In the same way that your car needs oxygen (mixed with fuel and a spark) to generate energy, so your cells need oxygen to generate their energy. One of the side effects is that this process releases free radicals, which are atoms or molecules that are missing an unpaired electron on their oxygen element.

Figure 3: The process by which a free radical, which lacks an electron, is put into a stable state by an antioxidant donating one of its electrons

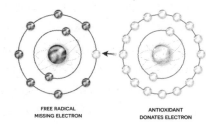

HOW ANTIOXIDANT
WORKS AGAINST FREE RADICALS

FREE RADICAL
MISSING ELECTRON

ANTIOXIDANT
DONATES ELECTRON

Do not worry if you are not of a scientific bent: all you need to know is that this lack of an unpaired electron makes these free radicals highly unstable, and as they bump around in the cells they either gain or lose an electron to other molecules. That process, known as oxidation, means our unstable free radical is now stable, which is good news. However, it had to get that electron from another molecule, which is itself now unstable and a free radical. This can unleash a chain reaction that can damage or even kill the cell.

The exchange of electrons ends only when an antioxidant donates its spare electron to the free radical, and puts the free radical into a stable state. That means no more bumping around inside the cell, and no more damage.

Oxidation – a heavy toll

To save you turning back to the chapter on the theories of ageing, here is a recap of some of what we learned about free radicals and oxidation. Oxidative damage goes on all the time in every cell of our bodies and around us too: you can see it in fruit when a sliced apple turns brown. You can see and feel it when the sun burns your skin. Oxidation causes plastic to become brittle and metal to rust. When we breathe in cigarette smoke, the oxidised metals we inhale are essentially rusting up our lungs, little by little.

Oxidation is responsible for many degenerative diseases, and many of the theories of ageing link to it. For example, the more we heat up our core temperature, the more oxidative damage occurs and the faster we could age. As our steroid hormones start to fail, we tend to accelerate oxidative damage. On the other hand, calorie restriction and intermittent fasting are associated with a reduction in inflammation and oxidative damage.

Inflammation is at the centre of modern illness, and oxidation is at the centre of inflammation: degeneration in the brain is due to inflammation, which is caused by free radical damage; free radicals also cause inflammation to our arteries, leading to diabetes and heart attacks, and inflame our lungs causing diseases such as emphysema. Sunburned skin has been oxidised, and that leaves those cells susceptible to skin cancer.

The heroes in this battle are antioxidants, as they neutralise free radicals and stop them from damaging us further. Glutathione and vitamins C and E are key antioxidants, as are our steroid hormones (DHEA, oestrogen and testosterone). Declining levels of those steroid hormones leave the skin more vulnerable to sun damage, which is one reason people burn more easily when they reach their forties and accumulate wrinkles faster. It is why too much sun at twenty might cause a small amount of redness, but the same exposure at seventy causes painful sunburn.

Indeed, your body has a host of antioxidants that it relies on to tackle free radicals and the damage they do to cell DNA. Among these are vitamins and steroid hormones, and we have also encountered an even more important substance called glutathione that is the cell's natural roaming antioxidant.

Then there is our protective system called superoxide dismutase, or SOD, that is our chief warrior against free radical damage, and which holds huge promise going forward. In the chapter on the theories of ageing I said it was not a good idea to flood the body with antioxidant vitamin supplements, because that might make the SOD system lazy – and this would reduce the body's ability to combat free radicals and therefore result in further damage.

But there are things we can do. Firstly, we know that exercise does a great job at stimulating our SOD system. Secondly, researchers have found that zinc, copper, magnesium and resveratrol (which is found in grape skins) are supplements that help to make SOD. The race is now on to find stimulators that will safely enhance our SOD system, and that should prove far healthier than overloading our body with antioxidants that could switch it off.

It could also provide breakthroughs for any number of inflammation-linked illnesses and conditions. Take the brain, for example, where one of the most exciting breakthroughs has seen psychiatrist Michael Berk show that depression, anxiety and bipolar disease all have their origin in inflammation. Instead of using lithium and other powerful drugs to counter mood swings in patients, Berk has had great success using N-acetylcysteine (NAC), an antioxidant that can cross the blood-brain barrier.[63] NAC has a number of independent functions in the brain and can also make glutathione, which we know is a key natural antioxidant. That means it has the ability to reduce brain inflammation, and it may prove useful in preventing conditions ranging from Alzheimer's to depression.

Regardless of whether we are talking about the brain, the arteries or the skin, free radicals and inflammation damage our bodies on a daily basis. Reducing catabolism relies heavily on making sure our antioxidant systems

63 Berk, M. et al. 'N-acetylcysteine for Depressive Symptoms in Bipolar Disorder. A Randomised Placebo-controlled Trial.' *Biol Psychiatry* (2008): 64, 6: 468–75.

are working as well as possible. To that end we are better off enhancing our body's *existing* antioxidant systems (the SOD system and the glutathione system) than by flooding it with vitamin supplements each day.

Glycation

The second factor that worsens catabolism in the body is glycation. My patients often ask me how this differs from oxidation – after all, both are linked to glucose (which is why sugar is so damaging to us). My answer is that we generate free radicals (which cause oxidation) when we *use glucose* to make energy in the cell; and we cause glycation when we *heat up glucose* in the body.

Glycation – turning up the heat

Glycation happens when we heat sugar in the body. Just as we finish preparing a crème brûlée – which means 'burnt cream' – by taking a blowtorch to the surface of that delicious dessert, so we can brûlée any part of our body if it has too much glucose and over-heats. Other examples of glycation are the browning on a cooked steak or fried onions. In short, glycation is the consequence of adding sugar to protein and turning up the heat.

If you want to see glycation in people, one of the easiest places is around the mouth of an elderly female smoker. As the protective oestrogen declines in menopause, female smokers become suscep-tible to this form of glycation damage. That hardened skin around the mouth is due to glycation, and is caused by the glucose melting itself on to the protein in the skin. The good news is that we can treat this.

One of the best ways to see glycation's damaging effects is by looking at the health effects of diabetes. Diabetics have too much sugar in the blood because they have a reduced ability to remove it, and one of the ways we can measure the damage this does is to look at their red blood cells: these are the oxygen-carriers in the blood, and in the laboratory we can see how sugar-coated, or glycated, they have become.

This measurement is known as the HbA1c level and, as explained in the chapter on inflammation and obesity, this figure *should* be around 5 per cent, which means one in twenty red blood cells are glycated. Small increments of just 0.1 per cent are warning signs, and if your HbA1c level is 5.5 per cent then you ought to cut sugar from your diet. If it is 6.3 per cent you should see your doctor as you might be pre-diabetic.

A diabetic who is not taking insulin might have an HbA1c of 20 per cent, which means one in five of his or her red blood cells are coated with sugar. Glycation causes damage throughout the body, including atherosclerosis, cataracts, kidney damage and strokes. What is happening is simply this: *diabetics are experiencing the same ageing from sugar excess that we all get, just much earlier and much faster.*

Thirty years ago, US researcher Anthony Cerami theorised that glycated proteins accumulate slowly in all of our organs causing gradual damage. He called them 'advanced glycation end-products', or AGEs: proteins that have become sugared, heated and then damaged. Because we have protein through-out the body, this damage can lead to problems of the arteries, brain function, immune system, DNA function, and enzyme and hormone activity.[64] And glycated proteins have been shown to play a key role in the development of cholesterol blockages of the arteries, leading to strokes and heart attacks.[65]

In short, glycation – which is the sugaring of proteins in our bodies – is dangerous and is happening to us all. But what can we do about it? The first step is to measure your HbA1c level, to see how glycated you are. If that level is above 5.0 per cent then you are slowly glycating; if it is above 5.5 per cent then you need to take action; if it is 6.3 per cent or higher you should ask your doctor to test for diabetes. It is also sensible to check your eyesight because worsening vision in your forties could be due to early cataracts, which are likely being accelerated by glycation. Having an eye test will clar-ify that.

64 Cerami, A. et al. 'Glucose and Aging.' *Sci Am* (1987): 256: 90–6.
65 Smith, M. A. et al. 'Advanced Maillard Reaction End Products are Associated with Peroxisome Proliferations.' *Chem Biol Interact* (1999): 1–3: 205–18.

The good news is that we can reverse glycation. How? Most obviously by cutting out sugar in our diet, because, logically enough, if there is no sugar then there can be no glycation. Given sugar's central role in inflammation of the arteries, obesity, diabetes and heart disease, and given that most of us consume far more sugar each day than is healthy, removing it from our diet is a sensible step. And by this I do not mean the sugar we add to our tea or coffee: as we have seen in previous chapters, manufacturers ladle vast quantities of sugar in to processed foods including soft drinks, bread, rolls, cakes, sweets, pasta sauces, biscuits – you name it. It is easy to see how much sugar has been added as nowadays you can just look at the nutritional table on the back of every tin or package.

An excellent second step is to take the correct antioxidants. Why? Because glycation, or sugaring of proteins, in the body is an oxidation reaction, so supplementing with the right antioxidants should help to prevent this. The following are among the most important antioxidants in the battle against glycation:

- Alpha-lipoic acid is the king of antioxidants in this fight. Scientists have shown that if you introduce AGEs (the advanced glycation end-products) to blood vessels, then the levels of vitamin C and glutathione will become depleted, resulting in atherosclerosis. But when alpha-lipoic acid was introduced to these now-damaged arteries, the glutathione and vitamin C levels were completely restored and glycation was halted.[66] (And while we are on the topic of alpha-lipoic acid, a great treatment for a smoker's hardened glycated top lip is – short of a plastic surgeon sanding it off in theatre – a good quality alpha-lipoic acid skin serum. Brands worth considering include RégimA, Environ and Perricone MD. Applying the serum nightly for three months to the top lip often reverses much of the hardening and damage.)
- Flavonoids, which are found in onions and berries, have been shown to reduce the glycation of haemoglobin – the oxygen-carrying

66 Bierhaus, A. et al. 'Advanced Glycation End Product-Induced activation of NF Kappa B is Suppressed by Alpha-lipoic Acid in Cultured Endothelial Cells.' *Diabetes* (1997): 47: 1481–90.

element in red blood cells – and therefore help to reduce the damage done by diabetes.[67]

• Once again we meet our old friend N-acetylcysteine (NAC). NAC helps to make glutathione in the body (as does alpha-lipoic acid) and, as we noted earlier, glutathione is essential when balancing sugar control in arteries. NAC has been shown to reduce insulin resistance in women with polycystic diabetic changes; it had a similar effect in tests on rats.[68]

• Green tea contains antioxidants and has been shown to improve sugar metabolism. It is therefore recommended for anyone who wants to improve their sugar metabolism and reduce glycation damage.[69]

The third step in the battle against glycation is to avoid eating burned food. Anything that is charred is full of glycated proteins, and eating these has been proven to accelerate ageing.[70] To put it another way: do not fry onions until they are dark brown; do make sure your fillet steak is rare; and do ask the chef only to sear your tuna. When it comes to cooking at home, grilling is better than frying, but if you have to fry then use an oil with a high smoke-point. Seed oils (such as sunflower oil and canola oil) are highly sensitive to heat damage and, when fried, release aldehydes, which are toxic. So do not use seed oils to cook.[71]

The fourth step is, as always, daily exercise, and this remains the one thing nearly everyone should do more of. It does not need to be three hours of

67 Asgary, S. et al. 'Antioxidant Effects of Flavonoids on Haemoglobin Glycosylation.' *Pharm Acta Helv* (1999): 73: 223–6.

68 Song, D. et al. 'Chronic N-acetylcysteine Prevents Fructose-induced Insulin Resistance and Hypertension in Rats.' *Eur J Pharmacol* (2005): 508: 205–10.

69 Masha, A. et al. 'Prolonged Treatment with N-acetylcysteine and L-arginine Restores Gonadal Function in Patients with PCO Syndrome.' *J Endocrinol Invest* (2009).
Nakagawa, T. et al. 'Protective Activity of Green Tea Against Free Radical and Glucose Mediated Protein Damage.' *J Agric Food Chem* (2002): 50: 2418–22.

70 Koschinsky, T. et al. 'Orally-absorbed Reactive Glycation Products (Glycotoxins): An Environmental Risk Factor in Diabetic Nephropathy.' *Proc Natl Acad Sci USA* (1997): 94: 6474–9.

71 Halvorsen, B. L. et al. 'Determination of Lipid Oxidation Products in Vegetable Oils and Marine Omega-3 Supplements.' *Food Nutr Res* (2011): 55.

punishing cross-trainer work; a thirty-minute gentle session in the gym or a daily one-hour walk if you are older makes a big difference. A regular exercise routine stimulates your anabolic hormones, raises your metabolism, uses up excess sugar from those biscuits that you had with your coffee and, in animal studies at least, has been shown to speed up the body's ability to reduce glycation.[72] The chances are that it does the same for humans.

CHANGING CATABOLISM TO ANABOLISM

As a child growing up in Cape Town, I remember how some of the dads would scoff at applying sunblock when sitting at the beach or working shirtless in the garden. For years this near-heroic 'no sunblock' approach appeared to cause few problems but, as we know, oxidation damages the skin. Sure enough, by the time they reached sixty – which is not old – the consequences of this carefree attitude caught up with them: sagging skin, and not much they could do to reverse it.

Of course we cannot stop ageing, and it would be arrogant to think we could. But we can prevent *premature* damage and at the same time give ourselves a chance at living the best life possible. I am convinced that if we could see how our shortfalls today would play out in the long run, we would be inspired to put in more effort. As one of my favourite phrases goes: 'If I'd known I was going to live this long, I'd have taken better care of myself.'

'Taking better care' involves less catabolism and more anabolism, and there is a lot we can do on both counts: two of the most effective anti-ageing measures are engaging in daily exercise and cutting out sugars. And, because we know chronic stress is one of our Three Horsemen, and we know that it drains our anabolic hormones – particularly our DHEA – rebalancing our anabolic-catabolic balance is key to getting us off the couch.

Failing to do so marks the beginning of the end: the lack of exercise further depletes the anabolic hormones, the muscles start to atrophy, the foggy thinking worsens, the abdominal fat and sagging skin accumulate and the person is

72   Boor, P. et al. 'Regular Moderate Exercise Reduces Advanced Glycation and Ameliorates Early Diabetic Nephropathy in Obese Zucker Rats.' *Metabolism* (2009): 58: 1669–77.

well on their way to being wheeled out of this world. By the time someone becomes a middle-aged couch potato, simply telling them to 'get out there and do some exercise' will not help, because they no longer have the hormones to carry them from the couch to the treadmill.

In my clinic, this is the moment many of my clients walk through the door. The list of issues is largely the same: they feel tired, life seems dull and flat, the sky is grey, their partner complains that they are increasingly irritable, and they lack the energy to exercise. In most cases the solution lies in rebalancing their anabolic and catabolic hormones – raising the levels of the former and going to war on the latter.

Once that is done, their brain finds its 'get-up-and-go' and my patients are able to make those vital lifestyle changes: exercising more and reducing stress. Those people who are successful at this in middle-age have every reason to be confident that they will, when elderly, have naturally good DHEA levels and optimal health. Bluntly put, those who continue with their stressful, low-exercise lifestyle will probably not.

Then again, we have known the importance of exercise for millennia as Plato's quote at the top of this chapter shows. And not only is it possible to change; it is vital, and anyone doing so will reap profound rewards. As one of my patients told me: 'It feels as though I've been given a second chance at youth, and this time I'm not going to waste it.'

Increasing irritability

People commonly get grumpier as they get older, and in many cases that is because their DHEA level is dropping: increased irritability and decreased ability to cope with change are indicators of low DHEA. Worse, this irritability often causes adrenalin to rise, which results in a spike in cortisol during the second half of the day, and this raised cortisol level is why the elderly often struggle to sleep.

Fortunately there are some excellent natural remedies that can help:

- To reduce stress: 5-HTP, a chemical compound that makes serotonin; sceletium, a southern African herb; saffron; camomile; rhodiola, also known as golden root or rose root; and vitamin B3.
- To support the adrenals: panax ginseng, also known as true ginseng; ashwagandha, which is an Indian herb; rhodiola; Cordyceps mycelium; vitamins B5, B6 and B12; and biotin.
- To reduce excessive evening cortisol levels: glutathione; N-acetylcysteine (NAC); phosphatidyl serine; vitamins B5, B6 and B12; and folate, which is found in spinach, broccoli and chicken liver.

ANABOLIC VERSUS CATABOLIC HORMONES: A FINAL WORD

Our body's workings are amazingly intricate, and our hormones are powerful chemicals. In this chapter we have seen that nature's design is for our anabolic hormones to start fading in our twenties as we begin the long decline into catabolism.

The key to a Younger for Longer life is boosting anabolism and reducing catabolism, but healthy ageing is not about taking lashings of anabolic hormones. Instead, our hormones work like an orchestra, and we will see time and again in the coming chapters how this hormone balance is essential to health. Once we get that balance right, energy and health should return.

One of the best predictors of successful ageing in the elderly is their ability to maintain muscle mass. Another key predictor is maintaining healthy levels of our anabolic hormone DHEA, because low DHEA levels are a sign of ageing and stress. And although growth hormone is an amazingly effective anabolic hormone, supplementing with it is not recommended because it might have the effect of lighting us up and then burning us out.

The two biggest markers of ageing are probably oxidative damage and glycation. It is far better to enhance our body's SOD antioxidant system to deal with oxidation than it is to take lots of vitamins; hormones such as DHEA also have a powerful antioxidant function, but their levels deplete as we age, exposing us more to this damage.

Glycation, which is the sugaring of proteins, is most obvious in diabetics but it affects us all and damages our arteries, brain, kidneys, eyes and skin. The most effective way to reduce glycation is to cut out sugar from our diet, but daily exercise helps too. When it comes to combating glycation, alpha-lipoic acid is the king of supplements.

Finally, once our cortisol level is higher than our DHEA level, we are moving down the slippery slope of ageing: worsening wrinkles, thinning muscle and spreading fat, to name but a few consequences. Reversing that hormone imbalance fixes this problem.

Key points
- The way to ensure an optimal Healthspan is to increase anabolism and decrease catabolism. That means maximising the activities that build us up and minimising those that break us down.
- Ageing well requires a good DHEA-cortisol balance, which means naturally high levels of DHEA and naturally low levels of cortisol.

Increase anabolism
- Exercise daily, because this tells our body to keep rebuilding bone and muscle.
- Optimise the anabolic hormones (testosterone and oestrogen), because they build us up.
- DHEA is our most reliable hormone when it comes to longevity; the longer we can maintain good DHEA levels, the longer we will stay healthy.
- Consume essential amino acids, particularly BCAAs (branch-chain amino acids) and glutamine, which is the king of amino acids and which is found in red meat and can be bought as a supplement. This ensures that we are giving our body the protein it needs to rebuild as we age.

Decrease catabolism

- Reduce stress. Doing that lowers the amount of cortisol (the stress hormone) that we produce, and less cortisol means less of our muscle mass will be converted to fat.
- Ensure the liver is functioning well, because this organ removes excess cortisol from the body.
- Enhance our internal antioxidant system to reduce the damage done by free radicals.
- Cut the amount of sugars and carbohydrates that we eat, because this will reduce the damaging effects of glycation.

Chapter 7

STRESS – THE THIRD HORSEMAN

Reality is the leading cause of stress amongst those in touch with it.

Lily Tomlin

Earlier in the book, I introduced my Three Horsemen of the Health-pocalypse, those big-ticket issues that cause us to live unhealthier and unhappier lives than our parents' generation. Two of the three were sugar and toxins, both of which we have covered. It is time to look at the Third Horseman: stress.

Most people know two things about stress: it is bad for us, and our fast-paced, modern lifestyle subjects us to too much of it.

Both are true, and the fixation of modern news and its extensive reach hardly helps. Despite plummeting levels of violent crime in the UK, for example – it is down two-thirds since the 1990s – the impression I get when I visit is that people believe it is worse than ever.[1]

Across the pond, half of the respondents in the American Psychological Association's annual survey say violence and crime is a big stress; even more worry about politics, work and finance. But the number-one issue, cited by nearly two-thirds of people, is the future of the country. More Americans today fear an attack on the nation than ever before.

Add to that the stresses of family, mortgage payments, health issues, commuting . . . the list goes on. Our lives today are full of stresses, some more obvious than others. Their debilitating aspects were apparent decades ago to

---

1 Flatley, J. 'The nature of violent crime in England and Wales: year ending March 2017.' The Office of National Statistics.

the late Hans Selye, a Canadian-Hungarian endocrinologist (which is medi-cal-speak for a hormone specialist) and Nobel Prize nominee, and a pioneer of stress-related research. He made an immense contribution to our understand-ing of stress hormones and the insidious effects of stress.

'Every stress leaves an indelible scar,' he wrote, 'and the organism pays for its survival after a stressful situation by becoming a little older.'

Stress is a silent killer, and a key part of its menace is that there are no warning signs like a headache or joint pain or a skin rash to show that our stress levels are dangerously high. We now know that stress leads to all the modern headline killers – heart attacks, strokes, cancer and diabetes. It also causes a weakened immune system.[2]

All of which is odd in a way, because our stress response is a safety mech-anism designed to *help* us – in its case, to escape danger. However, as we know, the modern world subjects us to too much of it, and I am sure Selye would not have been surprised to hear that I regularly see patients in their thirties who are exhausted, mysteriously putting on weight or repeatedly fall-ing ill. Invariably they have a stressful life, inevitably they struggle to get a good night's sleep, and without fail their blood results show their adrenal hormones are either revving high or have slumped.

In short, their body has exceeded its ability to keep them healthy.

What they need to do is to learn to pace themselves, to manage their stress, and to focus on sleeping better. But that is easier said than done, even though managing stress turns out to be one of the most important tasks to master in life. In our twenties we typically believe we are indestructible and burn the candle at both ends, but in later years we learn that is not true, and that working and play-ing too hard does hurt. Most of the successful professionals I know understand this, and they long ago learned how to pace themselves. It is this that has allowed them to stay successful. Those who disregard their health by putting the company, the children or the world first tend in the end to pay for it.

I would say that it is not selfish to look after yourself; indeed, it is essential if you want to help yourself and others. And although it is not the easiest of

2   Salleh, R. M. 'Life event, stress and illness.' *Malays J Med Sci* (2008): 15: 9–18.

tasks, the good news is that it is possible and that if we can get this right then we can expect to live a healthy life. If not our health will worsen. Why is that? We are about to find out.

> ### Sleep and stress
>
> The chapters on brain health will tell us much more about sleep, which – although still something of a mysterious process – is the cornerstone of good health. In many ways that is because sleep is the cornerstone of our *adrenal* health, and adrenal health is what this chapter is about.
>
> When we sleep, we manufacture cortisol, and it is this hormone that energises us during the day. We will see that restoring the body's natural circadian rhythm – sleeping well at night and being energised during the day – is central to optimising our adrenal health.

THE ADRENALS — THE LITTLE ENGINES WITH A BIG HEART

One giveaway sign of an excessively stressful life is that your levels of adrenal hormones are either too high or too low. The adrenal hormones are released, logically enough, by the adrenal glands, whose importance has long been understood in Chinese and Ayurvedic medicine. The former recognises the kidneys, on which the adrenals sit, as being the source of our life energy, or *jing*, and holds that we wither once our *jing* burns out. Ayurvedic medicine describes this energy as *prana*, and ranks it as important as oxygen; it focuses on quieting the mind with meditation, and supporting the adrenals with herbs such as ashwagandha.

Neither is that far off. I consider the adrenals as your body's brain outside its brain, and I regard these walnut-sized glands, which tip the scales at just a few grams, as the commander-in-chief of your body's hormones: they coordinate with the ovaries in women, the testes in men, the thyroid and the pancreas in both, and they are responsible for putting you on alert every time there is a suggestion of danger. If your adrenals were in the army, they would be Napoleon.

Most readers will be familiar with the description of adrenalin, one of the hormones produced by the adrenals, as the 'fight or flight' hormone. It is worth understanding what happens in our body to produce adrenalin. That process starts in the brain. The trigger, of course, is getting a fright: we encounter a situation that we assume is dangerous, and the brain sends a message directly to the adrenals, which release adrenalin. That wires us for action, giving us the heightened physical and mental alertness needed to make split-second decisions about whether to stand our ground or to run.

Animals display the same response to danger, but interestingly they are much better at dealing with it than we are, as primatologist and neurology professor Robert Sapolsky shows in his excellent book *Why Zebras Don't Get Ulcers*.[3] When a pride of lions chases zebras, Sapolsky writes, the herd's bodies flood with adrenalin to give them the best chance of galloping to safety. Once the pride has brought down one unfortunate zebra, the rest quickly settle to such a relaxed state that they can start grazing again and get on with life. We humans are unable to do that, and can remain on an adrenalin high for hours, days or even weeks. When it comes to dealing with stress, zebras are a long way ahead of us.

In the later chapter on the brain we will see how depression encourages us to push this adrenalin button to cheer ourselves up. But in this chapter we are going to find out just how damaging the effects of adrenalin can be, and how that holds true for another hormone released by the adrenal glands during times of stress: cortisol. This chapter will focus on both of these hormones and how they affect our health when our body is under stress.

Year by year, researchers are finding more evidence that stress is our biggest killer. Remember that we saw in the chapter on inflammation that the

3 Sapolsky, R. M. *Why Zebras Don't Get Ulcers: An Updated Guide to Stress, Stress-Related Diseases and Coping.* W. H. Freeman (1994).

killers in the developed world are no longer war, plague, malaria and water-borne diseases, but the chronic illnesses associated with unhealthy ageing: heart attacks, strokes and cancer. Research shows that stress is not only one of the most significant triggers of these diseases, but that *de-stressing* could be the single most significant thing we can do to ensure a healthy life.

But before we examine the stress hormones and how they operate, it is worth understanding just what happens to us when we produce too much or too little of these stress hormones. Not for the last time we will see that balance is key to a Younger for Longer life.

Adrenalin: in 2011 researchers showed that the effects of too much adrenalin range from turning our hair white to stimulating cancer. This happens because continuous adrenalin production activates two troublesome pathways in cells, and these pathways not only damage our DNA, they also block the essential (and boringly named) 'p53 system', which involves a gene that is best imagined as having a dual role as both medic and assassin. Without getting too technical, the p53 gene responds to stress by either repairing damaged DNA or, if that DNA cannot be fixed, killing the cell so that it does not become cancerous.[4] It is a phenomenal system, just as long as it keeps working properly. But if the p53 gene fails to repair or kill a damaged cell, then that cell can become overactive and can then transform into a cancer cell. In the less serious case of your hair colour, adrenalin's ability to prevent the p53 gene from fixing what has gone wrong means the pigment cells in your hair follicles die, and it is this that turns your hair white.[5] It is common knowledge that stressful events can turn our hair white, and now we know why. The key point is that stress prematurely ages us in part because too much adrenalin damages our DNA.

Excess cortisol: we will see later that too much stress can cause us to produce too much or too little cortisol. That is important because this hormone is vital in supporting our immune system and in combating inflammation in the

---

4   Lowe, S. et al. 'Control of Apoptosis by p53.' *Oncogene* (2003): 22: 9030–40.
5   Makoto, R. et al. 'A Stress Response Pathway Regulates DNA Damage Through B2-adrenoreceptors and B-arrestin.' *Nature* (online): 21 August 2011.

body. A 2008 study linked excessive cortisol with obesity and diabetes, even in teenagers.[6]

Insufficient cortisol: producing too little cortisol leads to weakened immunity and inflammation. A 2002 study showed that people with early rheumatoid arthritis had low levels of cortisol in their blood and had developed inflammation markers.[7] These markers can be detected with a simple blood test and they tell us that the body's white blood cells are starting to attack our joints, which causes redness, warmth or swelling.

In other words, we know that stress and excess adrenalin can damage our DNA, that stress and excess cortisol can cause obesity and worsen our diabetes risk, and that stress and insufficient cortisol cause inflammation. Simply put, *stress is associated with most of the modern chronic illnesses that damage our health and kill us*. And that is why we are devoting an entire chapter to it.

THE STRESS HORMONES

Our two key stress hormones, then, are adrenalin and cortisol, and both are produced in the adrenals. An easy way to check if you are running on stress is to consider this point: if you need coffee to get going in the morning and alcohol to wind down every night, then the answer is that you probably are.

Plenty of people do that, of course, and they seem to get by just fine, so why does it matter? Let us start with cortisol: this has a key role as our wake-up hormone, and if we burn up our stores of cortisol with too much stress then we will wake up each morning with too little of it, and we will feel exhausted. Instinctively many of us turn to the coffee machine for our caffeine hit (which you can think of as adrenalin in a cup) to get us going, and that works. For the rest of the day we run on stress and adrenalin. Unfortunately that means by the time we are ready for bed, our brain is still buzzing, so we cannot sleep.

6   Misra, M. et al. 'Higher Cortisol Associated with Greater Visceral Adiposity.' *Am J Physiol Endocrinol Metab* (2008): 295 (2).
7   Straub, R. et al. 'Inadequately Low Serum Levels of Steroid Hormones in Relation to IL6 and Tumour Necrosis Factor in Untreated Patients with Early Rheumatoid Arthritis.' *Arthritis Rheum* (2002): 654–62.

Instinctively we turn to the wine bottle knowing it will calm our busy brain and help us nod off.

Why is this coffee-alcohol routine so bad? Because running your life in a constant state of alert causes the overstimulated brain to send messages to the adrenals to act, and over time that can wear them down. Think of it in terms of your car: if you were to drive it by alternately switching between accelerating hard and jamming on the brakes, over and over and over again, it would eventually break down. That is what many of us are doing to our bodies every day.

It is unhealthy, and to better understand why we will look at how our adrenalin response is *meant* to work: every time you get a fright, the brain uses one or both of two systems to send the fight or flight message to the adrenals – the sympathetic nervous system and something called the ACTH stress hormone system.

This message sent from the brain triggers the adrenal glands to release an army of hormones: the two most important are cortisol (which is triggered by the ACTH system) and adrenalin (triggered by the sympathetic nervous system). Each has a number of things to do:

- Adrenalin instantly tells the body to release glucose into the bloodstream to provide the energy to escape, and it speeds up the heart-rate to boost our body's engine to get us away from the danger.

- Cortisol takes a little longer to kick in. It stimulates the brain, allowing us to think more clearly; it acts as an anti-inflammatory so that we do not feel any aches and pains should we need to fight our way out; and it releases glucose (but more slowly than adrenalin does) by squeezing it out of the liver, and then later by telling the muscles to convert protein into glucose.[8] Later we shall see how this final function – turning protein from the muscles into glucose – explains why producing too much cortisol has serious health consequences.

8 Khani, S. et al. 'Cortisol Increases Glucose-Genesis in Humans: Its Role in the Metabolic Syndrome.' *Clinical Sciences* (2001): 101: 739–47.

That, then, is the first part of the stress response – to provide the energy the body needs either to fight back or to run away, and to power the engine that needs to do that work. The second part requires the body to respond to any damage, and for this you could consider our adrenal hormones as the fire brigade – they scramble in response to the adrenalin alarm and for the next hour or two they rush around the body giving messages to its cells to repair whatever got damaged. One of these hormones is cortisol; the other two, for the record, are DHEA and aldosterone, and we will get to them later.

And *this* is why living a modern, stressed lifestyle is so damaging. Being in a constant state of hyper-vigilant stress means we produce firefighters all the time, and that has an effect. Just what effect depends on whether you were born with robust adrenals (a strong set of firefighters) or with weak adrenals.

People with robust adrenals respond to chronic stress – by which we mean 'long-term stress' – by secreting far too much of these firefighting hormones. That imbalance has consequences. Take cortisol, for example, one of whose functions is to tell the body to produce more glucose (see the box on page 224 for more details). This gives people with robust adrenals extra energy through-out the day, and allows them to complete Herculean amounts of work without getting sick or even needing much sleep. If it all sounds too good to be true, it is: the sinister side-effect is that this excess of glucose means they put on weight and are at risk of heart attacks and related problems. In my clinic, these are typically larger-than-life business people, big-bellied, full of confidence and unaware of the damage they are doing.

People with weak adrenals, on the other hand, eventually run out of one or more of these firefighting hormones, of which the most important is cortisol. Most mornings they wake up with a bit of energy (because we replenish our stores of cortisol when we sleep), but well before midday they feel tired and hungry because their cortisol stores are empty, which means there is no more cortisol telling their liver to release glucose. On top of that they lack the bene-fit of cortisol's anti-inflammatory properties, and that means they have a higher risk of inflammatory illnesses including sinusitis, hay fever, aches, arthritis and eczema.

Cortisol and the immune system

- It used to be thought, incorrectly, that cortisol suppresses the immune system; in fact it plays a vital role in boosting it. Studies have shown that in conditions of short-term high stress, cortisol can stimulate immune cells to go to a specific area and get to work;[9] even in conditions of long-term stress it has the ability to balance the immune response.
- That said, ongoing massive stress over a long period can exhaust numerous other hormones in the brain and the body, resulting in a higher risk of cancer. This is because chronic stress *plus* depression can combine to suppress the immune system, and this is due to a complicated interaction of serotonin, dopamine, acetylcholine (a neurotransmitter), growth hormone, prolactin, cortisol, DHEA and progesterone.[10] In other words, it is stress, with its effect on our hormones and neurotransmitters, that damages our immune system.
- Supporting the adrenal glands with small amounts of cortisol (as we will see later in this chapter) does *not* suppress the immune system and does not leave the patient more susceptible to coughs and colds – quite the opposite. In fact, doing this has an immune-boosting effect and helps people whose adrenals are not working as well as they should to beat a cycle of recurrent colds and inflammatory illnesses.

Adrenal strain is also called adrenal fatigue or, more properly, adrenal insufficiency. Whatever we call it, if we want to move beyond treating illness and focus on optimising our health then we have to deal with stress.

The sensible place to start is by measuring the levels of our hormones,

9 Dhabhar, F. S. et al. 'Acute Stress Enhances While Chronic Stress Suppresses Cell-Mediated Immunity In Vivo: A Potential Role for Leukocyte Trafficking.' *Brain Behav Immun* (1997): 11 (4): 286–306.
10 Reiche, E. M. V. et al. 'Stress, Depression, the Immune System and Cancer.' *Lancet Oncol* (2004): 5: 617–25.

including cortisol, and to do that we need to understand the adrenal glands better. That means it is time we met the person who pipped Hans Selye to the Nobel Prize in Medicine in 1950. His name was Philip Hench, and he shared it with two others for their work on, coincidentally enough, adrenal research.

Cushing's and Addison's

Two conditions that are linked to ultra-high or ultra-low cortisol levels are Cushing's disease and Addison's disease respectively. Both are rare, and both need to be treated by an endocrinologist.

Cushing's disease is found in people who have extremely high levels of cortisol, which results in scrawny legs and a big belly. Why? Because cortisol takes protein from the muscles to convert into glucose in the liver. Someone with Addison's disease, on the other hand, would have permanent exhaustion and a very poor immune system due to their abnormally low cortisol levels.

When I talk about excess or insufficient cortisol, I am not referring to those diseases. Instead I am looking at the average person whose lifestyle sees their adrenals constantly punished by ongoing, high-level stress. The adrenal strain that results – whether the adrenals push out too much hormone or too little – is not in itself an illness but it can lead to illness.

Compound E

In the 1930s and 1940s researchers were looking at the effects of chemical substances on the body, including understanding why adding stress hormones helped the performance of fighter pilots. That is where this story begins.

The research on stress hormones came about because the US military was trying to find ways to give fighter pilots an edge. Pilots' bodies undergo huge stresses, and the military reckoned that if it could work out which hormones helped them perform better under stress, it could synthesise that hormone to ensure a combat advantage.

It was while assessing pilots' stress reactions that scientists discovered a substance they christened Compound E, which was released by the adrenal glands. They noticed that the level of Compound E surged during the life-and-death battles of fighter pilots.

Compound E was later renamed cortisol and, because it was identified during the stressful conditions of flying fighter planes, the scientists assumed that this was *the* stress hormone. By the 1940s the Mayo Clinic was working to make an injectable form of adrenal cortex hormone for pilots in an effort to help them reach 45,000 feet without passing out. Rumour had it that Germany's Luftwaffe pilots were able to fly to these altitudes thanks to injections of adrenal extract, and US researchers believed adrenal cortex hormones would help keep a pilot's blood pressure high enough to stay conscious at extreme altitudes.

It took several more years before the researchers concluded that more than one hormone was present in a stress response. They worked out what we now know: that adrenalin is the stress hormone that helps a pilot's reaction time, and that after the adrenalin rush of battle, cortisol works as an anti-inflammatory to heal and reduce the pain of injury. (By then cortisol, not adrenalin, had earned the moniker 'stress hormone' and it has been unfairly tagged with that label ever since.)[11]

Prior to this work on adrenal hormones it was believed that rheumatoid arthritis, which we now know is an inflammatory condition, was an infection of the joints and was untreatable. That changed when two researchers at the Mayo Clinic presented papers suggesting that rheumatoid arthritis could be treated – not with an antibiotic, but with this strange substance produced by the adrenals called cortisol.[12]

It soon became apparent that cortisol was far more important than scientists had first thought: indeed, it was a wonder drug. Patients who were previously bedridden with arthritis could get up and walk. Those with asthma could breathe freely. Cortisol was lauded as the most significant discovery since

11 Jefferies, W. M. *Safe Uses of Cortisol*. Charles C. Thomas Pub Ltd, 3rd Ed (2004), pp. 3–9.
12 Hench, P. S. et al. 'The Effect of a Hormone of the Adrenal Cortex on Rheumatoid Arthritis.' Preliminary Report. Proc Staff Meet, Mayo Clinic (1949): 24: 181–97.

penicillin, and in 1950 the researchers – Hench, Edward Kendall and Polish-Swiss chemist Tadeusz Reichstein – were awarded the Nobel Prize for their work on cortisol and its application to rheumatoid arthritis. Selye missed out.

As it turned out those heady days of a miracle substance were drawing to an end. Reports started to pour in that high doses of cortisol caused serious side effects: swollen faces, weight gain, weakened bones, thinning skin, stomach ulcers, lowered immunity and cataracts. The wonder drug looked to have a dangerous underbelly, and by 1953 it was over: research was halted and cortisol was deemed to be a bad hormonal tablet that should be locked away and forgotten.[13]

But some scientists pressed on convinced that cortisol was misunderstood, and for forty years they tried to show that although cortisol was dangerous at high doses, low doses made it not only useful but essential for the many people with a mild cortisol deficiency.[14] Despite an array of studies in peer-reviewed medical journals backing up that view, other laboratories focused on the unacceptable side effects of high-dose synthetic cortisol. In the end, the naysayers won the day, which is why the medical community's largely negative view of cortisol persisted for so many years.

The cortisol studies

Once again, then, the secrets to good health and long life come down to balance. The truth about cortisol is that it will cause certain problems if it is too high, and it will cause others if it is too low. Plenty of reliable studies show what an *excess* of cortisol will do:

- A UK study on 3,000 patients showed chronic stress can increase cortisol levels and worsen depression.[15]
- A 2005 study showed excessive cortisol in humans causes nerve damage to the brain.[16]

13 Jefferies, W. M. *Safe Uses of Cortisol*. Charles C. Thomas Pub Ltd, 3rd Ed (2004), pp. 3–9.
14 Jefferies, W. M. 'Low-Dosage Glucocorticoid Therapy.' *Arch Intern Med* (1967): 119: 265–78.
15 Steptoe, A, et al. 'Depression and Elevated Cortisol.' *Am J Epidemiol* (2008): 167 (1): 96–102.
16 Lupien, S. et al. 'The Douglas Hospital Longitudinal Study of Normal and Pathological Ageing.' *J Psych of Neuroscience* (2005): 30: 328–34.

- Studies in rats have shown that exposing the brain to high cortisol levels over an extended period causes nerve endings in the brain to break down.[17]

These three studies looked at the problems associated with elevated cortisol levels in the brain, and their conclusions are as we would expect. After all, we know from the previous chapter that cortisol is a catabolic hormone, and that high levels of it will therefore cause catabolism – a breakdown of brain, bone and muscle.

On the other hand, a *deficiency* of cortisol causes a different set of problems, as the following studies showed:

- Asthma is a disease caused by inflammation, and babies with low levels of salivary cortisol tend to develop asthma and allergy as children.[18]
- Rheumatoid arthritis is another disease caused by inflammation, which is associated with low cortisol levels. This lack of cortisol leads to inflammation of the joints and an upset immune system, which can cause the body's immune system to misguidedly attack the joints.[19]
- A study of chronic fatigue patients showed they had *lower* salivary cortisol levels compared to patients who were depressed and compared to non-patients.[20]

In other words, if our cortisol levels are too low or too high we need to do something about it. Cortisol is a vital hormone: too much risks one set of problems linked to the breakdown of muscles or nerves or bones; too little risks another set based around inflammation and fatigue.

---

17 Swaab, D. F. et al. 'Elevated Cortisol in Rats Induces Neuronal Damage.' *Ageing Res Rev* (2005): 4 (2): 141–94.

18 Stenius, F. et al. 'Salivary Cortisol Levels and Allergy in Children: the ALADDIN Birth Cohort.' *J Clin Immune* (2011).

19 Hedman, M. et al. 'Low Blood and Synovial Fluid Levels of Conjugated Steroids in Rheumatoid Arthritis.' *Clin Exp Rheumatol* (1992) 10: 25–30.

20 Strickland, P. et al. 'A Comparison of Salivary Cortisol in Chronic Fatigue Syndrome, Community Depression and Healthy Controls.' *Journal of Affective Disorders* (1998): 47: 191–4.

In people with strong adrenal glands, elevated stress causes a high cortisol level which results in weight gain. In people with weak adrenal glands, elevated stress results in too little cortisol, which causes inflammatory problems.

The two faces of cortisol

We have grown up mistakenly believing that cortisol is *the* stress hormone and that it makes us fat. But in this chapter we have seen that, like other hormones, cortisol has two faces: one that reveals itself at low levels and another at high levels.

We know that people under stress divide into two groups: those who quickly run out of cortisol and become fatigued and sickly (they have weak adrenals), and others who produce too much cortisol, do not need to sleep much and put on weight (strong adrenals).

How do you know which you are? Short of doing medical tests, you can ask yourself a simple question: 'When I am stressed for a period of time, even though I eat the same amount of food, do I put on weight or do I lose weight?' If you put on weight with stress then you probably secrete too much cortisol. If you lose weight with stress, and perhaps get a sore throat or spastic colon, then you probably do not produce enough cortisol. Later we will see that a saliva test gives a reliable result.

THE TWO THEORIES OF STRESS RESPONSE

Let us delve more deeply into the stress triggers and look at a couple of theories to find out how scientists think this process works. Because we are talking about the fight or flight response, we will put one of our ancestors into the stressful situation of running into a lion.

The *traditional* stress response theory tells us that our hairy relative would get a fright, which is what we doctors call an acute stress reaction. Figure 1 shows how the brain sends a message along the sympathetic nerves to the middle (medulla) of the adrenal gland, which near-instantly releases adrenalin. Our ancestor's body goes into full alert, his or her muscles work quicker, any pain is dimmed, and glucose pours into the bloodstream. They are in fight or flight mode and ready for action.

That differs from ongoing stress, which we call chronic stress and which is something we city-dwelling types deal with all the time. This is the key difference between the two theories: traditional stress response theory tells us that chronic stress does *not* cause an adrenalin spike. Instead, in this situation the brain sends a message ordering the hypothalamus, a part of the brain that produces a number of hormones, to get to work. As Figure 1 shows, the brain releases ACTH, which flows to the adrenal glands, which release cortisol (and several other hormones) from the edge (or the cortex) of the adrenal glands.

Figure 1: Traditional stress response theory

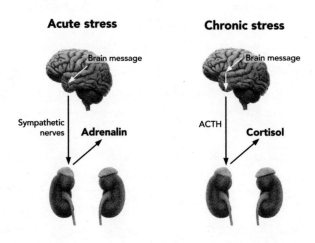

At the risk of hammering home the point, this fifty-year-old theory tells us that a situation of acute stress (encountering a hungry lion) causes us to produce an excess of *adrenalin* to prepare for fight or flight, whereas the chronic stresses of modern living mean we produce too much *cortisol* – and that, therefore, if we want to prevent the ravages of chronic stress then we must reduce the cortisol load on the body.[21] So far, so good,

21 Dunkelmann, S. S. et al. 'Cortisol Metabolism in Obesity.' *J Clin Endocrinol Metab* (1964): 24: 832–41.

except – like all good theories – this one has seen an important update, as Figure 2 shows.

Figure 2: Modern stress response theory

Acute and chronic stress

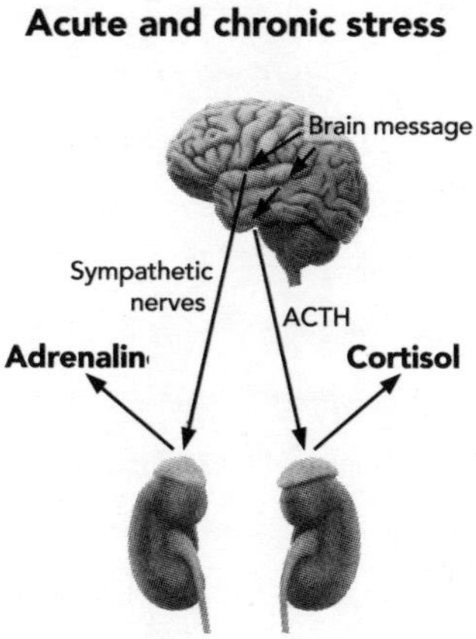

The modern stress response theory shows that in *any* stress response, whether acute or chronic, the adrenal glands will always release *adrenalin* AND *cortisol*. That might not sound like a big deal, but it is an important qualification and it makes more sense, for reasons I will go into shortly. First, we need to examine what happens.

Modern stress response theory tells us that every time the brain perceives danger it activates the sympathetic nervous system. The brain and adrenal gland then release hormones called catecholamines (in this case, adrenalin and noradrenalin), producing an effect similar to gulping down five cups of strong coffee. Our blood-sugar levels spike as the liver releases glucose from its stores, and in an instant we are wide awake, our pulse is rising and our blood pressure is increasing. Every nerve in the body is primed to react. This is the effect of adrenalin.

A split second later, however, the adrenal cortex is woken by this surge of adrenalin and forced to squeeze out an array of three healing hormones,[22] all of which are designed to relax us and heal us:

22 Szafarczyk, A. et al. 'Further Evidence for a Central Stimulatory Action of Catecholamines on Adrenocorticotropin Release in the Rat.' *Endocrinology* (1987): 121 (3): 121.

- Cortisol, which as we know reduces inflammation (hot, itchy areas) on the body. Cortisol also causes a gentle release of glucose from the liver in a process called gluconeogenesis, and – very importantly – it helps to switch off adrenalin, which is a key part of de-stressing.
- DHEA, which relaxes us and increases our immunity. These are vital steps as we wind down and perhaps need to stave off infection that we might have picked up if we were injured in the fight.
- Aldosterone, which retains water to keep our blood pressure up in case we get injured and are bleeding badly. This lowers the chance of dying because it ensures that blood continues to flow to the brain.

This is a superb system. It helps us to spring into action at the first sign of danger and then to relax and heal as fast as possible, with adrenalin and the three healing hormones working together to keep us healthy. For situations of acute stress such as getting into a fight with a hungry lion, it is essential that our body is flooded with the action hormone and the healing hormones. But, as we have seen, this response also kicks in for situations of chronic stress – the unceasing pressures of modern living – and that is bad for our health.

Stress: be more like a cat

Cats seem to have a particularly good brain for this: as anyone who owns a cat knows, they do not do stress. Anxiety seldom enters the world of our black cat who, unlike his owners, never sees the need to rush. When I come home after a day spent hitting and missing deadlines, he will be stretched out and purring in a sunny spot. He will come and say hello, eventually, but in his own time, and as if he is doing me the favour. This is the sort of stress management that would make Sapolsky proud.

I have no doubt that my cat's adrenals are in excellent order. Mine, on the other hand, are a weak point. Had I been born a century ago, pneumonia might well have carried me off in childhood. I am the not-so-proud owner of a collection of inflammatory problems including asthma, hay fever, sinusitis and eczema. My salivary cortisol test shows that I follow the trajectory you will see later in Figure 6: low cortisol in the morning, pushed higher during the day by stress, which leaves me late getting to sleep and tired the following morning. My adrenal gland is my Achilles heel and, because I recognise that a long, healthy life requires rebalancing my adrenals, I am motivated to help myself.

To that end I do not work past eight in the evening. Instead I play my guitar for a while, which brings benefits to the brain and reduces stress hormones. Next comes ten minutes of mindful meditation, which increases the slow brainwaves and will help me with sleep. I take 3mg of melatonin, which lets me sleep more deeply and lowers the chance that I will awake during the night.

Some years ago, during a particularly stressful period, I took a one-month course of low-dose hydrocortisone, which raised my cortisol levels, reduced anxiety, lowered inflammation and helped to rebalance my circadian rhythm. That meant I was energised during the day and sleepy at night. I then tried a variety of herbal adrenal supplements, with my favourite being a product by Metagenics called Licorice Plus, which works by keeping cortisol in the body for longer. That would be disastrous for anyone with high cortisol and high blood pressure, but – as I had low cortisol – it helped.

Although this is still theoretical, many researchers believe it is the case that every stress response causes adrenalin *plus* the healing hormones to come out, and that the traditional theory that suggests only cortisol is released during chronic stress is wrong. It means that if you are one of the many who live a stressful, caffeine-fuelled existence, then, under this chronic stress, you are pushing the adrenalin button continuously. Running is a great way to remove adrenalin, but if you are stuck in an office under huge stress then that is difficult, leaving you with adrenalin surges and no way to wash it out. This adrenalin will then squeeze your adrenals to release cortisol. If you are someone who releases too much cortisol, this chronic stress will likely cause you to put on weight; if you are someone who produces too little cortisol then it will likely make you thin, sickly and inflamed.

Hence my earlier question: 'Do you lose or gain weight when under sustained stress?' There are a number of tests we can do to test our levels of cortisol; however, as these vary throughout the day (as we shall see shortly), only the more expensive tests can measure those changes accurately. Here is a list of the most common methods for testing cortisol levels:

- A blood test. This is cheap and easy, but is unfortunately not very accurate. Also, blood is usually taken in the early morning, and not done repeatedly during the day, which means it does not show the variation of cortisol levels throughout a stressful day. This means that a blood test is not overly useful for people whose stress levels increase through the day.

- A synactin test involves injecting ACTH, the brain hormone that tells the adrenals to secrete cortisol, and measuring how much cortisol is released. This test is expensive and is usually done only if the endo-crinologist suspects you have Addison's disease, which means you have ultra-low levels of cortisol. That is a rare condition, however.

- A urine test can be helpful to test for cortisol levels over a 24-hour period. The test is expensive, and the patient needs to collect all urine over a 24-hour period, which is inconvenient, and which is mixed together over the 24 hours. If they secrete too much or too little overall, then this is useful. However, some people might have a spike of cortisol in the morning and feel exhausted as they run out of it in the afternoon; for them, this test will not be useful as those spikes and troughs will not be noticed.

- Finally there is a saliva test which is, in my opinion, the most useful. It is not cheap, however, and it does mean collecting saliva samples at four times during the day, which might not be convenient. The patient spits into a bottle at 7am, 11am, 4pm and 9pm on a given day and the laboratory then tests to see how their cortisol levels fared.

All of that raises the obvious question: how is your cortisol *meant* to fare? Figure 3 provides the answer. It shows how, in the morning, the stimulus of light makes your cortisol level shoot up. That wakes you, gives you a boost of glucose and makes you feel energetic and happy. As the hours pass, your cortisol level declines, and by the evening it is low and you feel sleepy. As it gets dark, your cortisol level drops further, and your body releases melatonin, the hormone that keeps you asleep. It is while you are sleeping that your body makes more cortisol for the next cycle.

This process is called our circadian rhythm, and it is the basis of being healthy. If you do not have a good circadian rhythm, you can largely guarantee that you are moving towards ill health. If you are energised during the day and sleep well for eight hours during the night, then your circadian rhythm is good and you have the basis of optimal health.

Figure 3: Normal cortisol response; the Y-axis represents the amount of cortisol in ng/ml

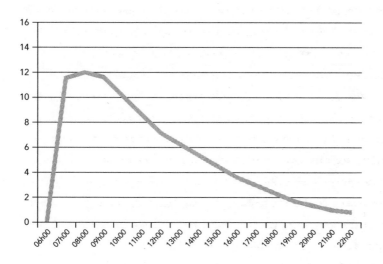

STRONG ADRENALS PRODUCING TOO MUCH CORTISOL

We saw earlier that people with robust adrenals produce excess cortisol when they encounter severe ongoing stress, and we will look at how that plays out on a daily basis. As soon as they wake they start to worry about deadlines, pushing out adrenalin and raising their cortisol to unhealthy heights (the dark line in

Figure 4). People like this are hyper-efficient and seem to run on stress and an array of stimulants from coffee to Red Bull to Coca-Cola and even cocaine. Their cortisol levels stay higher than average through the day, and at night, unable to switch off, they need alcohol or sleeping tablets to come down.

Should they wake at night, they start worrying and get a boost of adrenalin followed by a release of glucose and cortisol, which leaves them wide awake. They might get up at 3am or 4am to start their day, and then, if asked, tell people that is because they need only four hours' sleep a night. During the day they boost their performance with their stimulant of choice and get on with work.

As we have seen, this constantly high cortisol level leaves them at risk of obesity and metabolic syndrome – which, by way of a reminder, is that array of modern ills in the form of high blood pressure, increased blood sugar levels, excess fat around the waist, and too-high levels of cholesterol and triglycerides that increase the chances of diabetes, heart attacks and strokes.

Figure 4: Excess cortisol secretion; the Y-axis represents the amount of cortisol in ng/ml

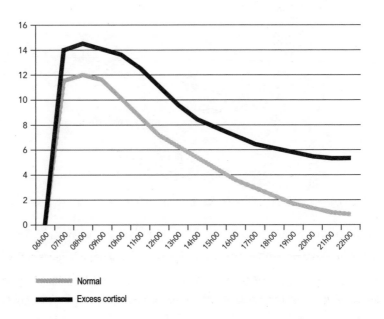

We saw earlier why constantly elevated cortisol levels cause weight gain: because cortisol ensures a constant trickle of glucose into the bloodstream, and when *too much* cortisol is released this trickle becomes a river. If the stress does not ease, then this river of glucose is stored as fat. The first place we notice it is around the belly but eventually this fat is stored everywhere and the person's weight will keep increasing.

We also saw the short-term benefits for people whose robust adrenals mean they push out too much cortisol under stress: they can burn the candle at both ends and not become ill, and they know that they will carry on when others around them collapse from exhaustion. In extreme settings, such as labour camps, it is often these people who survive because they have the reserves to stay healthier than others despite the harsh conditions. But most of us do not face such extremes, and instead our ongoing stress combined with comfort food results in weight gain and illness.

Figure 5: The five points where people with excess cortisol can prevent fat formation in a stressed adrenal gland

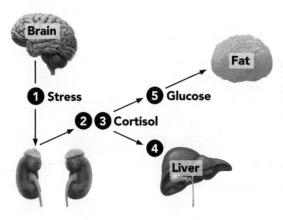

How should someone with robust adrenals turn this around? Figure 5 gives us some ideas. It shows how mental stress stimulates the adrenals, and how that leads to excessive cortisol, glucose release and fat formation. Sensibly enough, the solution lies in either decreasing how much cortisol we produce and/or increasing the removal of the cortisol that is in our system. The diagram shows the five points where people with overly robust adrenals can take action:

1. *Reduce anxiety or irritability*: this switches off the adrenalin response, which means the adrenals produce less cortisol and that means the body releases less glucose. Solutions here include regular exercise (which burns off anxiety); mindful meditation (which we will look at in the chapter on the brain); breaking up a stressful working day by taking a relaxing lunch break or, better still, a nap; attending counselling sessions to manage stress; and taking medication to reduce stress.

2. *Get the sleep-wake cycle right*: having too much cortisol in your system at bedtime results in a bad night's sleep and fat formation. Improved sleep is an indicator that you are calming your mind effectively. Regular exercise and meditation will help.

3. *Cut out coffee and other stimulants*: coffee and its ilk are adrenalin in a cup, and ditching these reduces excessive cortisol production.

4. *Detoxify the liver*: cortisol is removed via the liver, so the better the liver works the better that process will be. Among the solutions: stop consuming known toxins (alcohol, for instance) and take liver detoxifying tablets.

5. *Eat fewer starchy carbohydrates*: why do this? Because they convert to glucose, and we know that a surfeit of glucose gets converted into fat; that is particularly a problem for people with robust adrenals, because they already have too much glucose in their bloodstream.

The good news for these people is that if they can beat the overstimulation of cortisol, and if they can learn to recognise when they are redlining on stress and pull back from it, then their strong adrenal glands will help them to live a healthy, long life.

Weak adrenals producing too little cortisol

What about people on the other side of the coin – those whose adrenal glands do not produce enough cortisol? These are the fatigued and often thin people who have pushed their bodies through an extended phase of stress and whose cortisol is now relatively low. Their cortisol response generally falls into one of two types, as Figures 6 and 7 show.

Figure 6: Weak cortisol production, but still running on stress; the Y-axis represents the amount of cortisol in ng/ml

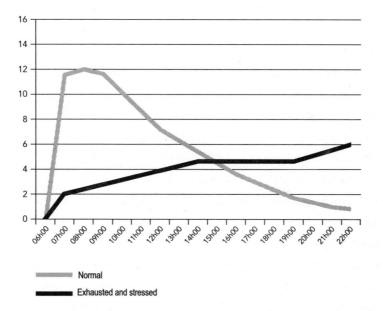

The darker line in Figure 6 shows the first type of what we call adrenal insufficiency: typically, someone like this had a normal cortisol response a decade ago, but years of burning the candle at both ends has taken its toll. Sleep no longer refreshes them, which means they do not rebuild their cortisol stores sufficiently at night. As the darker line shows, they wake up to a low morning cortisol level. However, a couple of coffees later their cortisol levels are climbing as their adrenals respond to the caffeine and the stress of the day.

By evening their cortisol is the highest it has been all day, and they feel surprisingly awake when they should be winding down. Of course that makes sleeping nigh on impossible so they self-medicate with a glass of wine as they sit in front of the computer enjoying their most productive hours, or simply slump on the couch watching television. Sleep comes eventually, but it is poor quality and insufficient, and they wake the following day exhausted and in need of a caffeine fix. Their circadian rhythm is upside down and they are on their way to becoming burned out.

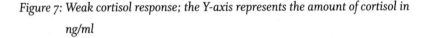

Figure 7: Weak cortisol response; the Y-axis represents the amount of cortisol in ng/ml

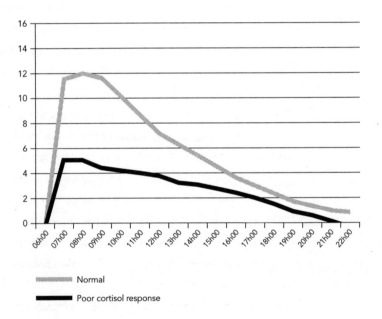

The dark line in Figure 7 illustrates the second and most exhausted type of adrenal insufficiency: after waking, this person still gets a boost of cortisol but generally less than half the normal amount. It means they wake up tired, and with already-low cortisol reserves. After that it gets worse: by mid-morning they have experienced an energy crash; they will have another in the after-noon as their post-lunch sugar levels dip, tempting them into a sugary snack.

Alternatively they might hit the couch for a nap, which is good news because it will help to rebuild some of their cortisol store, and that will give them a healthy energy boost for the afternoon.

Because cortisol is an anti-inflammatory, low cortisol levels like this often bring symptoms of inflammation such as hay fever (inflamed eyes and nose), spastic colon (an inflamed intestine), recurrent colds (an inflamed, compromised throat), joint and muscle aches (inflamed joints), dry and itchy skin (inflamed skin), asthma (inflamed lungs) or thrush. Although their low cortisol levels might not *cause* problems like asthma, arthritis or hay fever, those afflictions will certainly get worse when they are stressed and exhausted.

As always, the first step is to reduce any stress that might still be causing this exhaustion. After that we can add various supports that will help to rejuvenate the adrenal gland. People with adrenal insufficiency should consider six areas where they can take action – the first two are essential, and the others are listed in decreasing order of importance:

1. *Reduce anxiety and irritability*: we know anxiety causes cortisol spikes, and we know this reduces our stores of cortisol and leaves us tired and inflamed. Working to manage our anxiety through meditation, exercise, shorter office hours and getting back to nature helps to save our cortisol supply. Supplementing the adrenal hormones (cortisol, testosterone, DHEA and progesterone) is often very helpful in reducing anxiety. That said, anxiety can be deep-seated, and if natural measures do not work then the person might need to take medication for a time to break the cycle of worry.

2. *Better sleep*: we saw earlier that many people with weak adrenals get a spike of energy in the evening just as they should be settling in for a restful night. Because we manufacture cortisol when we sleep, it is essential to get an undisturbed eight hours of sleep a night, otherwise we will not have enough of it the following morning. That can be easier said than done, but if you cast your mind back to, perhaps, weekends away in the mountains, you might recall how physically active you were during the day and how you felt yourself nodding off

around the campfire by 8pm. One reason is that red and orange fire-light stimulates melatonin, which is our sleep hormone, whereas artificial lights and electronic screens have the opposite effect – their blue light blocks the release of melatonin, which undermines our natural circadian rhythm.[23] A few simple tricks work well: eat early and avoid excessive exercise in the evening (because that boosts cortisol, which wakes us up); turn on the night-shift mode on any screens used in the evening as that will filter out the blue light; do not use LED lighting in your bedroom or bathroom, because many LEDs emit blue light; and while you are at it, remove your television from the bedroom. If you still struggle to sleep, then calming the mind with meditation usually helps, as we shall see in the chapter on the brain. If those steps do not work then sleep supplements such as phosphorylated serine (a natural amino acid that we think assists in removing excess cortisol) and GABA (which slows down the brain) can help you to fall asleep, while melatonin and the amino acids 5-HTP and L-theanine will help to keep you asleep. I find these steps work for most of my patients, but inevitably not for all, and in those cases they need to follow up with a specialist who might prescribe medication to restore their sleep pattern. Sleep is essential for every aspect of our health, including restoring healthy adrenals, and the good news is that insufficient sleep is for most people simply a habit that has upset their circadian rhythm, and can be fixed.

3. *Measure and then balance the other adrenal hormones*: your DHEA, testosterone and progesterone might also have become depleted and, in my experience, gently replacing cortisol has a calming effect on the brain and accelerates the return to better health. We know that testosterone replacement in men improves mood and reduces

23 Figueiro, M. and Rea, M. S. 'The Effects of Red and Blue Light on Circadian Variations in Cortisol, Alpha Amylase, and Melatonin.' *International Journal of Endocrinology* (2010): ID 829351.

anxiety.[24] Other studies show that supplementing testosterone in women has the same effect. In the chapter on anabolic versus catabolic hormones we saw that supplementing with DHEA increases energy and reduces anxiety in men and women.[25] And the adrenal glands use progesterone to build other hormones including cortisol, as we will see in more detail in the chapter on women's health. Again we see the need for balance.

4. *Cut out coffee and similar stimulants*: although caffeine drinks stimulate cortisol release and make us feel good for a time, they burn up our remaining cortisol store leaving us tired and inflamed. Painful though it might be to cut out the caffeine, it is essential because each hit amounts to an adrenalin spike. For at least a few months your new friends should be water, non-caffeine herbal teas and red bush tea (known in South Africa as rooibos tea). And if you must have coffee, then drink decaffeinated, but know that it still contains a small amount of caffeine.

5. *Supplements*: these get a hard time in the media, but I find that my patients report good results from using these to restore adrenal function: the B-vitamins, panax ginseng, ashwagandha, Cordyceps mycelium and rhodiola. Although there is not a huge amount of convincing research in this area, these supplements have been used for countless generations in Chinese and Ayurvedic medicine, and I find them useful.

6. *Avoid sugary carbohydrates*: these work similarly to coffee – they briefly spike our energy and then, after those levels drop, leave us feeling exhausted. The solution is to eat healthily, as we saw in the chapter on nutrition.

---

24 Jung, H. J. et al. 'Effect of Testosterone Replacement Therapy on Cognitive Performance and Depression in Men with Testosterone Deficiency Syndrome.' *World J Men's Health* (2016): 34: 194–9.

25 Arlt, W. et al. 'DHEA replacement in women with adrenal insufficiency – pharmacokinetics, bioconversion and clinical effects on well-being, sexuality and cognition.' *Endocrine Research* (2000): 26: 505–511. Accessed at: http://www.tandfonline.com/doi/abs/10.3109/07435800009048561

STRESS: A FINAL WORD

Stress is directly implicated in all chronic illnesses from heart attacks to cancer: adrenalin switches off the p53 DNA-repair messenger that stops DNA from becoming cancerous; raised cortisol has been shown to trigger metabolic syndrome, by which we mean diabetes, heart attacks and strokes; depleted cortisol, on the other hand, leads to fatigue, infections and inflammation.

We can reverse these, in part by taking supplements to support the body and medications to rebuild and rebalance our hormones. But it is far more important to have the *desire* to change this stressed state in which we live. We need the motivation to change, to rebalance our lives and to release ourselves from our tendency to chase fleeting treasures.

Meditation gurus will tell you that either we control our thoughts or our thoughts control us. They are right, and one of the reasons that is important is because an ultra-busy life leaves us so fixated on the day-to-day that our brain fails to notice the stresses on our body. Adrenalin revs the body, the brain ignores the increasing fatigue, and the result is that we do not rest and recover. Fortunately we can retrain our brain to listen and, as we shall see in the chapters on the brain, the best way to do that is with mindful meditation, a process that requires no pills or injections, and is scientifically proven to work.

If you believe you control your thoughts (and perhaps you do), you can easily find out by focusing on a single picture in your mind for thirty seconds. If you can manage that without the day's concerns flooding in, then the chances are that you are in control. If like the rest of us you cannot, then it is never too soon to start learning how to help your brain listen better to the effects that stress has.

It is worth reiterating that stress is one of our Three Horsemen of the Health-pocalypse. It is directly implicated in all chronic illnesses from heart attacks and strokes to cancer, diabetes and a weakened immune system. Which of these you are at risk of getting depends partly on how your adrenal glands function:

- If you have robust adrenals, then running on adrenalin means your body will release too much cortisol. You will feel energised with the stress, but you will put on abdominal fat and fur up your arteries. The heart attack will be an unwelcome surprise.

- If, like me, you have weak adrenals then you will likely feel tired and anxious and be susceptible to various infections. Unless this is corrected you will not enter old age with a healthy DHEA level and you are unlikely to reach ninety.

Both of these conditions are reversible and, opposing though they seem, the treatment is the same – stress management. We need to switch off the trigger that is causing the problem and, more importantly, we need the motivation to change the stressed state in which we live.

It has to be said that some people are better at this than others, as I remember from a visit to Italy some years back. It was a sunny Monday morning and I saw a group of older men sitting outside drinking coffee, playing chess, laughing and watching the world go by. (No doubt their DHEA levels were excellent!) I turned to my Italian friend and told him that their's was a special moment. He smiled and replied that Italians have a phrase for that: *Il dolce far niente*, which means the joy of doing nothing.

Key points

- Stress accelerates disease and ageing, and every major stress leaves an indelible scar on our system. Mastering stress is central to our health and well-being.
- Stress directly affects the adrenals, which are the glands that produce the firefighters that heal the body after tense encounters. Our over-stimulated modern lifestyle means we do not turn off our stress switch as often as we should, and this unceasing stimulation causes further damage.
- If we have robust adrenals, constant stress causes our adrenal glands to release too much cortisol, leading to weight gain and the diseases associated with obesity.
- Weak adrenals and constant stress result in less and less cortisol being secreted, which causes fatigue and inflammation.

- A simple saliva test is probably the best way to measure our cortisol levels throughout the day.
- There are a number of ways to reverse the effects of stress, and these include: managing anxiety through exercise, meditation, less work and an outdoors life; getting eight hours of sleep every night, and ensuring that our circadian rhythm is functioning well; measuring and restoring our adrenal hormones; and cutting out caffeine drinks and sugary carbohydrates.

Chapter 8

Men's Health – The Decline and Fall of Marlon Brando

It's not the men in my life, it's the life in my men.

Mae West

There comes a time in the life of every ageing man when he is faced with the ultimate betrayal, a point where being dumped by a woman like Mae West pales in comparison with, to put it in the words of the eighteenth-century English poet Thomas Gray, that 'inevitable hour' when the body betrays itself.

Gray was talking about death, not about ageing – that moment when, as he wrote, 'the paths of glory lead but to the grave' – yet I believe it works for my comparison: the time in a man's life when the joy and bounce of youth is replaced with aches and pains, belly fat and sagging skin, failing eyesight, hair loss, exhaustion, erectile dysfunction, depression, forgetfulness and grumpiness. It is not only women who often feel they are becoming unattractive, unseen and irrelevant; men do too. As one of the songs in the musical *Chicago* put it, men become 'Mr Cellophane'.

'Manopause'

Pharmaceutical companies have focused for far longer on women than men, so it is not surprising that trumpeted solutions for women and ageing came first. In the second half of the last century the answer for women was thought to be found in hormone replacement therapy, or HRT. In the past decade or so, men too have been offered their own hormone-related solution: testosterone replacement. It has become a huge money-maker.

Readers who followed the purported HRT revolution for women might recall that this promised panacea did not materialise: in the 1990s it was suggested that all women entering menopause should take synthetic HRT tablets to optimise their health, but this idea collapsed after what looked to be the overwhelmingly negative results of a 2003 study. As we will see in the chapter on women's health, hundreds of thousands of women then stopped taking HRT, which inadvertently gave researchers the chance to study what happened next. What they found was that more women died over the next decade by avoiding HRT than would have died had they continued with it.[1] Since then the medical world has discovered natural products for HRT in women, which have contributed to better health and longevity. HRT using natural hormones, also known as bio-identical hormones, is the method I recommend to treat menopause in many women.

Sadly, and unnecessarily, the current approach to helping men through this crisis – by injecting ageing men with large doses of testosterone – has all the ingredients for failure that the so-called HRT revolution for women had twenty years ago. The good news is that it does not have to be this way: just as women now have a natural, healthier way to help them through menopause, so men have a better option than testosterone replacement, or TR. And that is what this chapter will look at.

Testosterone replacement, it should be said, started poorly when in the 1920s a Franco-Russian surgeon named Serge Voronoff provided an operation in which he inserted thin slices of monkey gland into the scrotums of wealthy ageing men. The idea was that the hormones from the monkey would rejuvenate the men, a view that a decade later was shown to be hopelessly optimistic. The medical community dismissed Voronoff's promise of renewed virility as a hoax.

---

1   Sarrel, P. M. et al. 'The mortality toll of oestrogen avoidance: an analysis of excessive deaths among hysterectomized women aged 50 to 59 years.' *Am J Public Health* (2013): 103: 1583–8.

Matters moved forward dramatically in 1939 when scientists Adolf Butenandt and Leopold Ruzicka were awarded the Nobel Prize for Chemistry for their work on sex hormones, including testosterone. After that the growth in testosterone treatment was somewhat pedestrian for half a century until, in the 1990s, ageing male baby boomers started seeking a solution to their flagging assets. The testosterone revolution has grown so rapidly in the intervening decades that *Time* magazine's cover story in one of its 2014 issues was an article titled, 'Manopause?! Ageing, insecurity and the $2 billion dollar testosterone industry'. The article noted that testosterone prescriptions had nearly trebled between 2007 and 2013 to 7.5 million, earning $2.4 billion in revenues in the US alone.

While that was clearly good news for the companies concerned, many doctors – myself included – are very concerned about this commercialisation of hormones. For example, a study released in 2010 showed that elderly men given testosterone treatment were at serious risk of a heart attack.[2] As with HRT, we cannot simply dish out testosterone in an unstructured way.

One of the problems about highlighting men's health is that we males do not see ourselves as being anything *but* fabulously robust. Scars and wrinkles are badges of honour, not shame; we do not suffer the challenges of menopause; and we are still fertile at seventy.

Or are we?

One of 2017's most disturbing statistics showed male sperm counts have declined worldwide: a meta-analysis of 195 studies showed that, on average, men have 49 million sperm per millilitre, down from 99 million just forty years ago.[3] In my clinic it is common to see sperm counts of 20 million or lower in couples who are struggling with fertility. What is the cause? We do not know for certain, but among the reasons suggested are high oestrogen levels in our environment, radiation from mobile phones kept in trouser pockets, and high stress. This should strike a note with every male, and make

2   Basaria, S. et al. 'Adverse events associated with testosterone administration.' *N Engl J Med* (2010): 363 (2): 109–22.
3   Levine, H. et al. 'Temporal Trends in Sperm Count: A Systematic Review and Meta-Regression Analysis.' *Hum Reprod Update* (2017): 1–14.

us realise that we also must take good care of ourselves if we want optimal health for ourselves and our unborn children. This chapter forms part of that effort.

What maketh a man?

When we think of a healthy young man, baby boomers might think of Marlon Brando in the 1953 film *The Wild One*; Generation X-ers, who grew up in the 1980s and 1990s, might visualise Brad Pitt in *Fight Club*; millennials might envision Zac Efron or Channing Tatum.

What they all have is good looks, of course, but also vigour, muscular physiques and great hair. And they have youth, with all the power that brings to us all. But by the time most men reach their fifties, they seem to get divided into one of two groups:

- Those who keep their hair but develop a belly and male breasts (moobs), and lose their libido.
- Those who lose their hair but retain their muscles and their libido.

Later we will see in detail why that happens. Briefly, though, it is because of our liver: we remove testosterone from the body via the liver and, by fifty, it is often tired. The result is that testosterone is processed into one of two products and, depending on which of these a man accumulates, he will develop moobs or become bald. Neither is a particularly attractive option.

Take Marlon Brando, for instance. Considered by some to have been the sexiest man of the twentieth century, even this god among us had, by the time he hit fifty, developed belly fat and sagging skin. He died at eighty, after decades spent battling his weight and an array of illnesses. For the sake of our categorisation, I would put Brando into the first category. Among those in the second category – those who lose their hair and keep their muscles – Sean Connery would be my pick.

Until recently there seemed to be limited interest in helping men with their depressing decline towards middle-aged collapse. When a man turned sixty-five, he could expect little more than a farewell handshake from his boss, and reassurance from his doctor that the prostate cancer he had just been diagnosed with would likely not carry him off. At the same time that his testosterone is dropping and his body is failing, many men go from being family provider to retiree. It is a significant psychological adjustment, and Thomas Gray's words start to become a haunting reality – 'the paths of glory lead but to the grave'.

Is there even such a thing as andropause – the male menopause – or is it just a case of the male ego struggling with mortality and grasping at anything that promises a return to youth? After all, men do not get hot flushes, so what are we complaining about? And do we really want to experience the misguided efforts that women went through with the dangers of synthetic HRT?

WHO SHOULD GET TESTOSTERONE REPLACEMENT?

I find it remarkable that the first World Congress on the Ageing Male was held only in 1998. Until that point it was felt that testosterone in men should be replaced only if the person's level was in the bottom 2.5 per cent of society. The remaining 97.5 per cent of ageing men might exhibit the symptoms of low testosterone – decreased libido, increased fatigue, anxiety, depression, muscle atrophy, pale dry skin and the rest – but they would not qualify for anything more than that firm handshake goodbye and some comforting words from their doctor.

With the rise in chronic illness, however, there has been a shift in medicine away from treating illness and towards ensuring wellness: preventing sickness rather than dealing with its consequences. This suggests that many more than just that bottom 2.5 per cent of ageing men with low testosterone might benefit from some sort of testosterone replacement.

It is worth stressing that we are not considering merely treating the illness of having almost no testosterone – a condition known as hypogonadism – but are looking to improve the health of men who have a low-to-normal testosterone level. For doctors, this is a fairly new concept and it is one that not all embrace, which I can understand. After all, if a treatment is likely to harm a patient then, all things being equal, it is probably better to do nothing.

While these debates continue, the global population is ageing, which is another way of saying that the proportion of older people is rising in both absolute numbers and relative to the number of younger people. Consider these figures: in 2015, there were 900 million people over sixty in the world. By 2050, the World Health Organization (WHO) reckons that will have reached more than 2 billion and, for the first time, the number of elderly people will outnumber children under five.[4] All of this tilts the social balance, and countries start to have more people drawing a pension than are paying in to support it, which in the absence of more taxation is financially unsustainable.

It becomes critically important to keep ageing populations healthy long before that point, and not just for ethical reasons. We know that people who maintain their health have fewer medical problems than those who do not, and that saves states money. In other words, there are good financial motivations too for countries to keep their adult populations healthy for as long as possible. Among those who have sounded that warning is the former head of the WHO who noted more than a decade ago that: 'In all countries, but in developing countries in particular, measures to help older people remain healthy and active are a necessity and not a luxury.'

So, having established that keeping older people healthy is a sensible proposition, the question for this chapter revolves around testosterone: does gentle rebalancing using natural, also known as bio-identical, testosterone lower the rate of chronic illness in men and extend healthy life? It is a key question, and this chapter will provide the answer. Before we get there, though, I want to recap two points:

- In the chapter on anabolic versus catabolic hormones we saw that low DHEA in elderly people is associated with worsening catabolism (breaking down of the body) and an increased risk of death. We also saw that supplementing with DHEA improves health, although it will not help someone to live longer.
- In the chapter on women's health, we will see how using bio-identical hormone replacement does help women to live longer and more healthily.

4   'Ageing and health.' World Health Organization. http://www.who.int/mediacentre/factsheets/fs404/en/

Free testosterone and total testosterone

First, though, what exactly *is* testosterone? Simply put, testosterone is a type of hormone known as an androgen, and this group of hormones (which also includes DHT that we will meet later) give so-called 'male' characteristics. As its name suggests, testosterone is made primarily in the testes, and it boosts confidence, strengthens the immune system, improves libido, builds muscle and reduces body fat.

It sounds fabulous, and men typically start their twenties with a high testosterone level, a healthy liver that can safely process and remove the testosterone that the body no longer needs, and a misplaced sense of immortality. That soon crumbles and, even in our thirties, our testosterone level can start to flag.

Typically we use a blood test to measure someone's testosterone level, and a laboratory will often give two results – the total testosterone figure and the free testosterone figure. There is a difference:

- Total testosterone: this shows the level of testosterone found in the blood sample, but it is important to know that not all of this testosterone is available. Quite a lot, in fact, remains bound to carrier molecules, and that can mean there is just a small amount of testosterone available to do the work of boosting a man's confidence, immune system, libido and muscles. In practice, then, a patient might have low libido, yet their total testosterone reading could be normal, and so they would not know there is a problem.

- Free testosterone: this is the level of testosterone that is *not* tied to the carrier molecules, and that therefore is available to do the work of boosting a man's confidence, immune system, libido and muscles. If someone's free testosterone level is low then there is no doubt they will notice the symptoms of low testosterone.[5]

5 Vermeulen, A. et al. 'The apparent free testosterone concentration: An index of androgenicity.' *J Clin Endocrinol Metab* (1971): 33: 759–67.

These levels decline over a lifetime: a man's total testosterone level can drop by about a third, but his free testosterone can halve.[6] That is why, as men age, they will feel the effects of low testosterone far more than their total testosterone level would indicate they should – which is why these days we measure both.

Unfortunately as the research stands at the moment there are still not enough good studies on free testosterone levels to draw any big conclusions. That will change in the coming years, but for now the total testosterone test is seen as being more stable, which is why we will use those studies to understand the dangers of low testosterone in men.

First we will see what is damaged when testosterone levels decline; after that we will see how health is boosted when testosterone is replaced.

Does low testosterone damage health?

As we have seen in this book, time and again it is the chronic illnesses that carry us off: weight gain (not an illness in itself, but obesity worsens inflammation which leads to illness), Alzheimer's, metabolic syndrome, diabetes and heart attacks tend to become far more common as we age. Could a falling testosterone level be partly to blame?

Since the start of the millennium a number of studies have looked at that:

- Weight gain: a trial in 2000 showed that a lowered testosterone level is associated with a raised triglyceride level, inflammation and weight gain.[7]
- Dementia: not long afterwards, two more studies showed that low testosterone was a significant risk factor in the development of Alzheimer's in ageing men.[8]
- Metabolic syndrome: another study showed very low testosterone

6 Kaufman, J. M. et al. 'Androgens in male senescence.' In Nieschlag, E., Behre, H. M. eds. *Testosterone action, deficiency, substitution.* Berlin, *Springer-verlag* (1998): 437–71. Liefke, E. et al. 'Age-related changes of serum sex hormones, insulin-like growth factor-1 and SHBG levels in men: cross-sectional data from a healthy male cohort.' *Clin Endocrinol* (Oxford) (2000): 53: 689–95.
7 Stellato, R. K. et al. 'Testosterone, SHBG and the development of type-2 diabetes in middle-aged men: prospective results from the Massachusetts Male Ageing Study.' *Diabetes Care* (2000): 23: 490–4.
8 Moffat, S. D. et al. 'Longitudinal assessment of serum free testosterone concentration predicts memory performance and cognitive status in elderly men.' *J Clin Endocrinol Metab* (2002): 87: 5001–193.

levels were strongly associated with causing metabolic syndrome. This is the recognised combination of a beer belly, raised blood pressure, cholesterol and high blood sugar. Metabolic syndrome is the most serious of the weight-gain patterns and is strongly associated with diabetes, heart attacks and strokes.[9]

- Diabetes: in 2007, the massive NAHANES III study showed a strong relationship between testosterone deficiency and diabetes. Importantly it showed that even low-to-normal testosterone levels are a risk factor for developing diabetes, which is one reason that men with a low-to-normal testosterone level should consider testosterone replacement, and not just the bottom 2.5 per cent of men.[10]

- Cardiovascular disease: in the same year, another study showed that low testosterone levels can contribute greatly to cardiovascular disease.[11]

- Chronic diseases: also in 2007, a study on 41,000 men showed that the lower their testosterone level, the more likely they were to die from one of a number of chronic diseases. One conclusion was that low testosterone levels could be used as a marker for cardiovascular disease.[12]

In other words, there is growing evidence that low total testosterone levels can worsen a man's chances of dying from one of the modern chronic illnesses, and is associated with dying younger.

Heart attacks are the most common of these chronic illnesses, and studies have shown a clear link between heart attacks and low testosterone. Why might that be? By way of a reminder, the chapter on inflammation showed us

9 Moffat, S. D. et al. 'Free testosterone and risk for Alzheimer's disease in older men.' *Neurology* (2004): 62: 188–93.
Braga-Basaria, M. et al. 'Metabolic syndrome in med with prostate cancer undergoing long-term androgen deprivation therapy.' *J Clin Oncol* (2006): 24: 3979–83.
10 Selvin, E. et al. 'Androgens and diabetes in men: results from the third National Health and Nutrition Examination Survey (NAHANES III).' *Diabetes Care* (2007): 30: 234–8.
11 Rosano, G. M. et al. 'Low testosterone levels are associated with coronary artery disease in male patients with angina.' *Int J Impot Res* (2007): 19: 176–82.
12 Khaw, K. T. et al. 'Endogenous testosterone and mortality due to all causes, cardiovascular disease and cancer in men. EPIC-Norfolk prospective population study.' *Circulation* (2007): 116: 2694–701.

that blockages in the arteries are mainly caused by inflammation of those arteries, and we know that inflamed artery walls are susceptible to small cholesterol packages creating blockages of plaque in these inflamed walls.

So, is low testosterone linked to blockages in the arteries? It turns out that the answer is yes. Low testosterone levels are associated with:

- Inflamed arteries: testosterone is anti-inflammatory, and men with low testosterone levels were shown in this study to have raised arterial inflammatory markers.[13]

- High cholesterol: men with low testosterone had higher blood cholesterol levels.[14] Why is that a problem? Because once an artery is inflamed, cholesterol is able to burrow into those inflamed walls and cause blockages.

- Formation of arterial plaque: this study put together both of the above studies and found that low testosterone levels are associated with arterial plaque formation and arterial blockages.[15] (This study was done on rabbits, as there are understandable ethical concerns about cutting open humans halfway through a trial.)

These three factors are the basis for cardiovascular disease that leads to heart attacks and strokes, and studies now suggest that testosterone deficiency is closely associated with cardiovascular risk. Low testosterone, then, does damage health.

Does testosterone replacement restore health?

We know that low testosterone levels are associated with the chronic illnesses of inflammation and in particular with cardiovascular disease. Now we need to turn to the second part, and see whether replacing testosterone can reverse this process.

We will start with arterial blockages, where studies have shown that testosterone replacement results in:

13   Malkin, C. J. et al. 'The effect of testosterone replacement on endogenous inflammatory cytokines and lipid profiles in hypogonadal men.' *J Clin Endocrinol Metab* (2004): 89: 3313–18.
14   Oppenheim, D. S. et al. 'Elevated serum lipids in hypogonadal men with and without hyperprolactinaemia.' *Ann Intern Med* (1989): 111: 288–92.
15   Hanke, H. et al. 'Effect of testosterone on plaque development and androgen receptor expression in the arterial vessel wall.' *Circulation* (2001): 103: 1382–5.

- Reduced arterial inflammation: testosterone replacement in men led to a lowering of inflammatory markers in the blood.[16]
- Healthier cholesterol levels: testosterone replacement in men improved the levels of healthy HDL cholesterol.[17]
- Reduced formation of arterial plaque: again, this study was performed on rabbits, but it showed that when the testosterone deficiency was corrected, the plaque blocking the arteries lessened, and the arteries opened up.[18]

What these studies show us is that a deficiency of testosterone leads not only to the woeful trinity of raised cholesterol levels, arterial inflammation and plaque formation, but that testosterone replacement can reverse all three.

That is good news, and it gets better, because testosterone replacement has also been shown to help other chronic inflammatory diseases: it helped men with metabolic syndrome safely improve their cholesterol level and sugar level, and to lose weight;[19] it helped men with type 2 diabetes, which is increasingly common, to reduce their insulin resistance and lower their body fat;[20] and it improved the mental functioning of men with Alzheimer's disease.[21]

These findings are remarkable, and show testosterone replacement could

16   Malkin, C. J. et al. 'The effect of testosterone replacement on endogenous inflammatory cytokines and lipid profiles in hypogonadal men.' *J Clin Endocrinol Metab* (2004): 89: 3313–18

17   Rubinow, K. B. et al. 'Testosterone replacement in hypogonadal men alters the HDL proteome but not HDL cholesterol efflux capacity.' *J Lipid Res* (2012): 53: 1376–83.
Nettleship, J. E. et al. 'Physiological testosterone replacement therapy attenuates fatty streak formation and improves high density lipoprotein cholesterol in the Tfm mouse.' *Circulation* (2007): 116: 2427–34.

18   Hanke, H. et al. 'Effect of testosterone on plaque development and androgen receptor expression in the arterial vessel wall.' *Circulation* (2001): 103: 1382–5

19   Hackett, G. et al. 'Testosterone replacement therapy improves metabolic parameters in hypogonadal men with type 2 diabetes but not in men with coexisting depression: the BLAST study.' *J Sex Med* (2014): 11: 840–56.

20   Dhinsa, S. et al. 'Insulin Resistance and Inflammation in Hypogonadotropic Hypogonadism and Their Reduction After Testosterone Replacement in Men With Type 2 Diabetes.' *Diabetes Care* (2016): 39: 82–91.

21   Cherrier, M. M. et al. 'Testosterone improves spatial memory in men with Alzheimer's disease and mild cognitive impairment.' *Neurology* (2005): 64: http://n.neurology.org/content/64/12/2063.full

bring profound health benefits for elderly men, particularly for those with chronic diseases. What is needed, though, are more human studies to show whether testosterone replacement will reduce heart attacks and help men to live longer.

What's the problem?

All of that amounts to a lot of good news, but, perhaps inevitably, it is here that we seem to hit a few bumps in the road. Some readers might recall that in 2014, the Food and Drug Administration (FDA) in the US cited two studies that suggested testosterone replacement in men worsened their risk of a heart attack.

The first looked at about 8,000 people who had both cardiovascular disease and low testosterone levels. Its initial results showed that men who received testosterone halved their risk of a heart attack compared with those who did not, which was positive. But after performing some statistical manipulation (which is permitted) the final results showed the opposite: the men who received testosterone now had nearly a one-third higher chance of a heart attack than those who received nothing.[22]

The second study showed that younger men who had previously had a heart attack and who had testosterone replacement increased their risk of another heart attack. It also found that men over seventy-five ran a higher heart-attack risk if they used testosterone replacement.[23]

As a result, the FDA concluded that testosterone replacement *worsens* cardiovascular health, and told manufacturers of testosterone to update their leaflets to warn patients that testosterone could cause cardiovascular problems.

But does it?

Following the FDA's concern about testosterone replacement, two reviews and one large study have been published that support testosterone replacement in heart-attack patients. The first was a meta-analysis of twenty-nine

22 Vigen, R. et al. 'Association of testosterone therapy with mortality, myocardial infarction, and stroke in men with low testosterone levels.' *JAMA* (2013): 310: 1829–36.
23 Finkle, W. D. et al. 'Increased risk of nonfatal myocardial infarction following testosterone therapy prescription in men.' *PLoS One* (2014): 9.

studies with about 120,000 men, and showed testosterone replacement was *not* associated with an increased risk of cardiovascular events.[24] The second was a review of all five meta-analyses done on the topic, and found that, over-all, testosterone replacement did *not* cause an increased cardiovascular risk.[25] The third was a 2017 study of 8,000 men, which again showed testosterone replacement did not worsen cardiovascular risk in men with low testosterone.[26]

I admit that it is difficult for people to know what to do with seemingly contradictory results, but as far as I am concerned the research done since 2014 tells me that testosterone replacement *is* safe in patients at risk of a heart attack. After all, meta-analyses, or studies of studies, are inherently more reli-able than individual studies.

However, we should still be careful when prescribing testosterone, and should ensure that:

- Patients get only as much testosterone as they are missing. Often they do not need a full vial of testosterone, and a blood test a month later will show whether they have too much or too little testosterone in their blood. Giving too much testosterone is clearly unwise and leaves people susceptible to side effects, as we shall find out.

- Doctors should measure the man's oestrogen level too. Why? Because, as we shall see, some men make too much oestrogen from testoster-one, and this worsens their heart-attack risk.[27] Giving testosterone without first measuring a man's oestrogen ignores this huge risk. We will see later how to correct it.

24 Patel, P., Arora, B., Molnar, J., et al. 'Effect of testosterone therapy on adverse cardio-vascular events among men: A meta-analysis.' American College of Cardiology 2015 Scientific Sessions (15 March 2015).

25 Corona, G. et al. 'Testosterone replacement therapy and cardiovascular risk: a review.' *World J Men's Health* (2015): 33: 130–42.

26 Cheetham, T. C. et al. 'Association of testosterone replacement with cardiovascular outcomes among men with androgen deficiency.' *JAMA* (2017): 177: 491–9.

27 Small, M. et al. 'Oestradiol levels in diabetic men with and without a previous myocar-dial infarction.' *Q J Med* (1987): 64 (243): 617–23.

How do men make testosterone?

Before we get into the subtleties of supplementing with testosterone, it is important to know how a man's body makes this hormone. The short answer is that men make testosterone from cholesterol, and testosterone is mostly made in the testes (although the adrenal glands make testosterone too).

As the chart shows, this is an involved process, but bear with me because by the end you will see why low testosterone pushes up cholesterol levels.

Figure 1: The pathway of testosterone formation

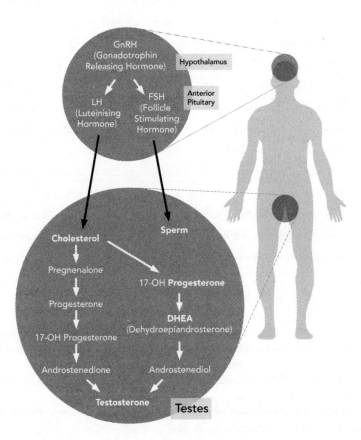

What it shows is the pathway by which testosterone is formed. The process starts with a brain messenger (known as luteinising hormone) telling the testes to start making testosterone from cholesterol.

The first thing that is important to note, then, is that the order to make testosterone starts in the brain, and specifically in an area of the brain called the hypothalamus. If the brain is stressed then that brain messenger, the luteinising hormone, that talks to the testes might get blocked, and that means the testes will make less testosterone.[28] Stress, then, is an important consideration.

The second is that testosterone is made from our old friend cholesterol in the testes and the adrenal glands. And most of the cholesterol our body needs is made in the liver. In other words, the liver has a doubly important role in the testosterone process: it makes the cholesterol that is then sent to the testes and adrenal glands to be turned into testosterone, and it later processes that testosterone safely.

Although our liver makes most of the cholesterol we need, some of it does need to come from our diet. For that reason we need to consume fats that our liver can then turn into cholesterol. Eating fish oil and saturated fats (these are mainly fats from animal products, but they are also found in coconut and palm oil) is one way to boost testosterone.[29] We can also help our liver by eating products such as eggs, animal liver and kidneys that contain cholesterol.

And while low-fat, vegetarian and vegan diets might have some benefits, they typically contain less in the way of saturated fats and so reduce that person's ability to make testosterone.[30] Men who follow those eating plans ought to ensure they get enough saturated fats from other sources.

28 Kirby, E. D. et al. 'Stress increases putative gonadotropin inhibitory hormone and decreases luteinizing hormone in male rats.' *Proc Natl Acad Sci USA* (2009): 106: 11324–9.

29 Volek, J. S. et al. 'Testosterone and cortisol in relationship to dietary nutrients and resistance exercise.' *J Appl Physiol* (1997): 82 (1): 49–54.

30 Wang, C. et al. 'Low-fat high-fiber diet decreased serum and urine androgens in men.' *J Clin Endocrinol Metab* (2005): 90 (5): 3550–9.

Statins and andropause

It is not uncommon that men going through andropause are prescribed statins to lower their heart-attack risk. Statins work by reducing LDL cholesterol (so-called 'bad' cholesterol), but they also lower HDL cholesterol, which is our good cholesterol. This is why men on statins are less able to make testosterone – because they have less cholesterol with which to make it in the first place.

One solution is to double up on fish oil supplements, as that will keep HDL levels healthy. Fish oil not only boosts testosterone; it also protects the heart.

Andropausal men who are *not* on statins, but who find their cholesterol levels are rising even as their testosterone levels are falling might want to resist the temptation of reaching for statins. Instead, it could be worth trying to supplement with testosterone, and then seeing whether their cholesterol level drops automatically. In many instances it will.[31]

Why is that? Because of the body's feedback mechanism. If the body is told to make more testosterone because the level of this hormone is low then it starts to make the building-block cholesterol to ensure it has the supplies to do so; but if the testes are for some reason failing to make testosterone, then the amount of cholesterol will start to accumulate, and the result is that the cholesterol level climbs. This feedback mechanism is a key reason why low testosterone levels in a man are often associated with high cholesterol.

If we replace testosterone, on the other hand, then there is no longer a need for the body to make cholesterol for testosterone, and the cholesterol level will drop.

The third point is that cholesterol goes through several stages before it is made into testosterone, and one of those stages is progesterone – as we can

---

31 Sadowski, Z. et al. 'Effect of testosterone replacement therapy on lipids and lipoproteins in hypogonadal and elderly men.' *Atherosclerosis* (1996): 121: 35–43.

see in the chart about testosterone formation. Why is that important? Because, like a game of snakes and ladders, hormones can convert into one or another hormone, depending on how the roll of the dice is going in your life. Under conditions of stress, for example, women use progesterone to make cortisol for survival. The same thing happens in men: instead of progesterone going down the pathway and making testosterone in a situation of chronic stress, it is instead converted to cortisol.

I see this in my clinic with high-stress male patients whose blood tests come back with both low progesterone *and* low testosterone levels. Part of their treatment might well involve supplementing with progesterone too, in order to help support both the formation of the stress hormones *and* testosterone.

All of this shows that the body needs three elements to make enough testosterone: a calm brain, because that sends the message to the testes to make testosterone; sufficient cholesterol, because cholesterol is the building block for testosterone; and a healthy adrenal gland, because testosterone is also made there, and if there is too much stress then these glands will make more cortisol and less testosterone.

TESTOSTERONE REPLACEMENT IN PRACTICE

Meet Richard (not his real name). He is a forty-eight-year-old patient who came to see me complaining of anxiety, low libido and a general lack of enthusiasm for life. A blood test showed his testosterone level was low and his cholesterol was a little high. Richard opted for a three-month testosterone injection instead of a testosterone cream.

After six months, Richard felt his libido had been restored, his anxiety was replaced with his more confident self and he was exercising. In short, life once again felt good. His blood tests showed that his testosterone level had returned to normal and that his cholesterol level had lowered on its own.

Richard's example shows what I regularly see at my clinic with male patients who have low to low-normal testosterone levels. Often enough, their problem is directly related to their liver.

How is testosterone removed from the body?

Figure 2: Pathway of testosterone metabolism

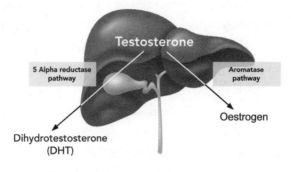

This figure shows how the liver metabolises, or processes and removes, testosterone. This system follows one of two pathways: on its way out of the body, testosterone is either pushed along the oestrogen pathway or it goes along the DHT pathway. A man's liver will use both pathways, but will tend to favour one over the other; which one it favours is determined by his genes.

The first pathway shows that testosterone is converted to oestrogen (thanks to enzymes known as P450 aromatase). Oestrogen then needs to be further metabolised in the liver before it is removed from the body. Men generally get the *first* half of this pathway right but, as the liver gets older, the second half falters. This is why some men accumulate oestrogen, the female hormone, and develop abdominal fat.

The second pathway looks like this: testosterone is converted (via a different enzyme called 5 α-reductase) to another androgen hormone called DHT, which stands for dihydrotestosterone.[32] DHT also needs to be processed further before it is removed from the body and, as with the mechanism of the first pathway,

32 Carruthers, M. *Androgen Deficiency in the Adult Male.* Taylor & Francis (2004) pp. 51–2.

men's ability to do this typically declines over the years as the liver ages. The result: some men accumulate DHT and lose hair on their heads.

Why is this so important? Well, that takes us back to the mystery we encountered near the beginning of this chapter: why men typically look fabulous at twenty, but – by the time they reach fifty – have developed baldness and hairy backs, or bellies and breast tissue? Simply put, it is because their liver becomes sluggish, and the two pathways that worked so efficiently to remove high levels of testosterone at twenty struggle to remove lower levels of testosterone at fifty.

The sluggish liver

As we have seen, a struggling liver tends to push testosterone only halfway along a pathway before it hits a bottleneck. The consequence is either an excess of DHT or too much oestrogen, the female hormone.

DHT is a very powerful testosterone, and it helps to maintain muscles, confidence and libido. Too much DHT, though, causes balding, a hairy chest and aggression.

DHT and the bladder

Excess DHT can also cause a swollen prostate, although that is not as bad as it sounds. This condition, known as BPH (which stands for benign prostatic hyperplasia), is very common, but it is not cancer.

It is, however, inconvenient, and means men cannot fully empty their bladder as they get older, which means getting up several times a night.

There is medicine available to treat BPH. Progesterone can also help, or a surgeon can re-bore a path that allows the urine to flow again.

Excess oestrogen, on the other hand, might allow a man to retain his full head of hair, but it also means he is likely to develop a beer belly and male breasts, and to suffer from low libido.

Male breasts, or 'moobs', are often due to high levels of oestrogen, the female hormone. Raised oestrogen in teenage boys, for instance, is often caused by an excess of oestrogens in the meat consumed, as well as that found in some plastic bottles and in recycled tap water. But when it comes to men around forty and older, a sluggish liver pathway is often to blame for this. That is the bad news. The worse news is that this problem compounds itself, because fat is able to manufacture yet more oestrogen from testosterone using the same metabolic pathway.

Excess oestrogen in men, then, is far more sinister than excess DHT, and is associated with:

- Prostate cancer: in the same way that oestrogen can cause changes in women's breast cells that can lead to breast cancer, oestrogen and testosterone can cause changes in men's prostate cells that can lead to prostate cancer.[33]

- Stroke: we know from studies carried out on women that oestrogen thickens the blood and increases the risk of brain clots. A 2007 study shows that men are just as much at risk of a stroke, and those men with high levels of oestrogen had double the risk of a stroke.[34]

- Atherosclerosis (thickening of the artery walls): studies show that raised oestrogen levels in men are linked with not only an increased risk of clotting, but also with greater risks of forming arterial plaque.[35]

- Heart attacks: this 1982 study adds weight to the two points above, and shows that raised oestrogen levels in men translate into an increased risk of heart attacks.[36]

33   Krieg, M. et al. 'Effect of aging on endogenous level of 5 alpha dihydrotestosterone, testosterone, Estradiol and Estrone in epithelium and stroma of normal and hyperplastic human prostate.' *J Clin Endocrinol Metab* (1993): 77 (2): 375–81.

34   Abbott, R. D. et al. 'Serum Estradiol and risk of stroke in elderly men.' *Neurology* (2007): 68 (8): 563–8.

35   Small, M. et al. 'Oestradiol levels in diabetic men with and without a previous myocardial infarction.' *Q J Med* (1987): 64 (243): 617–23.

Phillips, G. B. et al. 'The association of hypotestosteronemia with coronary artery disease in men.' *Arterioscler Thromb* (1994): 14 (5): 701–6.

36   Klaiber, E. L. et al. 'Serum estrogen levels in men with acute myocardial infarction.' *Am J Med* (1982): 73 (6): 872–81.

Clearly, no man would want his liver to be dominant along the oestrogen pathway; after all, the risks are significant. But the solution is not to take a fistful of tablets to drop the oestrogen level at all costs. Men need oestrogen; just not much. Very low oestrogen in men leads to lowered libido and, importantly, to osteoporosis and fractures.[37] As always, balance is key.

It is a shame that – despite the overwhelming evidence that it is important to keep men's oestrogen at a healthy low level – many pathology labs are unable to measure oestrogen accurately in men. In addition, many clinics are simply unaware that it is important to test men's oestrogen or why it is vital that men maintain a healthy liver. There is a long road ahead before knowledge of the issues surrounding men's health reaches the level it deserves. In the meantime, perhaps the most important thing we can do is to keep a healthy liver so that it can get rid of excess oestrogen as it is made.

Liver health

As we have seen, the liver plays a critical role in removing testosterone healthily from the body. In addition, many of us will have observed at our ten- or twenty- or even thirty-year school reunions that those friends who showed award-winning skills at drinking the rest of us under the table as students are now the ones sporting the biggest beer-bellies (courtesy of high oestrogen levels) or have deeply receded hairlines (thanks to their high DHT levels). For men in that situation, it is not safe simply to inject testosterone, because their liver will be unable to deal with it – as our next example shows.

We will call him Derek, and he is a jolly, fifty-something Capetonian who came to see me some years back. Derek tended to sweat easily, had a beer belly and complained that his libido had been problematic for five years. His blood tests showed that his levels of free testosterone and total testosterone were low, which indicated that he would benefit from testosterone replacement.

37 Mellstrom, D. et al. 'Older men with low serum Estradiol and high serum SHBG have an increased risk of fractures.' *J Bone Miner Res* (2008): 23 (10): 1552–60.

However, Derek's oestrogen levels were also very high (it was this that was causing his sweating), and that was a problem.

Why? Because putting Derek on a course of testosterone replacement would elevate his testosterone, but – given that he had a sluggish liver, as I could tell from his high oestrogen level – would simply mean Derek would make more oestrogen. And while more testosterone would help Derek's libido, it would also make him sweat more, cause him to put on more weight (because oestrogen causes fat formation) and that might even worsen his heart-attack risk.

After discussion, Derek agreed to go on a programme to support his liver and to take oestrogen-lowering tablets. After three months Derek had lost some of his excess weight, had stopped sweating profusely, and had trimmed his beer belly. Only after that was he given testosterone cream, and his libido improved without any nasty side effects.

WHAT TO DO?

Before giving testosterone, the first place to start is by working out whether a patient has a problem with high oestrogen or high DHT. Once I know that, I can help them to build their Younger for Longer life. In this section I will show you how that is done.

High oestrogen

If, like me, you are a middle-aged man who has raised oestrogen levels, then fixing that oestrogen issue is the first step before tackling low testosterone. We saw above that the liver is the central organ in this process, and in my clinic we would typically look at one or more of the following four steps to help:

- Do a liver detoxification programme: cut out alcohol, cigarettes, sugar and starches for two months, and do daily exercise to help remove toxins. Taking liver supplements will also help – among these are milk thistle, glutathione and the B-vitamins. For a refresher on this, see the chapter on toxins.
- Eat natural oestrogen-blockers: these are known as DIMS, which stands for diindolylmethane, and you can either take a supplement

(indole-3-carbinol) or eat the actual vegetable, for which read cauliflower, broccoli, kale and Brussels sprouts. Always buy organic, not least because pesticides are toxic and can make further oestrogens. (If you wondered why bodybuilders eat lots of broccoli, now you know: it reduces their oestrogen and therefore their body fat.)

- Anastrozole: if DIMS are not strong enough then speak to your doctor about prescribing a medical oestrogen-blocker. Very low-dose anastrozole, sold under the brand name Arimidex, taken once a week for a month, for instance, drops the blood oestrogen level quite quickly.

- Lose weight. Why? Because the liver is not the only part of the body that 'aromatises' testosterone in men to oestrogen: fat cells do too. When postmenopausal women 'aromatise' oestrogen, this process helps to keep their bones strong for the rest of their lives, which is a good thing. That is not the case for men: the more fat we have, the more we use that fat to 'aromatise' testosterone into oestrogen, which makes more fat, and so the problem continues. In other words, the less fat men carry, the lower their levels of oestrogen, and the lower the chance of making more fat.

High DHT

If, as a man, you are losing the hair on your head and growing more of it on your chest, then you might well have a sluggish DHT pathway; and if you measured your DHT level, you might well find it is high. However, this is an expensive test and is not done in many countries.

Fortunately, there is a workaround: I often find that men predisposed to form DHT do so mainly when they are stressed, and so I can get a good idea of their liver pathway by measuring the levels of three hormones that emerge during times of stress: cortisol, progesterone and DHEA.

A high DHEA level indicates that the person is under high stress; typically their DHT is also high at this time. To rebalance excess DHT I would (after a thorough examination, of course) likely recommend some or all of the following:

- Stress reduction: as we will see in the chapters on the brain, good sleep is the first step towards reducing stress. Daily exercise, meditation, counselling and natural mood-enhancers like saffron, GABA and 5-HTP are all useful to cut stress.

- Once again, we need to detoxify the liver. A cleaner liver helps to remove DHT faster, and so cutting out toxins from the diet (alcohol, sugar, cigarettes) is essential. Doing daily exercise is key too.

- Use natural DHT-blockers from natural products like saw palmetto, or by using progesterone cream. Progesterone is the body's natural DHT-blocker, but during stressful times it gets used up in the adrenal gland, which is one reason we tend to make more DHT when we are stressed. As a result, using a low-dose progesterone cream twice a week at times of stress can restore this balance.

- Medical DHT-blockers: if the natural products do not work well enough then I might recommend a patient uses 5α-reductase inhibitors (in the form of finasteride tablets) to block DHT formation. Finasteride, which is sold under the brand name Propecia, among others, is often used long-term by men who want to stop hair-loss. One problem with blocking DHT to that extent, though, is a lack of DHT, and that can make men depressed and reduce their libido. Once again, balance is key.

SUPPORTING TESTOSTERONE

While supplementing with testosterone can be useful for many men, there are ways to boost it naturally – and I always favour natural methods. The key lifestyle choice I would recommend is good sleep. Why? Because sleeping well lowers your stress levels, and that allows the brain to send the message to the testes to make testosterone. A good night's sleep, then, is the first step towards rebalancing testosterone.

The second is using supplements like zinc and vitamin D, because these are essential nutrients in forming testosterone.[38] (On that note, you might have read of a plant extract called tribulus terrestris that is widely used as a testosterone supplement; unfortunately there is little proof that it is effective.)[39]

The third is losing weight, which has been shown to improve testosterone levels in men and in women. As fat stores decline, testosterone levels climb.[40] The fourth is exercise, because high-intensity workouts boost testosterone. Next is diet, because eating healthy fats supports testosterone formation. [41]

Finally, many people will need a course of testosterone to reduce their anxiety, improve their energy and immune system, boost their libido and – perhaps most importantly – give them back their get-up-and-go. When it comes to prescribing testosterone, I far prefer natural testosterone to synthetic (man-made) testosterone. Why? Because as the chapter on women's health shows, long-term use of synthetic hormones might damage health.[42]

REPLACING TESTOSTERONE

In the event that I decide to put a patient through a course of testosterone replacement, my clinic sticks to using natural, or *bio-identical*, testosterone. As I said earlier, what we have learned about hormone replacement therapy, or HRT, in women (as we will see in the next chapter) is that it pays to be wary of synthetic hormones.

There are different ways to take testosterone, and the method I prefer is by using a testosterone cream or gel. This is applied to the skin, and the body then

38 Prasad, A. S. et al. 'Zinc status and serum testosterone levels in healthy adults.' *Nutrition* (1996): 12: 344–8.
Nimptsch, K. et al. 'Association between plasma 25-OH vitamin D and testosterone levels in men.' *Clin Endocrinol* (2012): 106–12.

39 Pokrywka, A. et al. 'Insights into supplements with tribulus terrestris used by athletes.' *J Hum Kinet* (2014): 41: 99–105.

40 Kim, C. et al. 'Changes in visceral adiposity, subcutaneous adiposity and sex hormones in the diabetes prevention program.' *J Clin Endocrinol Metab* (2017): 102: 3381–9.

41 Volek, J. et al. 'Testosterone and cortisol in relationship to dietary nutrients and resistance exercise.' *J Appl Physiol* (1997): 82: 49–54.

42 For example, see the Women's Health Initiative website: https://www.whi.org/about/SitePages/HT.aspx

absorbs the testosterone through the skin (in medical-speak, transdermally). Many testosterone creams or gels are made from natural testosterone, and it comes in different strengths – a doctor would decide which would best restore a low testosterone level. It is also important to do a blood test after using the cream or gel to make sure it is being absorbed, and that the dosage is working. That test should also, of course, measure the oestrogen level, as we saw earlier.

Two other options you might encounter are testosterone tablets and testosterone injections. I do not recommend testosterone in tablet form because it goes directly from the stomach to the liver, and that means the patient has a high risk of damaging their liver, developing breasts (because of the oestrogen that is formed), and losing their hair (because of the DHT that is formed). Testosterone tablets cause more problems than they solve.

Avoid at all costs

I cannot stress enough the dangers of 'juicing', or taking steroid hormones in unregulated quantities for often nebulous reasons (bodybuilding, for instance). Among the best-known of these products is nandrolone decanoate (sold under the brand name Deca-Durabolin).

Nandrolone decanoate, and its cousin nandrolone phenolpropionate (using the brand name Durabolin) are not testosterone, but a steroid hormone that acts like a strong testosterone. Medically it is useful to treat osteoporosis, among other conditions;[43] socially these have been massively abused by bodybuilders and some sportsmen.

The side effects these steroid hormones wreak on young lives is often terrible, and I can only warn people off them. Unless they have a medical condition that requires their use, they should be avoided.

43 Frisoli, A. J. et al. 'The effect of nandrolone decanoate on bone mineral density, muscle mass, and hemoglobin levels in elderly women with osteoporosis: a double-blind, randomized, placebo-controlled clinical trial.' *J Gerontol A Biol Sci Med Sci* (2005): 60: 648–53.

Testosterone injections are the other possibility, and there are two reasons some people prefer these to the creams and gels: they are convenient, because they are injected between once a fortnight and once every three months; and they can be stronger than the creams. The problem is that none of the testosterone injections uses natural testosterone, and that is because the body would remove it in a matter of hours, which would make them quite useless.

Because of that, manufacturers have got around this by attaching a chemical compound known as an ester to testosterone, which slows down its release into the blood. Different esters work at different rates:

- Testosterone propionate is the shortest acting, and peaks at about four days in the blood.
- Testosterone ethanoate is next: it peaks at about six days.
- Testosterone cypionate (under the brand name Depo-Testosterone) is the longest-lasting of these short-acting testosterones, and peaks at eight to ten days.
- Testosterone undecanoate (under the brand name Nebido, among others) does its work over a much longer period, being released over about two months. This gives a slow rise and fall of testosterone in the blood, and means there are few side effects.
- Finally, there are combination testosterones like Sustanon 250, which have four different testosterones that release at different times. The result is steady testosterone levels across a two-month period. However, Sustanon is no longer widely available in pharmacies in many countries.

In whatever form men take testosterone, it is essential to remember the purpose of doing so: it is simply to rebalance the body's orchestra of hormones; we are not trying to light up the sky with a testosterone rocket. What patients should feel is a gentle lifting of stress, a mild boost of energy and a normalisation of libido – helping them to get back to being active, which should then boost their hormones further and allow the body to correct any deficits naturally. At that point, they ought to stop testosterone support.

The final point to make is this: follow-up blood tests are important because they will show whether or not testosterone levels have returned to normal *and* that oestrogen levels have stayed low.

PROGESTERONE

You might have noticed that the hormone chapters in this book pay tribute to progesterone. In the chapter on stress, for example, progesterone was shown to be the helpful hormone that can be turned into cortisol allowing us to cope with pressure. In the chapter on toxins we saw that progesterone can help a man's DHT pathway to work more efficiently. We will spend nearly half of the coming chapter on women's health looking at the benefits natural progesterone provides menopausal women. And later, in the brain chapter, we will see progesterone return again as a natural brain-calming hormone.

Progesterone, then, has a big role to play in our lives, yet for many years the medical profession regarded progesterone and oestrogen as the exclusive domain of women, in the same way that we viewed testosterone as the domain of men. Things have changed: we now know testosterone is vital for women, and that oestrogen and progesterone are equally important for men.

We saw earlier that a high oestrogen level in men can contribute to obesity, heart attacks and prostate cancer, while a low level can result in osteoporosis. In short, oestrogen is a hormone that we should not ignore in men. That also holds true for progesterone. Remarkably, though, it is sold across the counter in some countries and is often seen as an unimportant player in the mix of male hormones. Nothing could be further from the truth.

Firstly, progesterone boosts the immune system. As we saw in the stress chapter (and will see in the women's health chapter), progesterone is released during the stress response and helps to maintain cortisol levels.[44] During

---

44   Herrera, A. Y. et al. 'Stress-induced increases in progesterone and cortisol in naturally cycling women.' *Neurobiol Stress* (2016): 3: 96–104.

acute stress this increase in cortisol and other stress hormones boosts the immune system.[45] Progesterone, then, not only helps to make our adrenal hormones; it also strengthens our immune system.[46]

Secondly, progesterone supports the brain. Men and women produce progesterone in the brain in similar levels,[47] and it is this hormone that reduces brain inflammation and helps to rebuild damaged brain cells.[48] Progesterone has a calming effect on the brain by activating GABA (which is the same neurotransmitter that Valium works its magic on).[49] Boosting low progesterone can be useful when we are stressed, because it not only calms the brain; it also improves sleep and balances the brain hormones.[50] Progesterone is also important in building healthy brain tissue,[51] and has been shown to help in the fight against Alzheimer's.[52]

Thirdly, progesterone protects the prostate gland, which can either enlarge under the influence of DHT or become cancerous – often due to oestrogen.[53] Both outcomes are typically the result of poor testosterone

45   Dhabhar, F. S. 'Enhancing versus Suppressive Effects of Stress on Immune Function: Implications for Immunoprotection versus Immunopathology.' *Allergy Asthma Clin Immunol* (2008): 4: 2–11.

46   Hall, O. J. et al. 'Progesterone-Based Therapy Protects Against Influenza by Promoting Lung Repair and Recovery in Females.' *PLoS Pathog* (2016): 12: e1005840.

47   Schumacher, M. 'Local synthesis and dual actions of progesterone in the nervous system: neuroprotection and myelin.' *Growth Horm IGF Res* (2004): 14 Suppl a: S18–33.

48   Stein, D. G. 'Progesterone exerts neuroprotective effects after brain injury.' *Brain Res Rev* (2008): 57 (2): 386–97.

49   Arbo, B. D. et al. 'Asymmetric effects of low doses of progesterone on GABA(A) receptor α4 subunit protein expression in the olfactory bulb of female rats.' *Can J Physiol Pharmacol* (2014): 92: 1–5.

50   Von Broekhoven, F. et al. 'Neurosteroids in depression: a review.' *Psychopharmacology* (2003): 165: 97–110.

51   Sitruk-Ware, R. et al. 'Progesterone and related progestins: potential new health benefits.' *Climacteric* (2013): 16 Suppl 1: 69–78.

52   Nilsen, J. et al. 'Impact of progestins on estrogen-induced neuroprotection: synergy by progesterone and 19-norprogesterone and antagonism by medroxyprogesterone acetate.' *Endocrinology* (2002): 143: 205–12.

Boomsma, D. and Paoletti, J. 'A review on the current research on the effects of progesterone.' *Int J Pharm Compd* (July/August 2002): (6) 4.

53   Stein, D. G. 'The case for progesterone.' *Ann NY Acad Sci* (2005): 1052: 152–69.

metabolism through the liver in older men, and supplementing with proges-terone helps in both cases. In the first scenario, progesterone blocks 5α-reductase, which therefore blocks the formation of DHT and prevents enlargement of the prostate.[54] In the second, progesterone competes with oestrogen at the oestrogen receptor site, and may also push cancer cells into apoptosis (cell death) and in that way reduce new cancer growth.[55] This ability of progesterone to remove damaged and cancerous cells by apoptosis has been shown to reduce prostate cancer in men, and to reduce breast and ovarian cancer in women.

Lastly, progesterone prevents balding. How? Because it is our body's natural DHT-blocker. We saw earlier that testosterone is removed via the liver, but it can get trapped in a sluggish liver in the form of DHT – and excess DHT leads to balding in susceptible men (and, for that matter, in women too). During stressful times our hair might thin for one or both of two reasons: because excess stress leads to excess DHT, and because excess stress causes our progesterone level to drop. Finasteride, which we encountered earlier, is a DHT-blocker that has been approved by the FDA to counter baldness. It is worth noting that bio-identical progesterone is also a natural DHT-blocker and therefore might help to reduce baldness too.[56]

This all sounds too good to be true, does it not? Surely we should just bathe in progesterone and enjoy the benefits? Well, by now you know that my answer is, as always, balance. Just as women do not require too much testos-terone to restore that balance, men do not need much progesterone to restore this balance.

One of the challenges in deciding what to do with managing progesterone

54 Mauvais-Jarvis, M. et al. 'Inhibition of testosterone conversion to dihydrotestosterone in men treated percutaneously by progesterone.' *J Clin Endocrinol Metabolism* (1974): 38 (1): 142–7.

55 Oettel, M. et al. 'Progesterone: the forgotten hormone in men?' *The Aging Male* (2004): 7: 236–57.

56 Cassidenti, G. L. et al. 'Effects of sex steroids on skin 5 alpha-reductase activity in vitro.' *Obstet Gynecol* (1991): 78: 103–7.

is that blood tests on their own are unreliable. That is why I typically look at several factors in combination, and this is perhaps best illustrated by looking at the example of one of my patients: Chad (not his real name), a fifty-something executive and weekend athlete.

Chad came to see me after his wife noticed he had become tired and grumpy and was no longer interested in sex, and indeed his blood results showed his levels of testosterone, progesterone and cortisol were low. Why might that be? Because Chad's body was buckling under excessive stress – in his case, his job and training too hard for those weekend sports events – and this depleted his cortisol levels, which knocked his progesterone levels and left him feeling tired.

Those, then, are the three factors I look for when assessing progesterone: fatigue, cortisol *and* progesterone. If all three are poor then there might be reason to give a man a little progesterone. In Chad's case, he applied a mild (5 per cent) testosterone cream each night, and a 3 per cent progesterone cream twice weekly. (His oestrogen level was normal, which is why he could start with a testosterone cream.) His energy, mood and hormone levels all improved, and after six months he stopped the progesterone cream.

I will end this section on progesterone by answering a question that my patients regularly ask me: if giving a little is helpful, then why not give a lot? I have yet to see studies on this, but it seems to me that too much progesterone for a man for too long can lower mood and libido. And that makes sense, because some DHT is important in many men for mood and libido, and blocking it excessively – which high levels of progesterone would do – for too long could well be counter productive. If we look at studies on finasteride, which is a powerful DHT-blocker, excessive use can reduce libido and lower mood in men.[57] Once again, balance is everything.

57   Singh, M. K. et al. 'Persistent Sexual Dysfunction and Depression in Finasteride Users for Male Pattern Hair Loss. A Serious Concern or Red Herring?' *J Clin Aesthet Derm* (2014): 7: 51–5.

THE FUTURE

Before we close this chapter it is worth taking a look at where the subject of men's health looks to be heading. A large amount of research has been carried out on developing SARMs, an acronym that stands for selective androgen receptor modulators. SARMs are drugs that mimic the effect of testosterone but do not attach to receptors on the prostate (and elsewhere); that means they might be able to provide the benefits of testosterone without the side effects and risks. The idea is that elderly men could enjoy improved physical function and better health without the long-term side effects to the prostate.[58] That said, the FDA has warned against using SARMs for bodybuilding,[59] and the jury is out on their future.

There is also rising interest in peptides – these are two or more amino acids that, when joined together, make certain hormones. Some hormones, like melatonin and serotonin, are made from the amino acid tryptophan, and – as we have seen – steroid hormones like testosterone are made from cholesterol.

The likes of growth hormones, on the other hand, are made from peptides. As we have seen in this book, giving growth hormone might make us feel and look stronger, but it also tends to burn us out. But this theory, which is fascinating yet which requires more proof for it to become widely accepted, is that if you took the peptide that coded just for building muscle and you injected it into an injured muscle, then you should get a powerful result and very few side effects.

Lastly, we need much more research on how testosterone affects our memory and brain. At this stage we know that: a deficiency of testosterone is connected to cognitive decline;[60] low testosterone levels predispose men to

58   Bhasin, S. et al. 'Testosterone therapy in adult men with androgen deficiency syndromes: An Endocrine Society clinical practice guideline.' *J Clin Endocrinol Metab* (1997): 82: 407–13.
59   'FDA In Brief: FDA warns against using SARMs in body-building products.' Press Release FDA (31 October 2017).
60   Moffat, S. D. et al. 'Longitudinal assessment of serum free testosterone concentration predicts memory performance and cognitive status in elderly men.' *J Clin Endocrinol Metab* (2002): 87: 5001–7.

Alzheimer's;[61] men with prostate cancer who are undergoing a treatment known as androgen-blocking therapy – which blocks the testosterone receptors, meaning testosterone is unable to do its job – have a worsened ability to recount memories and process information;[62] and some studies on memory have shown that supplementing with testosterone seemed to help some men, but in others that effect was less marked. Although we have learned a lot about testosterone in the past two decades, the coming years will teach us much more about this hormone and its effects on the ageing male.

MEN'S HEALTH: A FINAL WORD

Many governments know it makes sense to keep their ageing populations healthy rather than merely treating illnesses when they arise. As we have seen in this book, and will see again, natural hormone replacement therapy is a powerful treatment that can help to keep ageing people in optimal health.

Near the beginning of this chapter I said it needed to answer whether gentle rebalancing using bio-identical hormones would lower the rate of chronic illness in men and extend their healthy life. What have we seen? We know that low testosterone in men is associated with a raft of chronic problems, including metabolic syndrome, Alzheimer's, diabetes and heart disease. We also know that supplementing with testosterone helps to correct metabolic syndrome and diabetes, improves the effects of Alzheimer's, and reduces arterial plaque formation.

But the key, as always, is balance. We need to give an appropriate amount of testosterone depending on the person's circumstances, and we need to test the liver as well as the levels of oestrogen and progesterone to make sure that we are not going to cause more problems than we fix.

One of the newest studies about testosterone – it came out in 2018 – provides a good summary of what we know so far about testosterone

61 Moffat, S. D. et al. 'Free testosterone and risk for Alzheimer's disease in older men.' *Neurology* (2004): 62: 188–93.
62 Beer, T. M. et al. 'Testosterone loss and Estradiol administration modify memory in men.' *J Urol* (2006): 175: 130–5.

replacement: men with low testosterone levels who received testosterone injections over a decade had no serious side effects and had a better quality of life than those who did not take testosterone.[63]

However, unlike hormone replacement therapy in women and the consequences of DHEA levels in the elderly, we still lack definitive evidence that improving testosterone levels allows men to live longer. For now, perhaps it is enough to know that it does no harm, it improves the quality of life and, research shows, it reduces men's chances of suffering from chronic illnesses.

> Key points
> - Low testosterone is associated with the modern chronic illnesses such as heart attacks, diabetes and Alzheimer's.
> - Testosterone replacement has been shown to reduce arterial blockages, improve diabetes, and improve brain functioning in Alzheimer's sufferers.
> - Recent studies have shown testosterone replacement does *not* worsen heart-attack risk.
> - Men's natural production of testosterone improves when they have: a calm brain to send messages to the testes to make testosterone; a good supply of healthy cholesterol to make testosterone; and an unstressed adrenal gland that can make additional testosterone.
> - The liver is critical in removing testosterone from the body. As we age, the liver becomes sluggish, and that means testosterone is not removed efficiently. The result? Men either accumulate oestrogen, which causes moobs and a higher heart-attack risk, or their DHT level rises, causing balding and a thickening of the prostate gland.
> - A sluggish liver can be helped by using liver detoxification

63 Haider, K. S. et al. 'Long-Term Testosterone Therapy Improves Urinary and Sexual Function, and Quality of Life in Men with Hypogonadism: Results from a Propensity Matched Subgroup of a Controlled Registry Study.' *J Urol* (2018): 199: 257–65.

supplements (milk thistle, B-vitamins and glutathione), oestrogen-blockers (indole-3-carbinol, anastrozole) or DHT-blockers (saw palmetto, progesterone, finasteride).

- Among the ways men can naturally enhance their testosterone are sleep, exercise, eating healthy fats, losing weight, and taking zinc and vitamin D.
- Testosterone replacement can be done using natural testosterone creams or with short- or long-acting testosterone injections. There should be no place for testosterone tablets as these can cause liver damage and associated ailments.
- In men, progesterone boosts the immune system, supports the brain, prevents balding and protects the prostate gland.

Chapter 9

WOMEN'S HEALTH – MAKING FIFTY THE NEW THIRTY

> Thirty-five is a very attractive age. London society is full
> of women of the very highest birth who have, of their
> own free choice, remained thirty-five for years.
>
> *Oscar Wilde from* The Importance of Being Earnest

The transition from girlhood to adulthood is one of the key moments in every woman's life, and marks the time when the sex hormones start to dominate. As most parents can testify, the teenage years (for sons and daughters alike) can be heaven or hell; in most cases they are a mix of both.

As you might expect, my clinic sees its fair share of young women, with hormonal issues often the reason: from heavy, painful periods to polycystic ovaries; from mood swings to fertility issues. It would take an entire book to tackle those topics properly and – fascinating though they are – this is not that forum.

Instead, our focus is healthy ageing, and my intent is to examine what happens to a woman's hormones after the age of forty as she approaches menopause, another key moment, but this time when the sex hormones start to fade.

For many women, their conversations with doctors at this stage of their lives will involve the subject of hormone replacement therapy, or HRT, which is the science of rebalancing a woman's decreasing female hormones – oestrogen and progesterone – to support her body as menopause gets underway. During this time her oestrogen can halve and her progesterone can drop to near-undetectable levels. Changes of that magnitude, unsurprisingly, have a huge impact.

The solution – HRT – is so important that it will comprise the bulk of this chapter. Within that we will spend more time on progesterone than on oestrogen, because that is where the key medical conflicts arise, and that is where women can potentially most improve their health.

A central question around menopause is whether a woman should try to do something about it or should simply let nature take its course. In practical terms that leaves her with three options: do nothing; take bio-identical hormones for HRT; or take synthetic hormones for HRT. Each side has its proponents and, as we shall see, the answer depends largely on her situation. After all, we are all different.

HRT has proven a surprisingly controversial medical topic in the past few decades, so before we start I will introduce some of the key questions:

- Is HRT one of the greatest discoveries of the twentieth century or is it a curse? Or, to put it another way, will HRT help you to live longer, or will it cause you to die earlier? We looked at this in the chapter on anabolic versus catabolic hormones, and we shall return to it here in much more detail.
- If HRT is a good idea, then should you take bio-identical HRT or synthetic HRT?
- Should you start taking hormone replacement in your forties at the first sign of ovarian failure or should you wait until you are in the full flow of flushing – that is to say, when you are experiencing the menopausal symptoms?

In the world of hormone replacement, these are deeply contested subjects and, just when we start to think we have the answers, another study comes along that both muddies the waters and adds to our understanding. Just as the teenage hormonal shift can be disturbing to girls, so menopause can be disruptively upsetting to every forty-something woman; getting it right, though, can set her up for good health for the next forty years.

Menopause – the beginning or the end?

Menopause marks the beginning of the end of a woman's fertility, and can be seen as a depressing conclusion to one important stage of life or, possibly, as a new beginning.

Etymologically it comes from two Greek words: *men* (meaning 'monthly') and *pausis* (meaning 'cessation'). Menopause marks the end of a woman's periods, and is medically defined as occurring twelve months after her last period. It is one of the most obvious examples of the power that hormones exert over us.

There are, however, more colourful ways of looking at the subject. Suzanne Somers made the symptoms famous with her Seven Dwarves of Menopause: Itchy; Bitchy; Sleepy; Sweaty; Bloated; Forgetful; and All-Dried-Up. These cover most of the symptoms that women can feel as their sex hormones gear down. It can be an easy transition or, as Somers points out, it can be difficult. Given that women and men in their early fifties often struggle with fatigue, worsening wrinkles and brittle moods as a consequence of their significant hormonal shifts, it is little wonder that many couples are prone to divorce at this time.[1] Menopause (and, for men, andropause) affects people deeply, which is why being able to manage this passage of life successfully can bring great relief.

In theory, a woman can expect hot flushes to begin between the ages of forty-eight and fifty-two. Increasingly, however, I encounter distraught patients in their early forties with these symptoms. It is not clear why this is happening or even whether it is becoming more common, but I find myself wondering whether the stresses of modern life or the raft of toxins to which we are exposed might have something to do with it. Interestingly, research shows that the older a woman is when her menopause arrives, the healthier she can expect to be in later life.[2] Consequently, we would hope that hormonal support for women going through early menopause would extend their health in later years.

Away from the science, there is no question that menopause has attracted a vast amount of media attention in recent decades, not least because it affects women and couples so profoundly. There is a welcome cultural shift

---

1 'Divorce after 50 grows more common.' *The New York Times* (22 September 2013).
2 Gold, E. B. 'The timing of the age at which natural menopause occurs.' *Obstet Gynecol Clin North Am* (2011): 38: 425–40.

underway that tries to view menopause if not positively then at least less negatively. Take this quote by TV host Oprah Winfrey, for instance:

'So many women I've talked to see menopause as an ending – a loss of youth, autonomy and vitality. But I've discovered that the approach of menopause is a knock at the door that can prompt you to finally create the life you've always wanted. This is your moment to reinvent yourself after years of focusing on the needs of everyone else – your mate, your children, your boss. It's your opportunity to get clear about what matters to you and then to pursue that with all of your energy, time and talent.'

What to do about menopause?

You might think that among the many wonders of twenty-first-century medicinal advances – growing stem cells; mapping the human genome; any number of other significant steps forward – we would have solved the seemingly simple question of how to deal with hot flushes and middle-aged spread. You would be wrong. We in the medical profession are still fighting about how best to approach menopause.

That was not always the case. In the 1990s it seemed simple: as a young doctor, I would hand over HRT pills and fully expect that my patient would soon feel like a new woman. By 1999, an estimated 15 million women in the US alone were using HRT.[3] But then things changed: in 2002, the Women's Health Initiative (WHI) – the study-to-end-all-studies that was designed to showcase the wonders of HRT – seemingly concluded anything but.[4]

Within eighteen months of the WHI's results being published, a national survey estimated that around one-third of the women in the US on HRT had stopped treatment.[5] Over the next decade, researchers followed the health of these now HRT-free women and, by 2013, could show that the only thing

3 Hersh, A. L. et al. 'National use of postmenopausal hormone therapy: annual trends and response to recent evidence.' *JAMA* (2004): 291 (1): 47–53.

4 Pal, L. et al. 'The Women's Health Initiative: an unforgettable decade.' *Menopause* (2012): 19: 597–9.

5 Hersh, A. L. et al. 'National use of postmenopausal hormone therapy: annual trends and response to recent evidence.' *JAMA* (2004): 291 (1): 47–53d.

worse than taking HRT was *not* taking HRT: the follow-up estimated that between 18,000 and 90,000 women in the US alone might have died prematurely because they had avoided taking replacement oestrogen.[6]

That is very significant. If you recall from our chapter on anabolic versus catabolic hormones, oestrogen is one of our anabolic, or 'building up', hormones. In that chapter we saw that taking certain anabolic hormones as we age enhances our health and longevity; we will see that this is also true in the case of oestrogen.

For now, though, let us go back to the early 2000s when the results of that study meant many women were told their HRT pills were *not* good for them, which left them wondering what they could do to help their hot flushes. Back then, most HRT pills were made of synthetic hormones, which is why one popular alternative recommended using natural or 'bio-identical' HRT, known as B-HRT. Instead of using synthetic hormones, which the study had apparently shown were problematic, it seemed logical to use the exact – or bio-identical – hormones that the body makes. Logical though it seemed, B-HRT did not solve everything and, as we shall see later, there has been plenty of debate about B-HRT since.

Osteoporosis and HRT

Keeping bones strong is a major benefit for older women, and the WHI trial showed a 24 per cent decrease in bone fractures in women who took Premarin (the oestrogen tablet derived from horse urine).

On average just 2 per cent of women at menopause have osteoporosis, but by age ninety some two-thirds do. Once osteoporosis sets in, a woman who falls and breaks a hip has a one-third chance of recovering, a one-third chance of being bedridden for life, and a one-third chance of dying.

In short, osteoporosis is a serious issue, and preventing it is of

6   Sarrel, P. M. et al. 'The mortality toll of oestrogen avoidance: an analysis of excessive deaths among hysterectomized women aged 50 to 59 years.' *Am J Public Health* (2013): 103: 1583–8.

huge importance for older women. HRT plays a big part in preventing this risk, and so finding the healthiest possible long-term form
of HRT becomes an important consideration.

All of which is to say that there has rarely been such a swing in what we
doctors have advised patients. By way of a summary, our advice went like this:
in the 1990s we told women they should undergo HRT; in the 2000s we
pivoted 180 degrees and warned them off HRT. And now? Well, these days we
know for certain that some form of HRT is better than no HRT, but we are still
arguing about what would be most beneficial.

That said, I would urge you not to be disheartened, because this chapter will
show you some of the expected and unexpected benefits that B-HRT holds over
synthetic HRT, and will explain the controversies around it. My aim is to examine this subject to help readers decide the best approach for dealing with menopause. To that end, the logical place to start is not with the nineteenth-century
discovery of the sex hormones, but decades later – in the 1940s – when pharmaceutical companies began to mass-produce hormonal tablets.

Big Pharma's impact on menopause and health

In the years after World War II, the treatment for menopause was simple: a
woman took oestrogen to stop her hot flushes, and she took progesterone to
balance any negative effects that the oestrogen in the HRT tablets might have
on her uterus. If she had undergone a hysterectomy (the removal of her
uterus) then the procedure was even easier: she just took oestrogen to deal
with the hot flushes and did not need to bother about the progesterone.

It was around this time that a pharmaceutical company later called Wyeth
(and now owned by Pfizer) began making one of the most successful HRTs of
all time: Premarin. It was oestrogen extracted from pregnant horses (thus the
name: PREgnant MARes' urINe), and one pill per day caused hot flushes to
vanish, and probably strengthened bones and skin. The industry then did
what it sometimes does well and sometimes does badly: it conducted studies
in a bid to prove the effectiveness of HRTs.

By the 1990s these studies had become so convincing to so many of us doctors that pharmaceutical firms were able to embark on massive multi-country trials. The idea was that the results would prove so robust that nobody could argue with the outcomes, generating vast profits for the companies concerned and providing a foolproof medical solution for potentially billions of women. As we shall see, it did not work out that way.

Does oestrogen protect the heart?

It has long been known that younger women suffer significantly less heart disease than men of the same age, but that once they go through menopause their heart-attack risk rises and is as frequent as that of men.[7] Disturbingly, women who go through early menopause, defined as being before forty-six, are twice as likely as other women to suffer a heart attack or stroke.[8] That raises two questions:

Before menopause, does a woman's naturally high oestrogen level protect her from heart attacks?

The answer is a resounding yes. Oestrogen acts as an anti-inflammatory and is known to reduce 'harmful' LDL cholesterol in arteries.[9] The chapter on inflammation showed us that, for an artery to block, it first needs to become inflamed (which sugar, smoking and stress contribute to), and that assists inflamed or 'oxidised' LDL cholesterol to stick to the inflamed arterial wall. Too much of that blocks the artery and leads to a heart attack. However, oestrogen's anti-inflammatory and anti-LDL cholesterol abilities prevent that from happening and account in part for the lower heart-attack risk.

7 Barrett-Connor, E. 'Sex differences in coronary heart disease. Why are women so superior?' The 1995 Ancel Keys Lecture. *Circulation* (1997): 95: 252–64

8 Wellons, M. 'Early menopause associated with increased risk of heart disease, stroke.' *John Hopkins Medicine* (2012).

9 Campos, H. et al. 'Effect of oestrogen on very low-dose density lipoprotein and low density lipoprotein subclass metabolism in postmenopausal women.' *J Clin Endocrinol Metab* (1997): 82 (12): 3955–63.

Bourassa, P. et al. 'Oestrogen reduces atherosclerotic lesion development in apolipoprotein E-deficient mice.' *Proc Natl Acad Sci USA* (1996): 10022–7.

That said, oestrogen's main reason for preventing heart attacks appears to be because it relaxes the arteries. This improves blood flow and, over the long term, prevents plaque blockages in arteries.[10] The reason her heart-attack risk increases to that of a man of the same age once she reaches menopause is in large part because her oestrogen level halves, and that means she loses this protective advantage.[11]

After menopause, does oestrogen replacement protect women from heart attacks?

You would think it does, but it turns out that this is a much more complex question. Studies on animals strongly suggest that oestrogen replacement is beneficial: they show that oestrogen protects them from arterial blockages and heart attacks. But animal studies are not the same as human studies, and we had to wait until the 1990s for a large study called the Nurses' Health Study to show that HRT given to post-menopausal women gave them up to 50 per cent greater protection against heart attacks.[12] This was enough to make the 1990s the decade of HRT use.

The studies that followed, however, threatened to upend everything.

THE KEY HRT STUDIES

In 1996, researchers started the Heart and Estrogen/Progestin Replacement Study, known as HERS. It followed nearly 3,000 women, and was expected to show once

10   Mendelsohn, M. E. and Karas, R. H. 'The protective effects of oestrogen on the cardiovascular system.' *N Engl J Med* (1990): 340: 1111–801.
11   Barrett-Connor, E. 'Sex differences in coronary heart disease. Why are women so superior? The 1995 Ancel keys lecture.' *Circulation* (1997): 95: 252–64.
12   Grodstein, F. et al. 'Postmenopausal estrogen and progestin use and the risk of cardiovascular disease.' *N Engl J Med* (1996): 335 (7): 453–61.

and for all that an HRT combination of oestrogen plus progestin would significantly benefit women and, in particular, would reduce their heart-attack risk.[13]

That did not happen. By 2002, early results from HERS stunned the world when they showed that the combination had the opposite effect. *The New York Times* described the results as 'sobering', and concluded: 'HERS found that far from protecting women from heart attacks, the combination therapy actually increased their risk in the first few years of taking the drug'.[14]

Then came the largest of all these studies: the Women's Health Initiative (WHI). Like the HERS research, the WHI was expected to show that HRT was a healthy choice for menopausal woman.[15] To that end, the WHI study provided Premarin to 150,000 menopausal women across the globe to show how effective, beneficial and safe these tablets were. The early results that came out in 2004 were so unexpectedly bad that they put off hundreds of thousands of women from taking any form of HRT. The array of side effects saw the WHI study shelved that same year.[16]

It is important to look at this study to work out what happened, and that means starting with how it was structured. The participants were divided into two groups: those who had had a hysterectomy (meaning their uterus had been removed) and those who had not. Why this distinction? It comes down to the effects that oestrogen and progesterone have: oestrogen is effective at stopping hot flushes, but it also increases the risk of cancer of the uterus; progesterone, on the other hand, protects from that cancer.

For this reason the women in the first group received only oestrogen,

13   Blakely, J. A. 'The Heart and Estrogen/Progestin Replacement Study Revisited. Hormone Replacement Therapy Produced Net Harm, Consistent With the Observational Data.' *JAMA* (2000): 160: 2897–900.

14   'Hormone Replacement Study A Shock to the Medical System', *The New York Times* (10 July 2002). Accessed at: http://www.nytimes.com/2002/07/10/us/hormone-replacement-study-a-shock-to-the-medical-system.html?pagewanted=all

15   Grodstein, F. et al. 'Postmenopausal hormone therapy and mortality.' *N Engl J Med* (1997): 336: 1769–76.

16   Rossouw, E. et al. 'Lessons learned from the Women's Health Initiative trials of menopausal hormone therapy.' *Obstet Gynecol* (2003): 121: 172–6. Accessed at: https://www.ncbi.nlm.nih.gov/pmc/articles/PMC3547645/

because – as they no longer had a uterus – their body did not need the protective aspect that progesterone conveys. The women in the second group were
given both oestrogen and a synthetic form of progesterone called progestin.
Although progestin looks similar to progesterone, it is synthetic and therefore
different, and that would turn out to be important.

WHI Group 1: oestrogen-only HRT

For those of us who were following the WHI study, progress seemed a matter
of two steps forward and one step back: by 2004 we knew that taking the oral
oestrogen Premarin caused a nearly 50 per cent increase in blood clots. That
sounds frightening, but in practice it only meant a rise from fifteen clots to
twenty-two clots per 10,000 women. Overall, that is still not a big risk of
developing a blood clot, but the truth is that we do not want any clotting risk
at all. (The reason for this increased risk was that the oestrogen was taken
orally, and that meant it went from the stomach to the liver where a reaction
took place that saw the blood thickened; we will see later that using oestrogen
cream avoids that risk, and is today our first choice.)

The authors of the WHI study concluded three things: firstly, that taking
oestrogen orally worsened the risk of blood clots, which meant a higher chance
of a stroke or pulmonary embolism (which is clotting in the lungs); secondly,
that despite the fact that oestrogen is a natural artery-protector, oestrogen in the
form of Premarin did not help or worsen a woman's heart-attack risk; and
thirdly, that Premarin did protect against osteoporosis and hip fractures.[17]

In other words, the results were not that bad – they showed that oestrogen
taken as a tablet helped to keep bones strong, and neither improved nor worsened a woman's heart-attack risk. That said, it did increase her risk of a stroke
when taken orally. On the other hand, Premarin applied as a cream, not taken
as a tablet, stopped hot flushes, built up the bones and caused no ill effects,
making it a mildly beneficial anabolic hormone.

17 Anderson, G. L. et al. 'Effects of conjugated equine estrogen in postmenopausal women
with hysterectomy: the Women's Health Initiative randomized controlled trial.' *JAMA*
(2004): 291: 1701–12.

WHI Group 2: oestrogen and progestin HRT

This is where the wheels of the WHI really came off. This second group of women received oestrogen *and* progestin because they still had their uteruses. Adding progestin (of a type called medroxyprogesterone) saw the incidence of strokes increase 41 per cent, breast cancer rise 26 per cent and heart attacks 29 per cent.[18] This really was bad news, and it was the results in this progestin group that saw the study ended prematurely.

Little wonder that *The New York Times* headlined its article 'Hormone Replacement Study A Shock to the Medical System'. It was no less of a shock to investors in Wyeth, whose share price halved as the pharmaceutical juggernaut that prescribed pills for hot flushes ground to a halt.[19]

It was a rude awakening for those accustomed to the wonders of medicine. After all, many of the women in the studies had benefited from the emancipation brought by the invention of the contraceptive pill. Many questions were asked, perhaps none better than by R. K. Dubey of the Center for Clinical Pharmacology at the University of Pittsburgh's Medical Center, who wrote, in an article that made its purpose succinctly: 'What went wrong, and where do we go from here?'

Dubey concluded that the problem with the WHI trial was that it used the wrong oestrogen – equilin (which is extracted from horse urine) rather than human oestradiol; it used the wrong progesterone – synthetic provera instead of natural progesterone; and that oestrogen was given by the wrong route – orally, not through the skin.

The state of confusion was not limited to the US, where the study originated. At the time I was practising in the UK, and the fallout left my peers and me with little advice to offer women who came to our clinics suffering from menopausal symptoms. The media lost little time in offering their solutions, which ranged from yoga to exotic herbs like black cohosh.

---

18 Rossouw, J. et al. 'Writing group for the Women's Health Initiative randomized controlled trial.' *JAMA* (2002): 288: 321–33.
19 Accessed at: http://www.icis.com/resources/news/2002/07/17/177264/wyeth-shares-fall-11-to-new-low-on-hormone-drug-fears/

Two steps forward

The noughties, then, was a time of bad news in the world of HRT, but by 2012 matters began to move in the right direction when researchers released yet more studies.

Although many of the women on the WHI study had stopped taking HRT, some continued to do so, and scientists monitored many of them (and others) for the next eight years. They found that women who had previously been taking Premarin – the oestrogen tablet – were healthy, whereas women who had never taken HRT were dying prematurely. That told the scientists that although Premarin came with a clotting risk, as we saw earlier, *not* taking any hormone at all increased a woman's chance of dying earlier.[20] The conclusion is that oestrogen is protective for women, which matches my belief that this anabolic hormone helps women to live longer.

A small Danish study was also released around that time that took what we had learned from the WHI results and made some improvements. The WHI study had given HRT to women who were predominantly in their sixties; this study, on the other hand, gave HRT to women aged forty-five to fifty-eight whose menopause was just beginning. As part of that they also used a better progestin, this one called norethisterone. After a decade of using this combination of HRT, the women on the Danish study showed improved protection from heart attacks, and were not at increased risk of a stroke.[21] This was the start of a renewed move towards finding hormones that help women to live longer.

In summary then, we can say the following:

- Replacing hormones benefits menopausal women and, provided we choose the right ones, can be healthier than taking nothing.[22]

---

20   Sarrel, P. M. et al. 'The mortality toll of oestrogen avoidance: an analysis of excessive deaths among hysterectomized women aged 50 to 59 years.' *Am J Public Health* (2013): 103: 1583–8.

21   Schierbeck, L. L. et al. 'Effect of hormone replacement therapy on cardiovascular events in recently post-menopausal women: randomised trial'. *BMJ* (2012): 345: e6409.

22   Sarrel, P. M. et al. 'The mortality toll of oestrogen avoidance: an analysis of excessive deaths among hysterectomized women aged 50 to 59 years.' *Am J Public Health* (2013): 103: 1583–8.

- Natural oestrogen, which is called oestradiol, has proven to be a better choice than Premarin as it not only strengthens bones, but also protects from heart attacks.
- The dangerous element of HRT was shown to be the progestin, called medroxyprogesterone, that was used in the WHI trial; it was shown to lead to strokes, cancer and heart attacks.

My preferred approach to HRT

I am glad to say that our understanding of HRT has improved a lot, and it continues to do so. My clinic recommends that our menopausal patients take oestrogen as a cream (transdermally), because in this way the oestrogen does not get dumped into the liver, and that means avoiding an increased risk of blood clots.[23]

To that end, we also use only bio-identical oestrogen, which is called oestradiol. (Bio-identical hormones are also sometimes called 'natural' hormones to distinguish them from synthetic hormones.) Not only did the Danish study show that oestradiol was safe to use and was part of the solution in helping to prevent heart attacks, but because it occurs naturally in our blood we can easily measure it and keep it at safe levels. We cannot measure the levels of synthetic oestrogen in the blood, and that means we do not know whether the patient has absorbed too much or too little.

The final question to answer is whether women should use progestin, which is a synthetic progesterone, or a bio-identical progesterone.

Natural versus synthetic progesterone

Natural progesterone is called, logically enough, progesterone; synthetic progesterone is called progestin. We will see that they can have quite different effects on the body.

At the risk of stating the obvious, the majority of women on HRT have not had a hysterectomy and therefore still have their uterus. And so, if they are

---

23   Renoux, C. et al. 'Transdermal and oral hormone replacement therapy and the risk of stroke: a nested case-control study.' *BMJ* (2010): 340: c2519.

taking oestrogen (which worsens the risk of uterine cancer), then they need to take a progesterone too because that will protect against that risk.

The WHI study showed that the biggest problem with their HRT came not from oestrogen, but from the progestin (medroxyprogesterone), and it was this that caused a higher risk of breast cancer, strokes and heart attacks.[24] The Danish study showed that a different progestin (norethisterone) in younger women had a much better risk profile.[25]

What about natural progesterone, though? We know that oestrogen can stimulate uterine cancer, and so it is logical given that it stimulates the uterus to thicken – thereby preparing it for pregnancy – that *continuous* stimulation could increase the cancer risk. Progestins have a powerful effect on the uterus and they comfortably suppress any risk of this cancer. The concern with natural progesterone is that it is not strong enough to protect women from this risk in the standard dosage. In 2014, though, an excellent French study showed that, although natural progesterone given at a low dosage (100mg) is not strong enough to protect against uterine cancer,[26] it referenced other research that showed natural progesterone *is* protective when given at doses above 200mg.[27]

The same researchers carried out another study on 81,000 women that showed that while natural progesterone protects against breast cancer, progestins worsen that risk.[28] A meta-analysis in 2016 drew the same conclusions.[29]

24   Rossouw, J. et al. 'Writing group for the Women's Health Initiative randomized controlled trial.' *JAMA* (2002): 288: 321–33.

25   Schierbeck, L. L. et al. 'Effect of hormone replacement therapy on cardiovascular events in recently post-menopausal women: randomised trial'. *BMJ* (2012): 345: e6409.

26   Fournier, A. et al. 'Risks of endometrial cancer associated with different hormone replacement therapies in the E3N Cohort, 1992–2008.' *Am J Epidemiol Advance Access* (2014): 10: 1093.

27   'The effects of estrogen or estrogen/progestin regimens on heart attack risk factors in post menopausal women. The Postmenopausal oestrogen Progesterone trial (PEPI trial).' *JAMA* (1995): 273: 199–208. Accessed at: https://www.ncbi.nlm.nih.gov/pubmed/7807658

Moyer, D. L. et al. 'Micronized progesterone regulation of the endometrial glandular cycling pool.' *Int J Gynecol Pathol* (2001): 20: 374–9.

28   Fournier, A. et al. 'Unequal risks for breast cancer associated with different hormonal replacement therapies: results from the E3N cohort study.' *Breast Cancer Res Treat* (2008): 107: 103–11.

29   Asi, N. et al. 'Progesterone vs synthetic progestins and the risk of breast cancer: a systematic review and meta-analysis.' *Syst Rev* (2016): 5: 121.

Progesterone, it turns out, protects against breast cancer by modifying oestrogen receptors, and that slows down the growth effect that oestrogen has on breast tissue; less growth means less risk of cancer.

Our understanding of progesterone levels and a woman's heart-attack risk has also evolved in recent years. The WHI study showed that the progestin (medroxyprogesterone) given to women older than sixty worsened their heart-attack risk, whereas the Danish study showed that giving younger women (aged forty-five to fifty-eight) a different progestin (norethisterone) improved their heart-attack risk. And a much earlier study from the 1990s found that natural progesterone did a better job of protecting against the risk factors of heart disease.[30]

Finally, both progesterone and progestin have been shown to protect against ovarian cancer[31] – the seventh most common cancer in women.

Figure 1: Comparing progesterone and progestin

PROTECTIVE EFFECTS OF PROGESTERONE VERSUS PROGESTINS	
NATURAL PROGESTERONE	PROGESTINS
Protects against breast cancer	Worsens breast cancer
Moderately protects against cardiovascular disease	Mixed results
Protects against ovarian cancer	Protects against ovarian cancer
Above 200mg, protects against uterine cancer	Protects against uterine cancer

30 'The effects of estrogen or estrogen/progestin regimens on heart attack risk factors in post menopausal women. The Postmenopausal oestrogen Progesterone trial (PEPI trial).' *JAMA* (1995): 273: 199–208. Accessed at: https://www.ncbi.nlm.nih.gov/pubmed/7807658
31 Diep, C. H. et al. 'Progesterone action in breast, uterine, and ovarian cancers.' *J Mol Endocrinol* (2015): 54: R31–R53.

The chart above summarises progesterone and progestin, and shows clearly why the natural (or bio-identical) form of progesterone is either as beneficial or superior to progestin. Breast cancer is by far the most common cancer in women in the UK, being six times more prevalent than uterine cancer and nearly eight times more common than ovarian cancer.[32]

My conclusion is that wherever possible women should use natural progesterone.

THREE QUESTIONS

I am going to spend the rest of this chapter answering the three most common questions that I get asked. All three are excellent, because they require in-depth explanations, and this means that in just a few pages' time you will have a comprehensive understanding of HRT and the menopausal hormones.

The questions are:

- Is it safe *not* to take HRT during menopause?
- Does it ever make sense to start taking progesterone *before* the menopause begins?
- And – a question we have not yet even examined – why would I need to take the 'male' hormone testosterone during menopause?

Is it safe not *to take HRT during menopause?*

In the arguments so far about whether to take synthetic or natural hormones, we have so far ignored the third option: taking no HRT medication. In my opinion, if someone is suffering from hot flushes, low mood and is sleeping badly, then she would do well with some form of hormonal help. The HRT hormones also help to strengthen a woman's bones for future years. However, some women have much milder symptoms and choose not to take anything throughout their menopause.

Oestrogen has a vast array of tasks – from improving mood to overseeing

---

32 'Cancer incidence for common cancers.' Cancer Research UK. Accessed at: http://www.cancerresearchuk.org/health-professional/cancer-statistics/incidence/common-cancers-compared#heading-Two

pregnancy to making the skin glow, among others. One under-recognised job that oestrogen does is to prevent fat-formation around the midriff. American science writer Gary Taubes describes this in his 2010 book, *Why We Get Fat And What To Do About It*, in which he explains how the fat we eat is carried around the bloodstream in boats called lipoproteins. When these boats get to fat cells, an enzyme called lipoprotein lipase, or LPL, encourages the fat to enter the fat cells. When our LPL is active, we tend to be very good at packing away fat, and that makes us put on weight.[33]

Which brings us to oestrogen and one of its lesser-known roles – in this case, blocking LPL from doing its job.[34] Logically enough, the less able LPL is to pack away the fat in our fat cells, the less weight we will put on. We see this in teenagers: the oestrogen surge typically puts on the curves and, by blocking LPL, keeps her midriff hourglass-thin. But when menopause comes around and oestrogen levels drop, this lack of oestrogen allows LPL to come out and build that middle-aged spread, or the fatty deposits, around the abdomen. It is a common concern for menopausal women at my clinic: indeed, aside from the hot flushes, worsening abdominal fat is their next biggest worry.

Annoying though it is, middle-aged spread has a very important role in women. Once this fatty layer develops, the body will use it as an oestrogen-forming machine: it takes testosterone and converts it into oestrogen in the fat cells. This will then settle the hot flushes and give the woman enough oestrogen to strengthen her bones over the next forty years. Her middle-aged spread becomes a hormone factory that takes over from the ovaries, a sterling example of the genius of nature.

One of the touted benefits of HRT is that it prevents middle-aged spread.[35] That raises an obvious question: if a woman's fat cells are so important, then why

---

33 Rinninger, F. et al. 'Lipoprotein lipase mediates an increase in the selective uptake of high density lipoprotein-associated cholesteryl esters by hepatic cells in culture.' *J Lipid Res* (1998): 39 (7): 1335–48.

34 Price, T. M. et al. 'Oestrogen regulation of adipose tissue lipoprotein lipase – possible mechanism of body fat distribution.' *Am J Obstet Gynecol* (1998): 178: 101–7.

35 Sumino, H. et al. 'Effects of hormone replacement therapy on weight, abdominal fat distribution and lipid levels in Japanese postmenopausal women.' *Int J Obes* (2003): 1044–51.

take HRT in an effort to stop them from forming? My answer would be that many of my patients love the fact that applying oestrogen cream ends their hot flushes *and* stops them putting on weight,[36] but I would also say there is a perfectly sound argument that a woman who is healthy, who is not flushing much and who is not adding much body fat might prefer to avoid HRT medication and allow her body to produce the oestrogen it needs for the coming decades.

LPL and insulin

There is an important connection here between LPL, the shelf-packer for fat, and insulin, which does a similar thing by packing away glucose in our cells as fat. Briefly, insulin will sometimes team up with LPL and together these terrible twins work to accelerate fat formation.[37]

It works like this: if LPLs are pushing fat into cells, and you decide to knock back a sugary drink, for instance, then your body experiences a rush of sugar and then insulin, whose job is to pack away glucose as fat in our fat cells. This combination of insulin and LPL accelerates the fat-storing effect.

In the chapter on inflammation we saw that up to 80 per cent of people could have insulin resistance from eating too many carbohydrates. Studies suggest that women who enter menopause with even mild insulin resistance are the ones who put on the most weight when the flushes start.[38] It is wise, then, to be even more cautious about diet during menopause. Or, as one of my patients put it, to deal with menopause you need to halve your sugar intake and double your exercise.

36   Jensen, L. B. et al. 'Hormone replacement therapy dissociates fat mass and bone mass and tends to reduce weight gain in early menopausal women: A randomized prevention study.' *J Bone Miner Res* (2003): Vol 18: 333–42.

37   Sadur, C. N. et al. 'Insulin stimulation of adipose tissue lipoprotein lipase. Use of the euglycaemic clamp technique.' *J Clin Invest* (1982): 69: 1119–25.

38   Howard, B. V. et al. 'Insulin resistance and weight gain in post-menopausal women of diverse ethnic groups.' *Int J Obes Relat Metab Disord* (2004): 28: 1039–47.

Does it ever make sense to start taking progesterone before menopause begins?

We saw earlier that progesterone protects the uterus. However, it has many other roles than that, and a stressed woman in her forties can show signs of lowered progesterone long before she experiences her first hot flush. The effects of low progesterone are clear in the following three scenarios: heavy periods, mental irritability, and pimples and facial hair.

Heavy periods: women in their forties can find their periods become heavier and more erratic. This is because, while oestrogen causes the lining of the uterus to thicken, the lack of progesterone results in inflammation and heavy bleeding.[39] Boosting her progesterone reduces the amount of bleeding, restores her hormonal balance and decreases the risk of needing surgery on the uterus.[40]

Mental irritability: glutamate is a neurotransmitter that helps us to think fast, but too much stress or too much coffee cause the brain to release too much glutamate, and that excess irritates the brain. One of progesterone's functions is to remove glutamate, which means it has a significant calming influence on the brain.[41] Progesterone also stimulates GABA, which is a calming neurotransmitter (which is incidentally how drugs like Valium work).[42] Too much progesterone, however, can cause a person's mood to drop, because it stimulates an enzyme that breaks down our happy hormone serotonin.[43] In other words, although progesterone has a strongly calming effect on the brain, too much of it can lower our mood.

Pimples and facial hair: it is common that women in their early forties find they have more facial hair and are getting pimples. And while it is easy to assume that high testosterone is the culprit, in many cases blood

---

39 Maybin, J. A. et al. 'Menstrual physiology: implications for endometrial pathology and beyond.' *Human Reprod* (2015): 21: 748–61.
40 Maybin, J. A. et al. 'Medical management of heavy menstrual bleeding.' *Women's Health (Long)* (2016): 12: 27–34.
41 Smith, S. S. et al. 'Progesterone alters GABA and glutamate responsiveness: a possible mechanism for its anxiolytic action.' *Brain Res* (1987): 400: 353–9.
42 Wang, M. 'Neurosteroids and GABA-A Receptor Function.' *Front Endocrin* (2011): 2: 44.
43 Luine, V. N. et al. 'Gonadal hormone regulation of MAO and other enzymes in hypothalamic areas.' *Neuroendocrinology* (1983): 36 (3): 235–41.

tests show their testosterone level is in fact very low. The real problem is low progesterone. Why? Because progesterone is the liver's natural gateway that prevents certain testosterones from converting into the pimple-forming and hair-forming hormone DHT. If a woman has a low progesterone level, then her body is able to make more DHT, and that means more pimples and facial hair. Incidentally, this is also why some women notice pimples just before their period, because that is a time when their progesterone level drops. The solution is to supplement with natural progesterone.[44]

In other words, if a forty-something woman is starting to struggle with the worsening PMS symptoms of heavy periods, irritability, pimples or increased facial hair, then supporting with natural progesterone in the second half of her cycle can be helpful. In medical terms, as we saw earlier, menopause starts twelve months after a woman's final period. But the hot flushes start before her periods end, and it is at this time that many women start taking oestrogen to prevent those flushes, along with progesterone to protect the uterus. This stage of the transition is called the perimenopause.

However, it is common for women to suffer from what I refer to as the pre-menopause at a much earlier stage. Symptoms include worsening PMS or irritability before the period, heavy periods, fatigue, low mood, low libido and even a worsening of inflammatory conditions such as asthma and arthritis – and all of this in their early forties. Whereas her hot flushes are caused by declining levels of oestrogen, the other symptoms are typically due to faltering progesterone levels. That means it is important to understand better what progesterone does and, in turn, where it is made.

We will start by answering the second part first: progesterone is produced both by the ovaries and by the adrenal glands. Typically we view the role of progesterone made in the ovaries as being to help prevent cancer of the uterus, and we view the role of progesterone made in the adrenal glands as being to help make cortisol (as well as DHEA and testosterone) for the

44 Cassidenti, D. L. et al. 'Effects of sex steroids on skin 5 alpha-reductase activity in vitro.' *Obstet Gynecol* (1991): 78: 103–7.

adrenals.[45] But of course the body being as well designed as it is can use progesterone from either source for either of these tasks – and that is why this discussion is so important: because once a woman reaches menopause (and her uterus produces less progesterone), she might rely on her adrenal glands to make progesterone both for cortisol *and* for protection against uterine cancer. You can imagine that if her adrenal glands are tired then, as she reaches menopause and her progesterone is pulled in two different directions, she might start to exhibit some adrenal-related problems. Having less progesterone could see her produce less cortisol, and that could leave her at risk of worsening any inflammatory problems she already has, such as asthma or arthritis.

But is that what happens? The truth is that research on the topic of 'how does a low progesterone level affect the rest of the body' is scanty at best, which means proving this link is tricky. To see what the science says we shall look at three scenarios of illnesses that are linked to inflammation and low cortisol: asthma, arthritis and emotional stress. We shall see whether they worsen with low progesterone and whether they improve as we replace the progesterone.

Asthma

Asthma affects one in twelve adults in the UK, and it is not only life-threatening but common, which makes it doubly worth examining. One of asthma's characteristics is that it worsens as cortisol blood levels drop, so if we are correct in theorising that progesterone from the ovaries can assist in making cortisol in the adrenals, then we would expect an asthmatic woman's asthma to worsen during episodes of low progesterone.

That was indeed the finding of a 1996 study of 182 female asthmatics, which concluded that they were most likely to be hospitalised for an asthma attack just before their period when progesterone levels are typically at their

45 Payne, A. H. et al. 'Overview of steroidogenic enzymes in the pathway from cholesterol to active steroid hormones.' *Endocr Rev* (2004): 25 (6): 947–70.

lowest.[46] Other studies have shown a direct connection between progesterone and asthma: one showed that asthmatic women's breathing gets more difficult when their progesterone levels are at their lowest;[47] another showed that as menopausal women's progesterone levels dropped, their asthma attacks worsened.[48]

We already know that progesterone is converted into cortisol. Also these studies indicate that asthma is caused by low cortisol levels and that, at times like menopause – when the ovaries decrease their progesterone production – asthma will worsen. In other words, these studies seem to suggest that low progesterone causes low cortisol which worsens asthma.

All of these studies, however, are studies of association – they show a link, but they do not *prove* that low progesterone causes asthma (even though we know that progesterone is an anti-inflammatory and on its own will relax the lungs and improve asthma).[49] What we needed was a study that would show that adding progesterone would lead directly to the body using it to make more cortisol. However, two pieces of research have given contradictory results on that. One, published in 2001, showed that giving HRT to fifty-five asthmatic, post-menopausal women *improved their cortisol levels*, reduced their asthma symptoms and cut their need for cortisol inhalers.[50] However, a second published a few years later found that HRT did not improve asthma in menopausal women.[51]

46 Skobelov, E. M., Spivey, W. H. et al. 'The effect of the menstrual cycle on asthma presentations in the emergency department.' *Ann Intern Med* (1996): 156: 1837–40.

47 Hanley, S. P. 'Asthma variation with menstruation.' *Br J Dis Chest* (1981): 75: 306–8.

48 Barr, R. G., Wentowski, C. C. et al, 'Prospective study of postmenopausal hormone use and newly diagnosed asthma and chronic obstructive pulmonary disease.' *Arch Intern Med* (2004): 164 (4): 379–86.

49 Foster, P. S., Goldie, R. G., Paterson, J. W. 'Effect of steroids on β-adrenoceptor-mediated relaxation of pig bronchus.' *Br J Pharmacol* (1983): 78: 441–5.

50 Kos-Kudla, B. et al. 'Effects of hormone replacement therapy on endocrine and spiro-metric parameters in asthmatic postmenopausal women.' *Gynecol Endocrinol* (2001): 15: 304–11.

51 Barr, R. G., Wentowski, C. C. et al, 'Prospective study of postmenopausal hormone use and newly diagnosed asthma and chronic obstructive pulmonary disease.' *Arch Intern Med* (2004): 164 (4): 379–86.

Why might that be? One possible answer is that although progesterone improves asthma, the oestrogen in the HRT can worsen it. But the truth is at this stage we simply do not know. Medicine is, after all, a work in progress. Specifically, then, when it comes to giving progesterone to menopausal asthmatics, the evidence shows that it is probably helpful to do so, but we need more research to be certain.

Arthritis

Studies have shown that progesterone has a role to play in preventing other inflammatory illnesses like rheumatoid arthritis. Researchers have shown that a woman's rheumatoid arthritis improves during times of high progesterone,[52] and worsens during menopause when her progesterone levels are low.[53]

We know that progesterone is anti-inflammatory which will help her joints, and we also know that by boosting cortisol it improves our immune system.[54] However, at this stage we lack enough evidence to say that we should treat rheumatoid arthritis by using progesterone to boost cortisol levels.

Stress

There are few better ways to see how progesterone affects cortisol than by looking at the stress response. Stress has a huge impact on the ovaries and the menstrual cycle – for example, female students writing final exams can find their period stops for some months. Stress has an equally big impact on the adrenal glands, causing both cortisol and progesterone levels to rise.[55] This makes sense as both hormones are needed to repair the body and calm the brain after a stressful event.

52 Miyaura, H. 'Direct and indirect inhibition of Th1 development by progesterone and glucocorticoids.' *J Immunol* (2002): 168: 1087–94.
Hughes, G. C. 'Progesterone and autoimmune disease.' *Autoimmun Rev* (2012): 11: A502–14.
53 Sammaritano, L. R. 'Menopause in patients with autoimmune diseases.' *Autoimmun Rev* (2012): 11: A430–6.
54 Schulze-Koops, H. 'The balance of Th1/Th2 cytokines in rheumatoid arthritis.' *Best Pract Res Clin Rheumatol* (2001): 15: 677–91.
55 Herrera, A. Y. et al. 'Stress-induced increases in progesterone and cortisol in naturally cycling women.' *Neurobiol Stress* (2016): 3: 96–104.

The question here is whether ongoing physical or emotional stress exhausts cortisol, and then uses up progesterone in an effort to make more cortisol. A study of women aged eighteen to forty-four found that those who were under emotional stress had a much higher incidence of PMS, with more irritability, pain and swelling.[56] This suggested that emotional stress does use up cortisol, which causes the body to convert more progesterone to cortisol, and that this relative decline in their levels of progesterone means they suffer worse PMS.

Another study looked at women undergoing the physical stress of playing sport. We know that during a tough sporting challenge such as a long run on a treadmill, a woman's cortisol levels should spike to help her body cope with this stress, but that does not always happen. Researchers found that women who were suffering from PMS had low progesterone levels and, as a result, did not have a cortisol spike and performed poorly on the treadmill. However, after being given progesterone, their cortisol levels improved as did their sporting performance.[57] Giving progesterone allowed the body to use the hormone to make essential cortisol.

Summary

These studies suggest to me that low progesterone is associated with asthma, rheumatoid arthritis and poor sporting performance. Supplementing with progesterone, then, might improve cortisol levels – thereby helping inflammatory illnesses such as asthma – improve the stress response and in that way boost sporting performance. In other words, although progesterone has a key role in protecting the uterus against cancer, it also has a very important role supporting the adrenal gland and the immune system.

And that tells me that we need to be mindful to supplement progesterone in any pre-menopausal woman who already has adrenal insufficiency. And that, in short, is why I disagree with the standard HRT approach to

56 Accessed at: http://www.nih.gov/news-events/news-releases/prior-stress-could-worsen-premenstrual-symptoms-nih-study-finds

57 Roca, C. A. et al. 'Differential menstrual cycle regulation of hypothalamic-pituitary-adrenal axis in women with premenstrual syndrome and controls.' *J Clin Endocrinol Metab* (2003): 88: 3057–63.

menopause, which says that a woman who has had a hysterectomy should get *only* oestrogen, because she no longer has a uterus to protect. If her adrenal glands are robust and able to produce enough progesterone and cortisol then that would be fine. But everyone is different, and in this case withholding progesterone from a woman who has weak adrenal glands could increase her chance of developing or worsening asthma, rheumatoid arthritis and possibly other auto-immune diseases.

When doing a blood test for menopause, we doctors should always check the levels of a woman's adrenal hormones: cortisol, DHEA and testosterone. If any of these are low and she shows symptoms of adrenal insufficiency (which you can refresh yourself about in the chapter on stress), then her doctor should probably provide progesterone support.

I hope that this foray into the world of progesterone has shown why some women are lucky enough not to need any hormonal support during menopause, but that many will need some. I hope it has also made clear the reasons for the type of support they will need.

What we can say with certainty is that natural progesterone is superior to synthetic progestins, because it protects from breast cancer and heart disease. And at sufficient dosages it also protects against uterine cancer.

We also know that some women with strong adrenal glands and few menopausal symptoms will not need any support during the menopause. Others with weak adrenals or problems of asthma and arthritis might already be low in progesterone, and so withholding progesterone could worsen those conditions.

Outside of these key benefits, of course, progesterone is also a powerful hormone that calms inflammation in the body and the brain.

Why would I need to take the male hormone testosterone during menopause?

The third question I am often asked by patients starting HRT is whether they should take testosterone, and why.

After hot flushes and weight gain, testosterone deficiency is probably the most disturbing part of menopause. Low testosterone causes anxiety, low energy, flabby muscles and low libido; supplementing with testosterone often gives a woman a noticeable boost of energy and confidence (which is one reason it is abused by some men and women).

That said, there are some points worth noting about testosterone.

Testosterone and the adrenal glands: a woman's testosterone level, which is around a tenth that of a man's, varies throughout her cycle. It comes from two sources: her adrenal glands make testosterone throughout the month, and her ovaries boost the level on day fourteen when she ovulates. This boosts her sex drive, or libido, when she is at her most fertile. In other words, a woman relies on her adrenal glands to supply testosterone for most of the month. As with progesterone, if her adrenal glands are not working efficiently then she will have low testosterone levels through much of her cycle.

Testosterone and the contraceptive pill: younger women taking the pill often show a lack of testosterone, and they can as a result show signs of anxiety, low energy and reduced libido. A blood test will typically show very low testosterone levels – and it is often the pill that is to blame. A meta-analysis in 2014 showed it does not matter which pill (or combined oral contraceptive, to give it its medical name) is being used: the testosterone of the young women in the studies plummeted.[58]

Testosterone and libido: libido is central to what many people consider a happy and successful life. Decades of studies have shown that testosterone in men and women is key to their libido and to the intimacy this brings.[59] But, as men's and women's testosterone levels drop in their forties, their libido and joy for life can slide too. Research has shown that testosterone replacement for men and women improves their sexual enjoyment and intimacy with their partner.[60]

58 Zimmerman, Y. et al. 'The effect of combined oral contraception on testosterone in healthy women: a systematic review and meta-analysis.' *Hum Reprod Update* (2014): 20: 76–105.

59 Persky, H. et al. 'Plasma testosterone level and sexual behaviour of couples.' *Arch Sex Behav* (1978): 7: 157–73.

60 Goldstat, R. et al. 'Transdermal testosterone therapy improves well-being, mood and sexual function in premenopausal women.' *Menopause* (2003): 10: 390–8.

Testosterone, though, has a much more important role in a woman's health than being simply a 'feel-good' hormone. It is as important in women as it is in men, and is central to the health of the heart, the brain and the immune system.

Testosterone and heart health

Heart disease is the leading cause of death in women in the US, claiming about one in five lives, just ahead of cancer. However, heart attacks in women under fifty differ from those in men under fifty: in men of that age, a heart attack is usually because an artery blocks; in women under fifty, the spread of cholesterol in their arteries is usually more even – which is harder to detect, but which can result in the artery going into spasm, damaging the heart.[61] That changes once menopause starts: as her hormone levels drop, a woman's arteries start to clog in the same way that a man's arteries do, raising her chance of having a heart attack caused by an arterial blockage.

There are obvious lifestyle issues that affect the chances of having a heart attack in women over fifty – smoking, stress, sugar and bad fats are important there. But her hormones are implicated too. For instance, oestrogen has been shown to cause the release of nitric oxide, a chemical compound that protects pre-menopausal women from heart attacks.[62] Low oestrogen levels mean less nitric oxide is released, which increases a woman's susceptibility to heart attacks.

We have already seen that supplementing with natural progesterone might help to protect against heart disease.[63] However, the most important factor for post-menopausal women in terms of arterial blockages and atherosclerosis

---

61 Tun, A., Khan, I. A. 'Acute myocardial infarction with angiographically normal coronary arteries.' *Heart Lung* (2000): 29: 348–50.
Levit, R. D. et al. 'Cardiovascular disease in young women: a population at risk.' *Cardiol Rev* (2011): 19: 60–65.
62 Yang S. et al. 'Estrogen increases eNOS and NOx release in human coronary artery endothelium.' *J Cardiovasc Pharmacol* (2000): 36: 242–7.
63 'The effects of estrogen or estrogen/progestin regimens on heart attack risk factors in post menopausal women. The Postmenopausal oestrogen Progesterone trial (PEPI trial).' *JAMA* (1995): 273: 199–208. Accessed at: https://www.ncbi.nlm.nih.gov/pubmed/7807658

(which is the medical term for hardening of the arteries) is her declining level of testosterone.[64]

Testosterone and the brain

The brain is full of testosterone receptors, which in itself is a clue to just how important testosterone is to our brain health – in this case, as a hormone that reduces anxiety and depression. It is no surprise then that giving low-dose testosterone to depressed menopausal women has been shown to reduce their depression.[65]

It also helps with what we could call 'emotional flatness', which my female forty-something patients describe as being, well, if not depressed then not quite the person they were twenty years ago. In short, their mood is low, life seems less interesting and they lack the energy to do much – which is often due to depleted testosterone, as a simple blood test can prove. Once again, it is no great surprise that research has shown that boosting that low testosterone level back to normal improves their mood, sexual functioning and sense of well-being.[66]

A common problem that supplementing with testosterone can help with is to combat anxiety.[67] When patients tell me that they are easily irritated, I find that is often driven by underlying worry and anxiety. Supporting their testosterone by using a testosterone skin cream reduces irritability and anxiety.[68]

Lastly, low testosterone levels are associated with an increase in Alzheimer's in men (there are as yet no good studies on this in women) and poor memory

64   Golden, S. H. et al. 'Endogenous postmenopausal hormones and carotid atherosclerosis: a case-control study of the atherosclerosis risk in communities cohort.' *Am J Epidemiol* (2002): 155: 437–45.

65   Miller, K. K. et al. 'Low-dose transdermal testosterone augmentation therapy improves depression severity in women.' *CNS Spectr* (2009): 14: 688–94.

66   Goldstat, R. et al. 'Transdermal testosterone therapy improves well-being, mood and sexual function in premenopausal women.' *Menopause* (2003): 10: 390–8.

67   Miller, K. K. et al. 'Androgen deficiency: association with increased anxiety and depression symptom severity in anorexia nervosa.' *J Clin Psychiatry* (2007): 68: 959–65.

68   Hermans, E. J. et al. 'A single administration of testosterone reduces fear-potentiated startle in humans.' *J Biol Psychiatry* (2006): 59: 872–4.

in both.[69] But when menopausal women are given testosterone *and* the brain-protecting oestrogen, their memory improves.[70] In short, testosterone and oestrogen are integral to brain health.

A low level of testosterone in women going through menopause, then, is associated with depression, anxiety, poor memory and a lack of well-being. Supplementing with testosterone has been shown to improve mood, reduce anxiety and boost a sense of well-being.

Testosterone and the immune system

Patients sometimes ask whether a testosterone injection will help stave off winter's illnesses. The answer: probably not. Studies suggest testosterone does not help this aspect of the immune system and will not reduce the chance of getting a cold, bronchitis or pneumonia.[71]

That said, there is evidence that testosterone helps the immune system to combat auto-immune diseases, which is the catch-all term for when the immune system attacks the body. Studies have shown that replacing testosterone in menopausal women who have rheumatoid arthritis helps to reverse their illness.[72] That is also the case with another auto-immune disease called systemic lupus erythematosus, or SLE, which is commonly referred to as lupus. When researchers gave testosterone to SLE patients, this not only alleviated their pain and stiffness; it also reduced the number of antibodies that cause the disease.[73]

69 Moffat, S. D. et al. 'Free testosterone and risk for Alzheimer's disease in older men.' *Neurology* (2004): 62: 188–93.
Verdile, G. et al. 'Associations between gonadotrophins testosterone and B-amyloid in men at risk of Alzheimer's disease.' *Mol Psychiatry* (2014): 19: 69–75.
70 Wisniewski, A. B. et al. 'Evaluation of high dose oestrogen and high dose oestrogen plus methyl-testosterone treatment on cognitive task performance in postmenopausal women.' *Horm Res* (2002): 58: 150–5.
71 Naing, S. et al. 'Hypogonadism in chronic obstructive pulmonary disease.' *Curr Opin Pulm Med* (2012): 18: 112–17.
72 Booji, A. et al. 'Androgens as adjuvant treatment in postmenopausal female patients with rheumatoid arthritis.' *Ann Rheum Dis* (1996): 55: 811–15.
73 Naoko, K. et al. 'Testosterone suppresses anti-DNA antibody production in peripheral blood mononuclear cells from patients with systemic lupus erythematosus.' *Arthritis Rheum* (1997): 40: 1703–11.

Natural or synthetic testosterone?

The final point is whether there is much difference in using natural testosterone or synthetic versions of it – steroids such as Winstrol, Sustanon and Deca Durabolin, none of which, I hasten to say, is suitable for HRT.

When we replace testosterone in a medical situation, such as for women in menopause, we are assessing her low testosterone level and bringing it back up to normal using small doses of natural hormone. That is not the case among bodybuilders, who may be using high doses of these so-called 'roids named above to attain peak muscle and body-fat conditioning. Taking such high doses is thought to cause a range of ailments including: aggression;[74] heart attacks;[75] permanent masculinisation in women;[76] and, after stopping taking steroids, depression.[77]

Interestingly, when it comes to the immune system, synthetic steroids have been shown to behave oppositely to natural testosterone – synthetics suppress the immune system rather than boost it.[78] It is the case that low-dosage natural testosterone creams, gels or pellets that are put under the skin are the best way to help women.

TESTOSTERONE SUMMARY

The answer to the question 'should I take testosterone', then, is probably yes, if as a menopausal or post-menopausal woman your natural level of testosterone is low. Testosterone is in no way only a man's hormone: low testosterone

---

74 Pope, Jr, H. G., et al. 'Effects of supraphysiologic doses of testosterone on mood and aggression in normal men: a randomized controlled trial.' *Arch Gen Psychiatry* (2000): 57 (2): 133–40.

75 Santora, L. J. et al. 'Coronary calcification in bodybuilders using anabolic steroids.' *Prev Cardiol* (2006): 9 (4): 198–201.

76 Copley, L. M. et al. 'Consequences of use of anabolic androgenic steroids.' *Pediatr Clin North Am* (2007): 54 (4): 677–90.

77 Sample, B. R. 'Psychiatric effects and psychoactive substance use in anabolic-androgenic steroid users.' *Clin J Sport Med* (1996): 5 (1): 25–31.

78 Yofkova, I. et al. 'A decreasing CD4+/CD8+ ratio after one month of treatment with Stanozolol in postmenopausal women.' *Steroids* (1995): 60: 430–3.

in women is associated with heart attacks, depression, anxiety, poor immunity and low libido. Supplementing with small amounts of natural testosterone in a low-dose cream reverses many of these problems.

Clearly, too, high-dose testosterone or synthetic versions of it might well give great results in the gym, but I do not recommend those for anyone given their association with so many serious health problems. I would advise people to stay well clear of high-dose and synthetic testosterone.

WOMEN'S HEALTH: A FINAL WORD

Oestrogen, progesterone and testosterone are remarkable hormones that oversee the most important aspects of the female life – when a girl becomes a woman and, much later, when a woman loses her fertility.

When her hot flushes begin, a woman generally has three options ahead of her depending on how she is managing her journey through menopause:

No hormonal support: some women who have only mild hot flushes and who have healthy adrenal glands might not need any support. Their fat stores will take over the role of making oestrogen, and their adrenal glands will do whatever else is required to boost their testosterone and progesterone. Women following this route might well find that natural herbs like black cohosh and wild yam are all they need to support them gently through this time.

Conventional HRT: this remains a relatively cheap and simple solution (one pill per day) to the challenges of menopause. Some modern HRT treatments might work well without causing much harm for women who simply want a pill that stops their hot flushes for a year or two while the body gets used to this change.

Bio-identical HRT: this is my recommended solution for women who want to take the best care of their health. Using bio-identical hormones (preferably in creams or patches) allows her practitioner to measure the levels in the blood, and then adjust dosages to the optimum level. She can continue with this therapy for many years, and should expect that it will improve both her health and her longevity. Bio-identical HRT does cost a little more, and applying hormone creams is moderately more effort than taking one pill per day, but in my experience women feel far healthier on this path.

For most women, some form of HRT is useful, and indeed for them we have learned that the only thing worse than taking HRT is *not* taking HRT. What counts is to find the healthiest hormones available, which is what this chapter set out to do. By way of a summary, we saw that:

- We can measure the levels of natural hormones in the blood, but we cannot measure the levels of synthetic hormones. What this means is that supplementing with natural oestrogen, natural progesterone and natural testosterone allows your doctor to measure the levels of these hormones, and then calibrate the amount that you should take. That is personalised medicine at its best.

- Oestrogen should be taken via the skin, or transdermally to use the medical term, either as a cream or a patch. The problem with taking oestrogen in tablet form is that it goes first through the liver, which worsens the risk of clots and strokes.

- Synthetic progesterone, which is called progestin, is very effective at protecting the uterus, but worsens the risk of breast cancer; some progestins increase the risk of a heart attack. Natural progesterone, on the other hand, protects from heart attacks and breast cancer. A standard dosage (100mg) of natural progesterone is not strong enough to protect against the risk of uterine cancer caused by oestrogen, but using a higher dose of natural progesterone (200mg) does protect against that risk. That is why, for all the above reasons – being able to measure a woman's progesterone level, and the protection it affords against heart attacks and breast cancer – I far prefer using natural progesterone rather than progestin.

- Progesterone replacement not only protects the uterus; it is also used by the adrenal gland to make the hormones that help our immune system, which is why when women go through menopause they can suffer a worsening of immune disorders like asthma and rheumatoid arthritis. Replacing progesterone, logically enough, can improve these conditions. If a woman has had a hysterectomy then she would not *need* progesterone to lower her risk of uterine cancer, but she probably should take it to protect her body from a range of other ailments.

- Testosterone is not just a hormone for men. Twenty-year-old women can run low on testosterone if they are on the pill, and menopausal women can run out of testosterone before their hot flushes start – which leads to low mood, anxiety, reduced libido, a higher risk of heart attacks, and worsened immunity problems like rheumatoid arthritis. Supplementing with natural testosterone to return to normal levels helps many of these conditions.

Ultimately the aim of HRT should be to empower women to get through menopause, and not – as menopause educator Marie Hoag has put it – feeling as though 'oestrogen-deficient women are the walking dead'. And yet, to the detriment of many women, medical advice on HRT has changed dramatically and repeatedly over the past two decades.

Perhaps we should not be surprised: in the foreword, I recounted the words of my medical professor who told us young, eager students that within five years we would need to unlearn half of what we were cramming into our brains. His advice seems particularly apt for the world of HRT. At least today we seem to be back on the right track with HRT. Whether we can make fifty the new thirty remains to be seen, but we can certainly make fifty much more than tolerable, and that is a big step forward.

Key points

- Many women going through menopause suffer hot flushes and other unpleasant side effects, and will benefit from taking oestrogen and progesterone.
- In most cases it is better to use bio-identical oestrogen than synthetic oestrogen, and – to avoid blood clots and strokes – to take it as a cream or a patch rather than in tablet form.
- Synthetic progesterone, known as progestin, increases the risks of breast cancer and might heighten the risk of heart attacks, whereas bio-identical progesterone protects from those

ailments. Progestin has been shown to lower the risk of uterine cancer, which bio-identical progesterone at the standard dose of 100mg does not (although it does at 200mg).

- The risk of uterine cancer is far lower than that of heart attacks and breast cancer, so it makes sense for most women on HRT to use a bio-identical progesterone.
- Women who have had a hysterectomy should insist their blood is tested for adrenal fatigue; if their adrenals are stressed then they should seriously consider using progesterone as well as oestrogen for HRT to counter the risks of breast cancer and immune system problems.

Chapter 10

———

Your Skin – And Being Comfortable In It

Beautiful young people are accidents of nature,
but beautiful old people are works of art.

Attributed to Eleanor Roosevelt

The skin is the biggest organ in the body. If you were to shed yours and plop it on a scale, it would weigh around 3.5kg and measure about two square metres. And while many of us are concerned about the appearance of our skin, it is its function that is far more important: it protects us from dehydration, bacterial infection and sun damage, and it keeps heat and moisture in. The skin releases sweat to cool us down and it allows us the exquisite sensitivity of touch – one of our five senses.

Although the outer layer, known as the epidermis, is very thin it has a key role: protecting us from the outside world. The inner layer, called the dermis, is the business section; that is where the nerve endings, sweat glands and blood vessels are held; it is also where fibroblasts, elastin and collagen are found – three elements of the skin that, as we shall soon see, are essential to it maintaining its youthful vigour.

Trying to protect the skin, then, is common sense, as is helping it to heal. What surprises me is how many people do not do enough or, in many cases, anything at all to protect their skin from sun damage and premature ageing.

The purpose of this chapter is to show the different ways you can and should protect your skin and even restore it, using largely natural, wholly safe

Figure 1: The layers of the skin, and what is in each of them

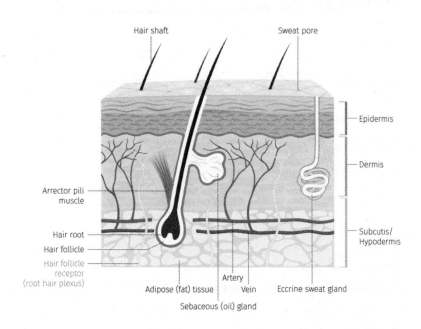

and entirely healthy methods. As you will see, the better you take care of your skin, the better you will be taking care of your overall health.

I will also explain why the best practitioners no longer focus on 'panel-beating' the skin with scalpels and old-style lasers, but instead work to strengthen its scaffolding and to generate new skin cells. In short, they use the best natural methods to encourage the skin to rebuild itself.

But before we get to that point, we should start by finding out just how poorly we used to understand the skin.

IN THE NAME OF BEAUTY

Gladys Deacon is today practically unknown, but at the turn of the last century she was an icon and was widely regarded as one of the most beautiful women alive. Among the countless men and women she dazzled was Wilhelm, the German crown prince, and the French novelist Marcel Proust. Proust wrote of her: 'I never saw a girl with such beauty, such magnificent intelligence, such goodness and charm.'[1]

Deacon became a duchess after marrying Charles, the 9th Duke of Marlborough, when she was forty (although by then they had been lovers for years). But tragedy had struck decades earlier, not long after they first met: in 1903, Deacon – in search of the perfect Grecian profile – had paraffin wax injected into the bridge of her nose. The results were catastrophic. Her body reacted to the toxin and she developed scars down her face as though a candle had dripped waxy lumps from her nose to her chin.

The belle of Europe eventually became a recluse and remained one for the rest of her long life. Stories of her sitting alone in front of the hearth trying to melt the paraffin deformation are surely apocryphal (although mental illness did run in her family). What is true is that the results scarred her face and her mind until her death, aged ninety-six, in a psychiatric ward in 1977.

Mutilation of the body in the name of beauty is nothing new; indeed, there are so many examples of the disasters of vanity that many people, men in particular, are too scared to admit they might consider doing anything for their skin lest they be viewed as shallow. And yet there is so much we can and should do, risk-free. After all, the skin is our body's barrier and does a phenomenal job protecting our health. In that role it gets exposed to the sun, to pollution, to injury and to general wear and tear. Why not help it to help us?

Thankfully, the demand in many parts of the world for the windswept effect of over-tightened facial surgery is for the most part gone, as are requests for over-inflated lips or for resurfacing lasers that produce a tight, whitened face. The trend is less towards invasive surgery and more towards natural aesthetic products. In that, TV shows like *Botched* (see box) have helped to move opinion towards gentler treatments.

1 Montgomery-Massingberd, H. 'The Duchess'. *The Spectator Archive*, (29 September 1978), p. 22.

The power of *Botched*

Nearly a century after Gladys Deacon dazzled Europe, British actress Leslie Ash, darling of the 1990's sitcom *Men Behaving Badly*, tried to preserve her looks by having silicone filler injected into her lips. (A filler is a gel that is injected into the lip or the nose or a crease in the skin in order to plump it out.)

Ash had undergone this procedure before without problem. But this time the surgeon used a different filler and Ash was left with swollen lips, described by the media as a 'trout pout'.

By the time the reality TV show *Botched* premiered in the US in 2014, the rise of celebrity culture meant the public was familiar with the extent to which those in the limelight would go to look youthful, and not always successfully. *Botched*, which covered the disasters of plastic surgery, was a hit: each episode drew about a million viewers.

Fillers have also come a long way since Leslie Ash's terrible experience, and a lot further since the days of Gladys Deacon. In short, the fillers we now use are much safer. That said, it is worth looking back at their history to see why that is, and why we can have confidence in those products that are available.

By the 1920s, the paraffin fillers that had been in use at the start of that century were largely rejected. In their place people were trying a plethora of other liquids, from vegetable oil to epoxy resin. All had disastrous effects. Next to emerge were liquid silicone fillers, whose heyday was between the 1940s and the 1960s. They were easy to inject, had a natural feel in the skin and seemed to be well tolerated. However, eventually these also showed problems similar to those found with paraffin fillers.

By 1965, the US Food and Drug Administration categorised silicone as a drug due to its lump-forming side effects, and stipulated that it must undergo proper medical trials before it could be accepted clinically. That testing never happened, although it was not until 1992, after numerous complaints and lawsuits, that the FDA banned the clinical use of silicone fillers.[2] Less than a decade later a new filler emerged that changed the industry.

Risky business

After decades of disastrous fillers, why would anyone invest in companies pursuing similar ventures? One firm that did was called Inamed; its core business was silicone in the form of breast implants and filler, which had been under the FDA's scrutiny since 1965.

The implants – essentially a silicone envelope filled with saline or a few hundred millilitres of silicone gel – were inserted into the breast to provide a realistic augmentation. But by the early 1980s patients were winning lawsuits on the grounds that the implants triggered rheumatoid arthritis and other auto-immune complaints. An FDA investigation about the safety of silicone implants saw silicone banned from cosmetic use in 1992.

Those were bad times to be a silicone manufacturer, and overnight Inamed and its competitors saw the market for their products disappear. Bristol-Meyers Squibb stopped making implants and focused its business on pharmaceutical products. Facing a multibillion-dollar class action suit, Dow Corning, king of silicone implants, in 1995 declared bankruptcy. By then just two players were left: Inamed and a firm called Mentor. Both were crippled by lawsuits and fighting a do-or-die battle to register their silicone implants with the FDA.

Mentor succeeded and survived; Inamed failed to get FDA approval and, in 2005, was forced to sell itself to Allergan, the up-and-coming giant of the aesthetics industry.

2 'Physicians to Stop Injecting Silicone for Cosmetic Treatment of Wrinkles'. Food and Drug Administration press release (1992).

Allergan is a name you might recognise as the firm that owns Botox, the brand it registered with the FDA in 2002 as the first injectable product for wrinkle reduction. Within a year of buying Inamed, Allergan did what Inamed had failed to do, and registered its silicone implants with the FDA.

But by then there was very little demand for silicone fillers. Prospective patients wanted natural products, and at the head of *that* queue was collagen, which is produced by the body's fibroblast cells and which is best thought of as the skin's scaffolding. The first collagen filler that had been registered with the FDA for cosmetic purposes was bovine collagen filler (which, as the name suggests, is from cows) back in 1981.[3] It seemed logical to put into the skin what the skin was trying to make anyway. But as you can probably guess, bovine collagen is not the same as human collagen, and some patients reacted to it by forming small lumps.

Saline fillers are another offering. These plump the skin for just a few hours but do not irritate it sufficiently to stimulate the production of enough collagen to get a beneficial effect.

Hyaluronic acid (HA) fillers

Perhaps the most important discovery in the world of fillers came in 2000 when researchers worked out the remarkable properties of hyaluronic acid. Also known as HA, hyaluronic acid is found naturally in our skin, is easy to produce and forms a gentle skin-filler that the body does not react against.

Indeed, HA was so successful that it sank the collagen filler industry overnight in the same way that silicone companies had disappeared a decade

3   Kontis, T. C. et al. 'The History of Injectable Facial Fillers.' *Facial Plast Surg* (2009): 25: 67–72.

earlier (see box on p. 320). Ironically for Inamed – by now owned by Allergan – its relatively unknown HA filler was rebranded as Juvaderm and eventually became the gold standard in the aesthetic market.

To understand why HA is 'the special one' we need to understand how a filler works. If you have a minor crease caused by a strong frown muscle, for instance, injecting Botox into the muscle will temporarily paralyse it and will smooth over the crease. However, if you have a deep wrinkle – perhaps around the mouth – then a specialist needs to inject a gel-like filler into that wrinkle to plump it out.

There is a lot more science to using filler to plump up the skin than meets the eye. Take, for instance, the example of what happens when a splinter gets under our skin: the body recognises it as a foreign object and attacks it. Specifically what happens is that the skin starts an inflammatory pathway (which we looked at in the chapter on inflammation) in which messengers tell skin cells to release large amounts of collagen to form a spider's web of scar tissue around the splinter. The body isolates and then rejects this foreign intruder.

Your body does exactly the same thing with silicone: it treats it as a foreign body, isolates it and rejects it. And, as Gladys Deacon learned to her cost, it does the same with paraffin and indeed with any of those successor fillers: these intruders cause the body to release large amounts of collagen, and it is that *excess* of collagen that causes the scars and granulomas, which are lumps of scar tissue buried deep within the skin.

Hyaluronic acid, on the other hand, does exactly what is needed: it is known as the 'Goldilocks' filler because it is not too strong and not too weak.[4] Indeed, like Baby Bear's porridge, HA is just right. It plumps up the creases in the skin, stimulates the right amount of collagen to keep the skin looking strong, and is very unlikely to cause the problems associated with other fillers.

---

4 Greco, R. M. et al. 'Hyaluronic Acid Stimulates Human Fibroblast Proliferation Within a Collagen Matrix.' *J Cell Physiol* (1998): 177: 465–73.

It is worth reiterating that HA is found naturally in our skin, where its primary role is to bind the collagen and elastin in the same way that jelly binds fruit and sponge in a trifle. It has other jobs too. As an antioxidant it helps to remove free radicals that would otherwise damage the skin.[5] It also works as an inflammatory marker, and it helps to heal wounds by stimulating the skin's superficial cells (called keratinocytes) and its deeper cells (called fibroblasts) to make more collagen scaffolding.[6]

That is so important that I will say it again: *HA helps to make more collagen, and collagen is the scaffolding that supports our skin.*

Much of modern aesthetics is built on collagen-stimulating effects: for example, a clinician could use a laser to do that, or, in a procedure known as mesotherapy, could make numerous tiny injections of vitamins into the skin; they could also needle the skin (which is ticklish more than painful), or they could introduce you to the so-called vampire facial in which growth factors extracted from your own blood are injected back into the skin; or you could simply apply high-quality vitamin skin creams on the skin (and in this chapter we will learn why that works). All share the same goal – to make more collagen and, importantly, to make just the right amount.

In short, collagen stimulation is the main pillar of skin rejuvenation, and much of the rest of this chapter will examine how different treatments achieve this.

But first we need to start with the basics; after all, nobody would begin to build their house by constructing the roof. One of the first questions I ask a new patient is what face cream they use. Too often they tell me that it is a cheap hydrating cream sold in their supermarket. And I will tell you what I tell them: before you start collagen treatment, you *must* treat your skin with a high-quality vitamin cream. Why, you rightly ask? Well, to explain that we need to understand how the skin works.

5 Ke, C. et al. 'Antioxidant Activity of Low Molecular Weight Hyaluronic Acid.' *Food Chem Toxicol* (2011): 49: 2670–5.
6 Chen, W. Y. and Abatangelo, G. 'Functions of Hyaluronan in Wound Repair.' *Wound Repair Regen* (1999): 7 (2): 79–89.

PROTECTING THE FIRST LINE OF DEFENCE

I want to take you back a couple of decades when, in my thirties, I examined my face under a Woods lamp. Simply put, a Woods lamp is a box with an ultraviolet light, and it shows up the irregularities in the skin that you often cannot see under normal light. For the first time, I saw how many pre-cancerous changes had evolved from years of windsurfing, hiking and general exposure to the sun.

I was determined to do something to reverse the damage before I started looking like the bruised prune that the Woods lamp was predicting or, worse still, developed skin cancer. I felt there had to be more I could do than simply slap on sun-protection creams, and it turned out that there was: despite years of medical training I had never heard of the extraordinary health benefits associated with certain vitamin creams. And so I turned my attention to them in an effort to understand how they could heal the skin damage and, intriguingly, how they might also prevent those changes from becoming cancerous.

The rise and rise of skin cancer

Skin cancer is both a serious problem and a growing one: despite our awareness of the importance of sun creams, skin cancer – and particularly malignant melanoma (see box) – has doubled in the UK since the 1990s and, at the time of writing, was the sixth most common cancer in men and the fifth most common in women.[7]

The following six theories help to explain the rise and rise of the major types of skin cancer.

Theory 1: the ozone layer

In the 1970s and 80s we realised that our stratospheric ozone layer was being harmed by everything from supersonic jets to aerosol cans.[8] The depleted

7 Cancer Research UK. Accessed at: http://www.cancerresearchuk.org/health-professional/cancer-statistics/statistics-by-cancer-type/skin-cancer#heading-Zero
8 Johnston, H. 'Reduction of Stratospheric Ozone by Nitrogen Oxide Catalysts from Supersonic Transport Exhaust.' *Science* (6 August 1971): 173 (3996): 517–22.
Molina, M. J., Rowland, F. S. 'Stratospheric Sink for Chlorofluoromethanes: Chlorine Atom-catalysed Destruction of Ozone.' *Nature* (1974): 249: 810–2.

Key types of skin cancer

There are three major skin cancers:

- Basal cell carcinoma;
- Squamous cell carcinoma; and,
- Malignant melanoma.

Basal cell carcinoma is generally easy to manage. Squamous cell carcinoma can be nasty if it spreads; however, it is predictable as it is caused by sun exposure and erupts in sun-exposed areas.[9]

That leaves malignant melanoma, which – although not the most common skin cancer – is the most feared, because it is the one most likely to kill us.[10] Unlike squamous cell carcinoma, malignant melanoma is unpredictable and does not necessarily occur in areas that have been exposed to the sun. Indeed, a great part of the reason why it has become more common could be because we have not properly understood what causes it, and therefore have failed to prevent it. That said, the last few years have seen significant research into malignant melanoma, and that has brought a better appreciation of how it is triggered.

ozone layer allows more ultraviolet light to penetrate the earth's atmosphere and damage our skin. By 1987 the Montreal Protocol was enacted, limiting the global production of ozone-depleting products, and over the next fifteen years the problem of ozone depletion stabilised.[11]

9 Armstrong, B. K. et al. 'Case-control Study of Sun Exposure and Squamous Cell Carcinoma of the Skin.' *Int J Cancer* (1998): 77: 347–53.
10 'Global, Regional and National Life Expectancy, All-cause Mortality, and Cause-specific Mortality for 249 Causes of Death, 1980–2015: A Systematic Analysis for the Global Burden of Disease Study 2015.' *The Lancet* (2016): 388: 1459–544.
11 'Ozone and UV: Where Are We Now.' Skin Cancer Foundation: 27 July 2009: http://www.skincancer.org/prevention/uva-and-uvb/ozone

That said, research has shown that reduced ozone is *not* the cause of malignant melanoma,[12] although it probably does explain the rising incidence of the other skin cancers. Studies reveal that, paradoxically, people who are exposed to the sun are often better protected from malignant melanoma than people who stay indoors. Why might that be? That brings us on to the second theory, which looks at the different components of ultraviolet light.

Theory 2: ultraviolet light

More than half of the sun's light is made up of infrared light, which we commonly call heat; another large chunk – more than 40 per cent – is comprised of visible light, which we can think of as the colours of the rainbow.

What we are concerned with here is what constitutes the last few percentage points. It is called ultraviolet light, or UV, and, despite being the smallest component, seems to inflict the most damage.

When it comes to ultraviolet light and skin cancer, we know that the different wavelengths (which are dominated by UVA, followed by UVB and UVC) have different effects.

- UVA typically damages DNA causing the skin to age.
- UVB generally causes the skin to burn.
- UVC damages DNA but it remains unclear whether UVC can penetrate the ozone layer.

At this stage, then, we are most concerned about UVA and UVB.

When ultraviolet light hits the skin, it affects the DNA of the cells, and a message goes out to build a wall of protective melanin. Some people show this off as a tan but melanin's real job is to shield us from further DNA damage and skin cancer. In other words, that golden tan means we have already paid the price with damage to cell DNA.

12 Godar, D. et al. 'Cutaneous Malignant Melanoma Incidences Analyzed Worldwide by Sex, Age and Skin Type Over Personal Ultraviolet-B Dose Shows No Role for Sunburn but Implies One for Vitamin D3.' *Dermato-Endocrinology* (2017): Vol 9, No 1: http://dx.doi.org/ 10.1080/19381980.2016.1267077

Twenty years ago, researchers thought only UVB was behind sun damage. They believed UVB burned the skin causing oxidative damage, which we refer to as free radicals. These free radicals then bashed their way into the DNA of the skin cells and damaged them – which is why UVB was seen as the main cause of skin cancer.[13] The oxidative damage associated with UVB is still seen as an important factor in worsening the risk for basal and squamous cell skin problems, but it is not seen as doing the same for malignant melanoma.[14]

Instead, recent studies indicate that malignant melanoma is triggered by exposure to UVA. This is because UVA *directly* damages the DNA of skin cells, which, it turns out, is much more serious than the oxidative damage caused by UVB.[15]

But for me the most interesting development is how UVA and UVB affect our levels of vitamin D, which we sometimes call the sunshine vitamin: UVA *breaks down* vitamin D levels in the skin; UVB *stimulates* them.[16] That is important because vitamin D defends us from skin cancer,[17] probably by activating T-cells whose job is to destroy any of our cells that have become cancerous or infected by a virus.[18]

It turns out that vitamin D deficiency is a big problem, with nearly half the world's population lacking enough of it.[19] Indeed, tests on my patients in

13   Brash, D. et al. 'A Role for Sunlight in Skin Cancer: UV-Induced P-53 Mutations in Squamous Cell Carcinoma.' *Proc Natl Acad Sci USA* (1991): 88: 10124–8.

14   Brash, D. E. 'UV Signature Mutations.' *Photochem Photo-Biol:* (2015): 91: 15–26: PMID:25354245: http://dx.doi.org/ 10.1111/php.12377

15   Cooke, M. S. et al. 'Oxidative DNA Damage: Mechanisms, Mutation and Disease.' *FASEB J* (2003): 17 (10): 1195–214: PMID:12832285: http:// dx.doi.org/10.1096/fj.02-0752rev

16   Lucas, A. et al. 'Increased UVA Exposures and Decreased Cutaneous Vitamin D3 Levels may be Responsible for the Increasing Incidence of Melanoma.' *Medical Hypotheses* (2009): 72: 434–43.

17   Nair, R. et al. 'Vitamin D: the 'Sunshine' Vitamin.' *J Pharmacol Pharmacother* (2012): 3: 118–26.

18   Von Essen, M. R. et al. 'Vitamin D Controls T-cell Antigen Receptor Signaling and Activation of Human T-cells.' *Nat Immunol* (2010): 11: 344–349: PMID:20208539: http:// dx. doi.org/10.1038/ni.1851

19   Alshishtawy, M. M. 'Vitamin D Deficiency. A Clandestine Endemic Disease is Veiled No More.' *SQUMJ* (2012): 140–52.

sunny South Africa regularly show even their levels are too low. Your first thought might be to sunbathe to boost your vitamin D levels, but that will not work as much as you might want because sunlight is made up of both UVA and UVB – and we know that UVA breaks down vitamin D. The best solution is to have a blood test to find out your vitamin D level, and then supplement with tablets if needed. (Your medical practitioner should be well placed to give advice on quantities.)

UVA and UVB, then, have mixed effects. But is there evidence that one is worse than the other? Indeed there is: a 2009 study revealed that being exposed to UVA alone is worse than being exposed to *both* UVA and UVB. The researchers showed that fair-skinned people working indoors who were exposed solely to UVA lights had a higher incidence of malignant melanoma than those working outdoors, who were exposed to sunlight's UVA and UVB.[20] Why was that? Because those working indoors did not get the vitamin D stimulation conveyed by UVB, and were exposed solely to UVA's damaging effects.

To summarise Theory 2, then: malignant melanoma is triggered specifically by UVA damage. UVB might cause free-radical damage but it is UVA that directly damages our DNA, and it is UVA that lowers the levels of protective vitamin D. When it comes to the skin cancer epidemic, there can be little doubt that indoor ultraviolet lights and some types of sunbed have much to answer for.

Theory 3: defective DNA repair system

Why is it that we might be vigilant about overexposure to the sun yet still be susceptible to skin cancer, while plants and reptiles can sunbathe all day and never look the worse for wear? After all, have you ever meet a sun-damaged cactus?

Bear with me as I explain how this revolves around how the body tackles damaged DNA: this process is known as nucleotide excision repair, or NER,

---

20   Lucas, A. et al. 'Increased UVA Exposures and Decreased Cutaneous Vitamin D3 Levels may be Responsible for the Increasing Incidence of Melanoma.' *Medical Hypotheses* (2009): 72: 434–43.

and it cuts out damaged DNA and repairs it.[21] Most of the time the NER system works just fine but there is one type of DNA damage that it *cannot* fix, and that is known as thymine dimers.[22]

If, like me, you studied biology at school then you might recall that each DNA strand is made up of four bases: A, G, C and T. The 'T' in that sequence stands for thymine, and a thymine dimer is the term used to describe what happens when two damaged thymine units join up. For reasons that we do not need to go into, our NER system cannot fix DNA that is damaged to this extent. That is important because a cell damaged this much cannot read its own DNA, and that means it could become a cancer cell.

So much for our human failings. The reason plants and reptiles do so much better is that they have an extra defence against damage from ultraviolet light. It is called the photolyase enzyme (a type of protein) and it can repair all DNA damage including thymine dimer damage.[23]

Lucky plants and reptiles, I hear you say. Well, the good news is that photolyase has been shown to reduce pre-cancerous skin changes in humans,[24] and some skin-cream companies now add photolyase to their sunblock as added protection against skin cancer. Later we will see that some high-quality vitamin creams are also able to act like photolyase.

In short, this theory holds that we develop skin cancer because, unlike a cactus, we do not have photolyase enzymes, and that puts our skin's DNA at risk of irreparable damage from ultraviolet light.

21 Daya-Grosjean, L. 'Xeroderma Pigmentosum and Skin Cancer.' *Adv Exp Med Biol* (2008): 637: 19–27.

22 Leibeling, D. et al. 'Nucleotide Excision Repair and Cancer.' *J Mol Histol* (2006): 37 (5–7): 225–38.

23 Weber, S. 'Light-Driven Enzymatic Catalysis of DNA Repair: A Review of Recent Biophysical Studies on Photolyase.' *BBA* (2005): Vol 1707: 1–23.

24 Milani, M. et al. 'Efficacy of a Photolyase-Based Device in the Treatment of Cancerization Field in Patients with Actinic Keratosis and Non-Melanoma Skin Cancer.' *G Ital Dermatol Venereol* (2013): 148: 693–8.

Theory 4: damage from infrared light

Heat can damage the skin – think of how your skin would react if you held it over an open flame, for instance. The name given to this is *erythema ab igne*, or EAI, a combined Greek-Latin phrase that broadly translates as 'redness from fire'. Colloquially it is known as granny's tartan or fire stains, and it comes from spending too much time close to a heat source such as a fire. What happens is that the heat damages the DNA of the exposed skin leaving scarred red-brown skin that is mildly prone to skin cancer.[25] You can get the same effect from too-warm hot-water bottles and even from balancing your laptop computer on your legs for extended periods.

We saw earlier that more than half of the sun's light is comprised of heat waves, which we call infrared, and which we divide in different categories. Infrared A, or IRA, is the most dangerous and can cause sun damage down to the dermis layer; that damage is worsened when IRA is accompanied by ultra-violet light.[26] And although sunblock creams reflect ultraviolet radiation, they give no protection whatsoever from IRA heat.

When researchers exposed the buttocks of twenty-three volunteers to IRA heat equivalent to that which reaches us from the sun, they showed this caused collagen in the skin to break down,[27] and they found that the skin's antioxidant system designed to protect us from this damage was depleted. They theorised that putting antioxidants into the skin to combat infrared heat *and* applying sunblock to counter the ultraviolet light would protect us from skin cancer.

Later we will see which vitamin creams can be absorbed into the skin to help this process. In summary, though, this theory suggests that we should not ignore infrared heat damage if we want to beat skin cancer.

---

25 Rudolph, C. M. et al. 'Squamous Epithelial Carcinoma in Erythema Ab Igne.' *Hautarzt* (2000): 51: 260–3.

26 Kligman, L. 'Intensification of Ultraviolet-Induced Dermal Damage by Infrared Radiation.' *Arch Dermatol Res* (1982): 272: 229–38.

27 Schroeder, P. et al. 'Infrared Radiation-Induced Matrix Metalloproteinase in Human Skin: Implications for Protection.' *J Invest Dermatol* (2008): 2491–7. Accessed at: https://www.ncbi.nlm.nih.gov/pubmed/18449210

Theory 5: pollution causes ozone damage to the skin

Studies have shown that sooty particulate matter from car fumes damages the skin, worsens wrinkles[28] and is associated with skin cancer.[29] This is in part because soot directly irritates the skin, and in part because soot stimulates the formation of damaging gases.[30]

Ironically, given the lack of ozone in some parts of the stratosphere, car fumes cause a build-up of ozone all around us at ground level.[31] That is a problem because ozone, a gas comprised of three oxygen atoms (its formula is O3), is highly unstable and releases free radicals that irritate the skin until our natural antioxidant systems clean them up.

Fortunately it seems there is something we can do: one study grew human skin cells and exposed them to ozone. As expected, the O3 damaged the cells. However, once they were fortified with vitamin C, vitamin E and ferulic acid (a compound found in the cells of many plants), they were protected from this ozone damage.[32] (This study was funded by a cosmeceutical company, but it has been published in peer review journals and its findings seem legitimate to me.)

Theory 5, then, contends that car fumes and other pollution sources contribute to skin cancer by creating ozone, which irritates the skin. The solution? Washing one's face every night to remove the soot and then applying antioxidant serum.

28   Vierkotter, A. et al. 'MMP-1 and 3-Promoter Variants are Indicative of a Common Susceptibility for Skin and Lung Aging: Results from a Cohort of Elderly Women (SALIA).' *J Invest Dermatol* (2015): 135: 1268–74.

29   Farmer, P. B. et al. 'Molecular Epidemiology Studies of Environmental Pollutants. Effects of Polycyclic Aromatic Hydrocarbons (PAHs) in Environmental Pollution on Exogenous and Oxidative DNA Damage.' *Mutat Res* (2003): 544: 397–402.

30   Huls, A. et al. 'Traffic-Related Air Pollution Contributes to Development of Facial Lentigines: Further Epidemiological Evidence from Caucasians and Asians.' *J of Invest Dermatol* (2016): 136: 1053–6.

31   Manning, W. J. et al. 'Ozone and Levels in European and USA Cities are Increasing More Than at Rural Sites, While Peak Values are Decreasing.' *Environ Pollut* (2014): 192: 295–9.

32   Valacchi, G. et al. 'Vitamin C Compound Mixtures Prevent Ozone-Induced Oxidative Damage in Human Keratinocytes as Initial Assessment of Pollution Protection.' *PLoS ONE* (2015).

Theory 6: human papillomavirus (HPV) causes malignant melanoma

A decade ago I would not have bet on this theory but an array of studies now supports it. HPV is a sexually transmitted virus that damages the DNA of the cells in a woman's cervix and can trigger cervical cancer. So far, so logical. However, it turns out that HPV can also travel around the body and cause exactly the same DNA damage to skin cells that UVA causes.[33]

HPV is by no means the first virus to be implicated in causing cancer: Epstein-Barr virus, for instance – which is one of the herpes viruses and which most people carry – was the first to be shown to cause some types of cancer.[34] Overall, as much as 15 per cent of cancers could be caused by viruses,[35] and it is worth noting that the biopsies of some people with melanoma have contained HPV.[36] It is thought that this might explain why women in particular are prone to getting melanoma in non-sun-exposed areas.[37]

Making sense of the theories

The issue of skin cancer has generated a wealth of research over the decades, which has in turn given us a far greater understanding of its causes.

We now know that UVA exposure not only damages DNA directly, thereby causing melanomas, but also destroys vitamin D whose job it is to wake up that part of the immune system that removes cancerous and virally infected cells.

We also know that both infrared heat and air pollution damage the skin.

33   Lai, D. et al. 'Localization of HPV-18 E2 at Mitochondrial Membranes Induces ROS Release and Modulates Host Cell Metabolism.' *PLoS One* (2013): 8 (9): e75625. eCollection 2013: PMID:24086592: http://dx.doi.org/10.1371/journal. pone.0075625

34   Prabhu, S. R. and Wilson, D. 'Evidence of Epstein-Barr Virus Associated with Head and Neck Cancers: A Review.' *J Can Dent Assoc* (2016): 82: g2: http://www.jcda.ca/g2

35   Parkin, D. M. 'The Global Health Burden of Infection-associated Cancers in the Year 2002.' *Int J Cancer* (2006): 118 (12): 3030–44.

36   Dreau, D. et al. 'Human Papillomavirus in Melanoma Biopsy Specimens and Its Relation to Melanoma Progression.' *Ann Surg* (2000): 231 (5): 664–71.

37   Godar, D. et al. 'Cutaneous Malignant Melanoma Incidences Analyzed Worldwide by Sex, Age and Skin Type Over Personal Ultraviolet-B Dose Shows No Role for Sunburn but Implies One for Vitamin D3.' *Dermato-Endocrinology* (2017): Vol 9, No 1: http://dx.doi.org/ 10.1080/19381980.2016.1267077.

And, in perhaps the biggest surprise, we know that the human papillomavirus can damage skin cells in much the same way as UVA does.

All of this provides plenty of tips on how to avoid skin cancer. For example:

- Avoid artificial ultraviolet lights.
- Test (and boost, if necessary) your vitamin D levels.
- Practise safe sex, and screen to see whether you have contracted HPV.
- Apply high-quality vitamin skin creams.

As we will shortly see, the evidence is clear when it comes to skin creams: these are *not* a matter of vanity but are essential for the health of your skin, whether you are a man or a woman.

But it makes no sense to slap on the first cream you see advertised, because thousands are useless and some are harmful. Instead it is essential to understand what works and why, and only then to go out and buy what is best. So with that said, let us turn to the fascinating world of skin creams.

THE WORLD OF SKIN CREAMS

Broadly speaking there are two skin types: dry and oily. Having oily skin means you might suffer from pimples, particularly during your teenage years; on the positive side it means you are generally well protected from wrinkling when you get older, unlike your dry-skin peers.

Until recently, skin creams were targeted largely at this latter group, and they helped them do what people with oily skins enjoyed free of charge: they kept the skin hydrated and protected.

There is now growing research about the natural protection that the surface layer of oil provides, and how fortunate oily-skinned people are. In short, it seems this specialised oil layer keeps the moisture in and the soot and bacteria out.[38] As we age, however, this protective oil layer recedes and the surface layers of the skin are damaged. If you are born with dry skin, then this can happen from an early age.

---

38   Wertz, P. W. 'Lipids and Barrier Function of the Skin.' *Acta Derm Venereol* (2000): 208: 7–11.

Helping to hydrate the skin has for decades been a core principle of the likes of Clarins, L'Oréal, Estée Lauder – indeed, pretty much any cosmetics company you can name. But since the 1990s, new insights – particularly in the realm of vitamins – has seen dozens of new brands and thousands of products from what are known as cosmeceutical companies. Some of the better-known are Dermalogica, Perricone MD, Dr Sebagh, Obagi, SkinCeuticals (which is now owned by L'Oréal), Environ, Lamelle and RégimA, but there are many more.

And as we are about to see, the world of skincare has moved far beyond simple hydration; these days the best products incorporate vitamins and compounds that, when applied to the skin, penetrate to the deeper layers to work their magic.

Why not just swallow vitamins?

The simple answer is that swallowing, for example, a vitamin C tablet does not do much in terms of protecting us from wrinkles and skin cancers.[39] Putting vitamin C or vitamin A directly on to the skin has a much more profound effect, as we shall see shortly.[40]

That said, two vitamins are useful in tablet form: vitamin D (which we encountered earlier) and vitamin E.

Vitamin E tablets help to reduce the chance of getting sunburned, and they ensure fewer skin cancer markers in the skin (those thymine dimers[41] again). Vitamin E makes the skin operate more like that of a cactus or a reptile, and these tablets have a place in protecting our skin.

39   Jackson, M. J. et al. 'UVR-Induced Oxidative Stress in Human Skin in vivo: Effects of Oral Vitamin C Supplementation.' *Free Radic Biol Med* (2002): 33: 1355–62.
40   Telang, P. S. 'Vitamin C in Dermatology.' *Indian Dermatol Online* (2013): 4: 143–6.
41   Placzek, M. et al. 'Ultraviolet B-Induced DNA Damage in Human Epidermis is Modified by the Antioxidants Ascorbic Acid and D-alpha-tocopherol.' *J Invest Dermatol* (2005): 124: 304–7.

Vitamin C serum

We can thank the late American dermatologist, academic and researcher Dr Sheldon Pinnell, who founded SkinCeuticals in 1994, for highlighting the powerful effects of antioxidants that are able to cross the skin (known as 'transdermal antioxidants') in protecting our skin from sun damage.

In the 1970s Pinnell studied the role of collagen in the skin and the effects of antioxidants on the skin, and spent much of his career contributing to this topic. As professor of dermatology at Duke University in the 1990s, he selected a base of 100 antioxidants to study. Most, it turned out, could not cross the skin barrier. However, vitamins A and C could, and the latter eventually became his favourite transdermal vitamin.

Sheldon also looked at other elements found in the natural world, and found two substances that plants use to protect themselves from sun damage: ferulic acid and phloretin.[42] We encountered ferulic acid earlier; we have not yet mentioned phloretin. The combination of these two has proved to be phenomenal, as we will shortly find out.

First, though, I will start by outlining the remarkable properties of vitamin C serum:

- It protects us from skin cancer.
- It protects our skin from photo-ageing, a term that refers to the wrinkles and discolouration caused by sunlight.
- It protects our skin from infrared heat damage.
- It stimulates new skin-cell formation – and as part of that, it stimulates the formation of new fibroblasts, which are key to skin health.

Pinnell showed that vitamin C serum should play a central role in our skin-care regimen. This is how he came to that conclusion.

---

42   Pinnell, S. R. et al. 'Topical L-ascorbic Acid: Percutaneous Absorption Studies.' *Dermatol Surg* (2001): 27: 137–42.

Protects from skin cancer

In 2003, Pinnell published a study that showed what happens when you take pigskins, apply vitamin C serum and vitamin E serum to them, and place them under (in this case artificial) sunlight.

He found that each serum helped to protect the pigskins from sunburn, but that when used in combination they performed significantly better with regards to sunburn and the formation of thymine dimers.[43] (Earlier we saw that our NER system cannot repair thymine dimers; this is why measuring the number of thymine dimers in the skin indicates our level of sun damage.)

Priming the skin with vitamin C serum does for us what photolyase enzymes do for plants: it provides protection from thymine dimers and so protects us from skin cancer.

Protects from photo-ageing

Five years later, Pinnell released another key study. This time he used ten (living) humans with pale, sensitive skin to make his point about the power of vitamin C. He applied vitamin C serum along with ferulic acid and phloretin to their backs for four days and, after that, exposed them to the sun. As before, when combined with these other ingredients, the effects of vitamin C were significantly enhanced.

Just as Pinnell expected, his human guinea pigs burned in the places where vitamin serum had not been applied, and had very little sunburn in areas where it had been. When he examined their skin, he found fewer thymine dimers where the skin had been treated, which meant the combination of vitamin C, ferulic acid and phloretin had provided their skin with the ultimate protection from DNA damage.[44] Pinnell was not surprised; after all, he had concluded as much during his earlier study on pigskins.

43 Pinnell, S. R. et al. 'UV Photoprotection by Combination Topical Antioxidants Vitamin C and Vitamin E.' *J Am Acad Dermatol* (2003): 48: 866–74.
44 Pinnell, S. R. et al. 'Protective Effects of a Topical Antioxidant Mixture Containing Vitamin C, Ferulic Acid and Phloretin Against Ultraviolet-Induced Photodamage in Human Skin'. *J Cosmet Dermatol* (2008): 7: 290–7.

Where it gets interesting is that this combination of ingredients *also* gave protection from photo-ageing (which is ageing due to sun damage), and it does this by protecting the skin's collagen. By way of a reminder, collagen is the scaffolding that keeps our skin strong, and typically we do not want it to break down. When it does, this breakdown process is coordinated by wound-healing enzymes called MMPs (which stands for matrix metalloproteinases). MMPs go to work when, for instance, a scar is being remodelled into healthy tissue (the scar has too much collagen, which is why it looks lumpy) or when the skin is damaged by the sun.

Why does this matter? Because exposure to the sun causes a surge of MMPs. These attack the collagen and break it down, and it is this process that eventually results in saggy skin. Pinnell showed that adding his combination of vitamin serum to his subjects' skin protected them from sunburn and from sagging collagen breakdown. In short, the serum prevented the skin from premature photo-ageing.

By 2008, Pinnell had concluded from these and other studies that the combination of vitamin C with other antioxidants has a powerful effect in protecting us from sunburn, skin cancer and premature ageing of the skin, and should be part of our skin protection regimen.[45]

Protects from infrared heat damage

If you have ever strapped on a set of infrared goggles you will know that every-thing around us emits heat – some things give off a lot (fires, lasers, a cup of tea); others much less (a chair, a flower, Snuffles the hamster). The amount of infrared heat that Snuffles generates is of no concern, but the heat that reaches us from the sun, for instance, is both significant and damaging.

It is in this area – infrared heat damage – that we see the collision of three of the most significant names in vitamin skincare – Pinnell and a couple called Albert and Lorraine Kligman.

45   Pinnell, S. R. et al. 'A Topical Antioxidant Solution Containing Vitamins C and E Stabilized by Ferulic Acid Provides Protection for Human Skin Against Damage Caused by Ultraviolet Irradiation.' *J Am Acad Dermatol* (2008): 59: 418–25.

In 1982, Lorraine Kligman published an important paper on the damaging effects of infrared heat on the skin.[46] Pinnell followed that up a decade later and showed that adding vitamin C serum to the skin protects it from the damage caused by infrared heat.[47] As we will shortly see, those findings would prove important in sun protection and when heating the skin using medical lasers.

Stimulates new skin-cell formation

Earlier we learned that the skin's fibroblast cells are responsible for building collagen, which provides the skin's scaffolding, and that they repair the damage caused by injuries. In aesthetic medicine, we use this knowledge to stimulate the fibroblasts to do more of what they are good at: building more collagen and repairing damage.

There are plenty of ways to stimulate fibroblasts: we can use vitamin creams; we can use a skin-roller (which has dozens of fine needles that lightly puncture the skin); we can put threads into the skin; and we can laser the skin. We could even punch the skin with a fist, although the pain factor means I do not recommend it. All of these methods have the same effect – they cause an inflammatory response that tells the fibroblasts to make more structural collagen.

Unfortunately, as we get older we end up with fewer fibroblasts, and those we do have get lazier, which is one reason why our skin sags as the years go by and our collagen-depleted skin struggles to hold together its youthful shine. We are born with around 10 billion fibroblast cells; by the time we turn forty that number has halved, and by seventy we could have as few as 1 billion active fibroblasts.

But all is not lost: we can still stimulate the skin to wake up those fibroblasts and get them to do more work, although inevitably the results will be better with 5 billion cells than with 1 billion.

46 Kligman, L. 'Intensification of Ultraviolet-Induced Dermal Damage by Infrared Radiation.' *Arch Dermatol Res* (1982): 272: 229–38.
47 Pinnell, S. R. et al. 'Topical Vitamin C Protects Porcine Skin from Ultraviolet Radiation-Induced Damage.' *Br J Dermatol* (1992): 127: 247–53.

Logically, the holy grail of skincare would be this: getting the body to make *more* fibroblast cells rather than pushing the worn-out remaining fibroblast cells to build more collagen. In 1994 Pinnell showed that was possible. In his study, Pinnell compared infant skin with elderly skin. As you would expect, the elderly skin had fewer fibroblasts, and those fibroblasts were not building much collagen. That is, until Pinnell introduced vitamin C serum. Rejuvenating elderly skin with vitamin C caused it to respond just as well as the infant skin: it not only produced more collagen than before, it regenerated sluggish fibroblasts too,[48] raising the possibility that we could make new skin cells. We will come back to this topic when we look at growth factor and stem-cell stimulation of the skin.

What to make of the evidence

Vitamin C serum can: protect us from skin cancer; protect us from sunburn, from the damage from ultraviolet light, and from the sun's infrared heat damage; stimulate collagen formation to strengthen ageing skin; and rejuvenate old fibroblasts to rebuild the skin.

But before slathering your body in vitamin C serum for the rest of your life, remember what you learned earlier in the book about supplementing with vitamins: we saw that, although vitamins can protect us from free radical damage, using them continually might switch off our own SOD (superoxide dismutase) antioxidant system. And, once we have unplugged our powerful SOD system, we are more susceptible to free radical damage.

What to do? As yet there are no studies about the continuous long-term effects of using vitamin C on the skin and on the skin's SOD system. However, the principle remains the same, which is why I recommend using vitamin C serum for a couple of weeks, particularly when you are exposed to the sun, and then stopping for a week to allow your SOD system to recover.

48 Pinnell, S. R. et al. 'Effects of Ascorbic Acid on Proliferation and Collagen Synthesis in Relation to the Donor Age of Human Dermal Fibroblasts.' *J Invest Dermatol* (1994): 103: 228–32.

Beyond vitamin C

Other vitamins and supplements have shown benefits for skin health, and three of the main contenders are:

Vitamin B5

This is a skin hydrator and is therefore vital for everyone, but particularly for people with dry skin.

Alpha-lipoic acid

We met this powerful antioxidant earlier in the book, where I listed it as a contender in my list of five favourite supplements. It is thought to stimulate collagen[49] and to have an antioxidant effect[50] by clearing away damaging particles in the skin. Most usefully, it helps to reverse glycation, which is easily pictured as the hardened skin around a smoker's mouth, and it reverses premature ageing in sun-damaged skins.[51]

Resveratrol

I include resveratrol because in recent years this big-league antioxidant garnered a lot of media attention. However, it has struggled to live up to its promise. In a laboratory setting, resveratrol applied to a tumour has beneficial anti-cancer effects. Outside the laboratory, resveratrol should stimulate and boost our internal antioxidant system (the SOD system), and in theory this should help us, particularly if overuse of vitamin C has made our SOD system sleepy.

49   Han, B. et al. 'Transdermal Delivery of Amino Acids and Antioxidants Enhance Collagen Synthesis: In Vivo and In Vitro Studies.' *Connect Tissue Res* (2005): 46: 251–7.

50   Thomas, S. et al. 'Stability, Cutaneous Delivery and Antioxidant Potential of a Lipoic Acid and Alpha-Tocopherol codrug Incorporated in Microemulsions.' *J Pharm Sci* (2014): 103: 2530–8.

51   Beitner, H. 'Randomized, Placebo-Controlled, Double Blind Study on the Clinical Efficacy of a Cream Containing 5% Alpha-Lipoic Acid Related to Photoageing of Facial Skin.' *Br J Dermatol* (2003): 149: 841–9.

How best, then, to take it? If we swallow resveratrol it typically gets metabolised before reaching the skin. And although transdermal use of resveratrol has shown promise, it still has some distance to go to convince people of its efficacy.[52] In short, the jury is out on resveratrol.

Vitamin A cream

Earlier I said that Pinnell had found two vitamins able to cross the skin barrier. We have delved into the benefits of vitamin C – which has, I grant you, an impressive resumé – but in the world of dermatology it is the other transdermal vitamin, vitamin A, that is royalty.

Our story starts in 1969 with Albert Kligman, someone who – despite controversial testing practices involving US prison inmates – is regarded as the father of vitamin dermatology.

The common form of vitamin A is called retinol, which you might see in slightly amended form as retinol acetate, retinol palmitate and, most notably, retinoic acid. It was the last of these, retinoic acid, that Kligman put on the map in 1969 as the first effective vitamin-cream treatment for acne.

Acne is caused by the blockage of the sebaceous glands in the top layer of the skin; Kligman showed that his cream, which he named Retin-A, destroys that top layer of dead cells and causes the lower layer of living cells to replicate. Clearing out that dead top layer unblocks the sebaceous glands and so clears up acne.[53]

Back then, skin studies tended to come down to doctors slapping potions on patients then sitting back to see what happened. Kligman's approach of applying three different creams to three groups of patients and then comparing them against the performance of a neutral cream and documenting the

52   Ahmed, N. et al. 'The Grape Antioxidant Resveratrol for Skin Disorders: Promise, Prospects and Challenges.' *Arch Biochem Biophys* (2011): 508: 164–70.
53   Kligman, A. M. et al. 'Topical Vitamin A Acid in Acne Vulgaris.' *Arch Dermatol* (1969): 469–76.

results showed an unusual level of scientific rigour. Proving that this metabolite of vitamin A could treat acne was exciting news, and over the next five years retinoic acid treatments were shown to remove warts and to treat psoriasis (which is an illness of thickened skin), age spots and skin cancers. Retinoic acid worked on warts, psoriasis and age spots by sanding down the surface of the skin, and it worked on skin cancer by altering the DNA expression of cancer cells.[54]

No other cream could show retinoic acid's promise, and there were even suggestions that it might reverse sun damage in ageing skin. The downside was that retinoic acid tended to burn sensitive skin: after applying it at night, people might wake the next morning with a dried, pink skin. If Kligman could conjure a gentler version of retinoic acid, then that might prove to be the first cream to improve sun-damaged skin.

Like many a sensible man, Kligman turned to his wife, and he and Lorraine drove the research. By 1981 they had shown that retinoic acid could reverse sun damage in the skin of mice.[55] Three years later they went back into the laboratory and showed that retinoic acid could reverse sun damage in human skin.[56] Importantly, they also showed how retinoic acid works: by removing the broken elastin fibres in the skin and rebuilding structural collagen.

By 1986 the couple had mapped out what happens to skin as it ages and how retinoic acid could reverse that. Specifically, they showed that ageing skin has a thickened surface layer of dead cells with the following consequences: the dead cells suffocate the living cells below, and cause the turnover of living cells to slow down; living cells are not only sluggish but show abnormalities; and ageing skin has blotchy pigmentation patches.

---

54 Meyskens, F. L. et al. 'A Phase-1 Trial of All-Trans-Retinoic Acid Delivered Via a Collagen Sponge and Cervical Cap for Mild or Moderate Intraepithelial Neoplasia.' *J Natl Cancer Inst* (1983): 71: 921–5.

55 Kligman, L. H. and Kligman, A. M. 'Histogenesis and Progression of Ultraviolet Light-Induced Tumours in Hairless Mice.' *J Natl Cancer Inst* (1981): 67: 1289–97.

56 Kligman, L. H. and Kligman, A. M. 'Topical Retinoic Acid Enhances Repair of Ultraviolet-Damaged Dermal Connective Tissue.' *Connect Tissue Res* (1984): 12: 139–50.

Sun-damaged skin looks dry and dull with thickened plaques and patches of pigment. The Kligmans were able to show that treating such skin with retinoic acid sanded off that layer of thickened dead cells; sped up the turnover of cells living beneath that outer layer, resulting in stronger, normal-looking cells; removed excess pigment; increased collagen in the dermis; and increased the number of arteries bringing nutrients to the skin.

The result was skin that had a healthy, hydrated and strong appearance – with the best results from those who had the most sun damage.

But even patients who had good-quality skin to start with showed improvement after treatment.[57] In a small follow-up study in 1993, they found that the skin of elderly people who did not have sun damage also improved when they applied retinoic acid to their skin.[58]

Vitamin A cream, and particularly the retinoic acid version of it, is probably the most studied vitamin cream that we have. It has been shown to:

- Treat acne effectively.
- Remove precancerous age spots.
- Remove skin cancer cells.
- Effectively reverse the ageing effects of sun damage.

Indeed, most of us should use retinoic acid on a regular basis. Most of us do not, though, and that is possibly because the earlier versions of this form of vitamin A could leave our skin looking dried out and sensitive – due to the acid's skin-peel effect on the surface of the skin, which is known as the 'retinoid reaction'. We can get around that by using less powerful versions of vitamin A such as retinol, retinol acetate and retinol palmitate, but we will not get quite the same result. The good news is that cosmeceutical companies have these days found ways of delivering retinoic acid through the skin without irritating the surface. In short, to protect our skin we ought to use some form of high-quality retinoic acid.

57   Kligman, A. M. et al. 'Topical Tretinoin for Photoaged Skin.' *J Am Acad Dermatol* (1986): 15: 836–59.

58   Kligman, A. M. et al. 'Effects of Topical Tretinoin on Non-Sun-Exposed Protected Skin of the Elderly.' *J Am Acad Dermatol* (1993): 29 (1): 25–33.

Combating ageing skin

We have talked a lot about older skin, but what exactly do we mean by that: what is it that makes skin *look* old? It is, of course, obvious to the eye: it is easy to tell that a twenty-year-old has younger-looking skin than a fifty-year-old. But apart from the wrinkles, it can be tricky to explain exactly *what* makes a fifty-year-old's skin look fifty.

Figure 2: The layers of the skin

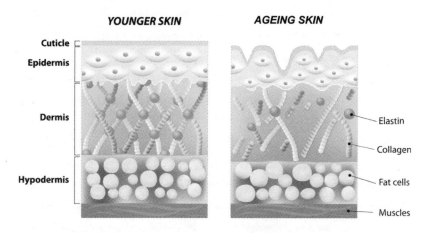

To do that, we need to look again at the skin. As we can see, it is made up of three layers: the outer layer called the epidermis, the inner layer called the dermis, and a base layer called the hypodermis. The epidermis is there to protect us from the elements; the dermis is the workhorse of the skin, building the collagen scaffolding and containing the nerves, arteries and sweat glands; the hypodermis is comprised of fat and connective tissue.

Five key elements cause our skin to age, and understanding these allows us to work out which treatments to use to slow that process. We will start from the outermost layer and work our way in:

- Dead cells accumulate: a layer of dead cells protects the outer wall of the skin. It is the job of an enzyme called cathepsin-D to break down these dead cells, shed them and stimulate the living cells underneath to blossom. But as we age, our levels of this enzyme decline and the cell turnover process stalls. As a result, the layer of dead surface cells builds up, and the living cells underneath become sluggish and abnormal. In our fifty-year-old's skin, this appears as roughness and dullness.

- Pigment cells clump together: just below the dead outer layer is the main part of the epidermis. It holds the pigment cells and, as we saw in the section on skin cancer, these cells make the protective pigment called melanin that shields us from sun damage. In the twenty-year-old these cells are spread evenly throughout the skin, but as the years pass some of them clump together causing dark areas, while other areas become pale where the cells are absent. The result is that our fifty-year-old's skin starts to look pigmented and mottled.

- Collagen starts to thin: next, we have the dermal layer, which is full of fibroblast cells that make the collagen that are the skin's scaffolding. As the collagen within the dermis depletes, we start to develop fine wrinkles. The weakened scaffolding also results in thread veins popping up as red patches on our skin. Rebuilding collagen is the mainstay of modern skin treatments with various stimulants ranging from needles to lasers, as we saw earlier.

- Hyaluronic acid levels decline: within the dermis we also find most of the hyaluronic acid, or HA. This substance holds together the structures of the dermis in the way that jelly holds the fruit in a trifle. However, as our levels of HA lower through our life, our skin dries out and looks wrinkled. Modern fillers work by plumping up the dermis with this natural gel.

- The fatty layer dwindles: just below the skin is the fatty layer called the hypodermis or sub-dermis, which also contains some collagen structuring. As this weakens we develop deep wrinkles and sagging, particularly of the jowls and around the eyes.

TACKLING THE FIVE ELEMENTS

The solution to minimising skin ageing, then, is a range of techniques that tackle each element. My clinic uses five common methods to excellent effect.

1. *Skin peels*

Peeling the skin sounds dramatic, but in truth it can – and should – be mild. Peeling lessens the roughness and dullness of the skin, and is necessary because, as we age, our levels of cathepsin-D drop, causing the dead surface of our skin to thicken.

Modern peels, which are much gentler than their equivalents of even a decade ago and require little or no downtime for the patient, remove this dead surface of skin, stimulate the living cells beneath, even out some of the pigmentation and let the skin glow.[59]

2. *Pigmentation*

If, like me, you are an outdoors person then you will not be able to prevent pigmentation from returning next summer, but you can improve it by doing the following:

- Use gentle skin peels to strip off the surface pigmentation.
- Apply high-quality vitamin C serum and vitamin A cream to block new pigment from forming.
- Use skin lasers to vaporise the deeper pigmentation.

3. *Fibroblasts*

We can improve the fine lines associated with ageing by stimulating the fibroblast cells that manufacture the structural collagen. We saw earlier that one way to stimulate fibroblasts is by using vitamin C serum, vitamin A cream and by injecting small amounts of hyaluronic acid filler into the dermis.

---

59   Kligman, A. M. et al. 'Salicylic Acid Peels for the Treatment of Photoaging.' *Dermatol Surg* (1998): 24: 325–8.

There is another way to increase collagen: using growth factors. These are proteins or hormones that your body produces, and that you can also find in a bottle. They work like this:

- Any trauma to the skin – from a needle to a fist – causes the skin to release growth factors that stimulate collagen to heal the wound with a small scar. Instead of having to look for a needle or a fight every time we want to strengthen our wrinkled skin, we can simply apply a cream that contains the appropriate growth factors identified by science as stimulating collagen.

- Useful though bottled growth factors are, those made by your body are stronger and better. To achieve that, many of my patients use a skin-roller that has dozens of tiny needles on it. Rolling this across the skin makes multiple tiny pinpricks in the skin and stimulates a face full of growth factors. And although it sounds painful, the sensation is merely ticklish.

- Finally, you can go one better than using a skin-roller in a process known as Platelet-Rich Plasma therapy, or PRP, which uses your own growth factors. A medical practitioner draws some of your blood, spins it to extract the activated growth factors, and injects those back into your skin. PRP is affectionately known as the 'vampire facial', and has been shown not only to stimulate collagen but also to stimulate the holy grail of skincare – new fibroblasts.[60]

4. Hydration

A dry skin is one that lacks moisture. Turning this around means adding moisture, and there are several ways to do this: use high-quality hydrating skin creams; balance the menopausal hormones[61] in women and testosterone in men; and inject tiny drops of hyaluronic acid (HA) filler just under the skin, which refills the dermis with HA and hydrates the skin.

60 Hara, T. et al. 'Platelet-Rich-Plasma Stimulates Human Dermal Fibroblast Proliferation via a Ras-Dependant Extracellular Signal-Regulated Kinase ½ Pathway.' *J Artif Organs* (2016): 19: 372–7.
61 Brincat, M. P. 'Review: Hormone Replacement Therapy and the Skin'. *Maturitas* (2000): 35: 107–17.

5. *Deep tissue weakness*

The fifth method to reduce deep wrinkles and sagging jowls requires working with the skin's third layer: the hypodermis or sub-dermis. Injecting filler into the sub-dermal layer irritates the skin into manufacturing collagen, which, as we know, strengthens this deep layer.

Another technique, called 'threading', sees the practitioner insert very thin threads into the sub-dermal layer. This pulls back the skin and irritates the sub-dermal layer into producing more collagen.

Fat transfer and stem cells

So far, we have encountered two 'holy grail' treatments for skin rejuvenation that stimulate and form new fibroblasts: vitamin C serum and PRP. There is a third method too, and it is to my mind the most exciting.

It involves something called a fat transfer procedure in which a doctor removes a small amount of fat from your love handle and injects it back into the skin of your face. This not only acts as the ultimate natural filler; it also improves skin quality by stimulating new collagen[62] and, most rewardingly, stimulates stem cells in the skin to develop into new skin cells.[63]

Modern techniques mean that not only is the fat removed more gently; the stem cells can also be infused with fibroblast growth factors to encourage more of them to develop into fibroblasts.[64] The result is a skin that is gently plumped up and looks younger.

---

62 Damour, O. et al. 'Improvement of Skin Quality After Fat Grafting: Clinical Observation and an Animal Study.' *Plast Reconstr Surg* (2009): 124: 765–74.

63 Edward, W. et al. 'The Stromal Vascular Fraction of Autologous Fat Graft Induces Proliferation of Epithelial Progenitor Cells in Healthy and Cancer-Containing Breast Tissue In Vitro.' *Plast Reconstr Surg* (2014): 134: 51–2.

64 Jiang, A. et al. 'Improvement of the Survival of Human Autologous Fat Transplantation by Adipose-Derived Stem-Cells-Assisted Lipotransfer Combined with bFGF.' *Scientific World Journal* (2015): 968057.

Why does it work? Because tucked in between fat cells are millions of stem cells. Over the last twenty years technology has evolved to harness these stem cells and use them to regenerate tissue in the body: they can be injected into the skin for a younger look; they can be injected into the knee joint to rebuild cartilage; and they can be injected into the blood from where they travel to the body's organs and replace damaged tissue.

SKIN LASERS

The word 'laser' stands for Light Amplification by Stimulated emission of Electromagnetic Radiation, and it is this technology that underpins the last item we shall examine in our quest for better skin health. Lasers have garnered plenty of bad press in recent decades, yet even if they are not your thing I would encourage you to read this section and understand the fascinating progress we have made in turning light energy into skin healing.

A century ago, Albert Einstein unpacked the 'Stimulated emission' part of the 'laser' mouthful. Einstein theorised that electrons could be stimulated to emit a light of one particular wavelength or colour – and that is precisely what lasers are all about. It took another four decades before Columbia University graduate Gordon Gould jotted on scrap paper his ideas for building a laser. From that point lasers evolved rapidly, and today are used in areas including: reading barcodes, CDs and DVDs; scanning documents; weapons; and hospitals.

For our purposes, medical lasers are employed to focus energy to vaporise different targets on the skin.

The way it works is straightforward. Earlier we saw that sunlight is made up of different wavelengths. More than 40 per cent is visible light, and this covers the spectrum from violet to red (the colours of the rainbow) and has a wavelength of between 400 nanometres and 700 nanometres. Each colour has a different wavelength – violet is around 400nm, for example, moving all the way through the rainbow to red, which is around 650–700nm.

Figure 3: The visible light spectrum

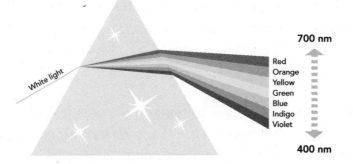

A laser simply splits white light into the colours of the rainbow (and more), and then focuses one wavelength on to the skin. The longer the wavelength chosen – with red being the longest of the visible spectrum – the deeper the laser can penetrate the skin.

We use this feature in two ways:

- We can vary the depth at which the laser heats the skin and in that way penetrate light into the top (epidermis), the middle (dermis) or the sub-dermis.

- And we can choose a specific wavelength and focus the heat on only one structure in the skin that absorbs that wavelength colour. For example, we could choose a laser wavelength of 650nm, which our eyes will see as red. Anything red on the skin will attract all the heat of the 650nm laser and be vaporised. This is useful for targeting red pigmentation or for removing superficial red veins.

Using a laser, then, allows us to choose the depth to which we shoot the wavelength and the structure that we are targeting.

The evolution of lasers

Given the value of lasers, it is worth exploring how far they have evolved since their early days and what it is still worth being cautious about.

Intense Pulsed Light

Readers might have encountered an Intense Pulsed Light machine, known as an IPL, in a beauty salon. Where a laser employs just one wavelength, IPLs use a multitude of wavelengths, and this allows them to target multiple problems on the skin.

Strictly speaking, an IPL is not a laser but it looks like one, acts like one and is often referred to as one.

Early lasers were used to rejuvenate the skin by delivering 'controlled thermal damage', medical-speak for heat. As we saw earlier, heat causes skin inflammation, the release of growth factor and, thus, collagen formation. But we also know from the section on skin cancer that *too much heat* damages the skin. So, a bit of heat can stimulate collagen, but too much heat tends to break down the skin. As in so much of life, balance is key.

By the 1980s, medical-laser companies recognised this danger and developed techniques to prevent the skin overheating. Instead of releasing a continuous stream of energy, these new machines pulsed the beam of light, which meant less heat entered the skin. These machines were aptly named 'pulsed dye lasers'.

Pulsed dye lasers were later followed by Q-switch lasers that did much the same thing: they pulsed energy to reduce heat and achieve selective heat damage. Studies from those days showed that reducing the heat to the skin stimulated collagen and did not damage[65] or weaken[66] the skin. Despite these measures to reduce heat, some people worried that *repeated* mild heat from lasers would one day be seen to do more harm than good.

Using the heat in a laser to achieve one result and reducing the heat to achieve another is best illustrated by the not-so-snappily named Nd:YAG laser. This laser can both remove keloid scars (it *uses* heat to break down

65   Kuo, T. et al. 'Collagen Thermal Damage and Collagen Synthesis After Cutaneous Laser Resurfacing.' *Lasers Surg Med* (1998): 23: 66–71.
66   Schomaker, K. T. et al. 'Thermal Damage Produced by High Irradiance Continuous Wave CO2 Laser-Cutting of Tissue.' *Lasers Surg Med* (1990): 10: 74–84.

scar tissue) and can rejuvenate skin (by *reducing* heat to stimulate collagen formation).

Figure 4: Collagen formation and destruction in the skin

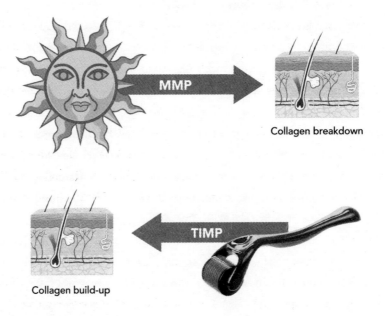

To explain how it does this we need to understand how keloid scars form. Earlier we saw that a wound-healing enzyme called MMP (matrix metalloproteinase) is responsible for breaking down excess scar tissue. Similarly, an enzyme called TIMP (tissue inhibitor of metalloproteinase) *inhibits* the MMP enzyme and therefore is responsible for building up scar tissue. So, MMP breaks down scar tissue, and TIMP builds it up. And because scar tissue is made up of collagen, MMP breaks down collagen and TIMP builds it up.

Figure 4 shows how this works: the heat from the sun stimulates MMP in the skin, and this breaks down collagen. An activity such as rolling micro-needles across the skin stimulates TIMP and builds up collagen.

Some people are born with an excess of one of these enzymes: those with too much TIMP will not wrinkle much through life, but if they scar they will build too much scar collagen which will form a keloid lump. On the other hand those with excessive MMP will not scar badly, but they will not make enough skin collagen as they age and – particularly if they are exposed to the sun – will tend to develop a wrinkled skin.[67]

How does this relate to our Nd:YAG laser? Simply enough, applying infra-red light (which is heat) from the Nd:YAG laser to a keloid scar or an acne scar in someone who produces too much TIMP will stimulate their skin to release excess MMP, and that will break down and thin the collagen in the keloid scar in just a few sessions.[68]

But if we put a Q-switch on to this same Nd:YAG laser, we can remove most of the heat. Now, instead of stimulating MMP, the Nd:YAG will mainly stimulate the production of TIMP, which builds collagen. This treatment is useful for patients who lack sufficient TIMP to build collagen in the skin.[69]

Lasers – the unloved cousin?

At my clinic, I regard lasers as invaluable: we use them to remove pigments, acne scars, thread veins and unwanted hair; to tighten sagging jowls; and to target wrinkles.

And yet they are not as popular as I would have thought. They are not cheap either, with machines costing around $100,000, which means many practitioners cannot afford them. It seems that one reason for the lack of uptake is the public's suspicion of anything 'too medical', and in the case of lasers that is in part due to

67 Kligman, L. H. 'Photoaging. Manifestations, Prevention and Treatment.' *Clin Geriatr Med* (1989): 51: 235–51.
68 Ogawa, R. et al. 'Nd:YAG Laser Treatment of Keloids and Hypertrophic Scars.' *Eplasty* (2012): 12: e1.
69 Ye, X. et al. 'Investigation of the 1064 Q-Switched Nd:YAG Laser on Collagen Expression in an Animal Model.' *Photomed Laser Surg* (2012): 30: 604–9.

the skin damage done in the 1990s by so-called 'ablative' lasers. However, poor medical practice with modern machines has also had an effect: chatrooms list cases of laser damage to skin, while TV shows like *Botched* encourage people to be sceptical of the industry.

That said, it is important to be cautious because it is difficult to apply a laser to the skin without delivering *some* heat. This mild infrared heat might not directly cause an MMP surge and collagen breakdown, but it has been shown to cause free radical damage to the skin, and this stress – with repeated laser use in a dry, fragile skin – can damage collagen.[70] In truth, any laser machine – from the venerable Nd:YAG[71] to the gentle IPL machines[72] – has the potential to increase free radical damage in the skin. And that is even more the case if the patient has a dry skin (as opposed to an oily skin), because a dry skin is generally already inflamed and therefore at a greater risk of oxidative damage from even a small amount of heat.[73]

What does all that mean in practice? Simply that someone with dry skin should exercise more caution when it comes to laser treatments and should ensure that their skin is prepped appropriately beforehand. How might they do that? As we saw earlier, Pinnell showed that applying vitamin C serum protects the skin from mild heat damage,[74] even if a strong laser is used on the skin.[75]

70 Schroeder, P. et al. 'Infrared Radiation-Induced Matrix Metalloproteinase in Human Skin: Implications for Protection.' *J Invest Dermatol* (2008): 2491–7. Accessed at: https://www.ncbi.nlm.nih.gov/pubmed/18449210.
71 Guzey, M. et al. 'Increase of Free Oxygen Radicals in Aqueous Humour Induced by Selective Nd:YAG Laser Trabeculoplasty in the Rabbit'. *Eur J Opthal* (2001): 11: 47–52.
72 Sorg, O. et al. 'Effect of Intensed Pulsed Light on Lipid Peroxidises and Thymine Dimers.' *Arch Dermatol* (2007): 143: 363–6.
73 Elias, P. M. et al. 'The Aged Epidermal Permeability Barrier: Basis for Functional Abnormalities.' *Clin Geriatr Med* (2002): 18: 103–20.
74 Pinnell, S. R. et al. 'Topical Vitamin C Protects Porcine Skin from Ultraviolet Radiation-Induced Damage.' *Br J Dermatol* (1992): 127: 247–53.
75 Elford, E. L. et al. 'Treatment of Photoaged Skin Using Fractional Nonablative Laser in Combination with Topical Antioxidants.' http://www.struckmd.com/pdf/Combo_Tx_ePoster_ASLMS_2012.pdf

(This study was also funded by cosmeceutical companies, with all the potential conflicts that can bring; that said, I find its conclusions compelling.)

In short, lasers are a key part of the aesthetic practitioner's arsenal: they remove pigment, unwanted hair and thread veins with ease; they reduce scarring in oily skins; and they rejuvenate ageing skins. Importantly, though, if you have a dry, ageing skin then you need to be cautious when using a laser as the damage from the heat could outweigh the benefits. At my clinic, PRP and needle stimulation of the skin are often the preferred choice when rejuvenating a dry, older skin; laser is typically preferred when rejuvenating an oily, pigmented skin.

YOUR SKIN: A FINAL WORD

Like the rest of the body, the skin is in a constant state of rebuilding, and it is only when this repair system of inflammation, growth factors, fibroblasts and collagen-building fails that we start to scar and wrinkle. Trying to fix this with the wrong products – as Gladys Deacon and others learned to terrible cost – can be disastrous.

After decades of experience I can tell you that the most important thing we can do for our skin is not surgery, it is not Botox and it is not a laser treatment. The most important thing is to apply good-quality vitamin products with sun protection factor at the beginning of the day, and at the end of the day to wash off any pollutants and apply a good-quality vitamin A cream.

Whether we blame the depleting ozone layer, ultraviolet light, a lack of vitamin D, infrared heat, pollution or HPV for rising skin-cancer rates is an argument that will resound for years. There is evidence for all of them, but the argument that stands out is the one that shows how well vitamin serums and creams work to prevent skin cancer and DNA damage from the sun. Adding these to our skincare routine ties in with an important trend in aesthetic medicine in recent years: to steer away from over-tightened faces, and to raise awareness of more natural skin treatments.

But be aware: using a sun-protection cream is not enough.

Key points

- Fibroblast cells are the workhorses of the skin: they build the collagen that holds the skin's structure. We are born with billions of fibroblasts, but they deplete in number and effectiveness through life.
- Vitamin C and vitamin A creams protect us from skin cancer, stimulate collagen to reverse wrinkles, and, in the case of vitamin C, stimulate the awakening of fibroblast cells.
- Although stimulating collagen is one solution for an ageing skin, the future lies in treatments that rebuild our fibroblasts. There are three ways to do this: vitamin C serum, vampire facials (PRP treatments), and fat transfers using stem cells.
- We should all use *high-quality* vitamin creams on our skin, but just because the cream states that it has vitamins in it does not make it worth using. Ask a good skin practitioner what they recommend.
- If our skin needs help to repair itself, options include home treatments such as gentle skin peels and needle stimulation.
- Other help is available from the aesthetic world and includes fillers, PRP, fat transfer, lasers and plastic surgery repair. These treatments have become gentler and safer over the years, and modern aesthetic doctors and surgeons ought to be as much artists as physicians in treating their patients.

Chapter 11

THE BRAIN, PART 1 – MUCH MORE THAN IQ

> The mind is everything. What you think, you become.
>
> *Attributed, perhaps inaccurately, to the Buddha*

When I look at this page, everything that happens – from my ability to focus on the words, to the muscles that allow my eyes to turn, to my interpreting the squiggles on this page – is thanks to my brain. Reading is an activity that most of us take for granted, and is just one of countless activities the brain computes every day.

Without my brain I am nothing. If I damage it, the rest of my body crumbles like a sandcastle in a storm, so it makes sense to do everything in our power to feed and protect this vital organ. This chapter will show not only how easily we can damage the brain, but how marvellous life is when we optimise it. In some important ways healthy ageing starts with the brain, and if we do not get this right then we will not get much else right either.

BRAIN DAMAGE

Concussion is the brain injury that most coaches try to avoid at all costs in their athletes. Swedish studies have shown that a single blow to the head in childhood is associated with worse grades at school and a greater potential for depression later in life.[1] Various studies have shown that repeated concussions are even more damaging:

[1] Fazel, S. et al. 'Long-term Outcomes Associated with Traumatic Brain Injury in Childhood and Adolescence: A Nationwide Swedish Cohort Study of a Wide Range of Medical and Social Outcomes.' *PLOS Medicine* (2016): http://dx.doi.org/10.1371/journal.pmed.1002103

- American football players with *recurrent* concussions are susceptible to suffer from depression later in life.[2] Why? Because repeated blows to the head scar the brain in a particular pattern called chronic traumatic encephalopathy (CTE), although we can only know for certain whether someone has suffered this by doing an autopsy after their death. Disturbingly, a study of 111 dead professional American football players who had suffered depression showed 99 per cent of them had the CTE scars to prove it.[3] Among the most recent was ex-NFL star Aaron Hernandez, who hanged himself in 2017 aged twenty-seven while serving a life sentence for murder; CTE researchers at Boston University said his was 'the most severe case they had ever seen'.[4]

- Boxers with multiple concussions also show permanent brain damage in the form of CTE.[5] Interestingly, those who carried the dementia gene (called APOE e4) were shown to be more susceptible to brain damage from concussions than those who did not.[6] They were not necessarily more susceptible to concussion, but once concussed, their brain did not heal as well as people without the gene and, six months later, they displayed more brain damage.[7]

- Even low-contact sports can be fatal: twenty-nine-year-old soccer player Patrick Grange died from chronic brain damage simply from repeatedly heading the ball.[8]

2   Guskiewicz, K. M. et al. 'Recurrent Concussion and Risk of Depression in Retired Professional Football Players.' *Med Sci Sports Exerc* (June 2007): 39 (6): 903–9.

3   Mez, J. et al. 'Clinicopathological Evaluation of Chronic Traumatic Encephalopathy in Players of American Football.' *JAMA* (2017): 318: 360–70.

4   See, for example: www.bbc.com/news/world-us-canada-41356137

5   Ryan, A. J. 'Intracranial Injuries Resulting from Boxing.' *Clin Sports Med* (January 1998): 17 (1): 155–68.

6   Jordan, B. D. et al. 'Apolipoprotein E Epsilon4 Associated with Chronic Traumatic Brain Injury in Boxing.' *JAMA* (1997): 278: 136–40.

7   Zhou, W. et al. 'Meta-analysis of APOE4 and Outcome After Traumatic Brain Injury.' *J Neurotrauma* (2008): 25: 279–90.

8   See, for example: 'Brain Trauma Extends to the Soccer Field' by John Branch. *The New York Times* (26 February 2014).

- Recurrent blows to the brain are also believed to cause another illness called motor neurone disease (MND).[9] In this illness the nerves that tell the muscles to work become diseased and hardened, and so the muscles stop working and wither. The person becomes wheelchair-bound, struggles to breathe and usually dies of a lung infection. Perhaps the best-known MND sufferer was the late physicist Stephen Hawking, although in his case the disease was caused by genetics.

These days, as awareness of brain damage in sports personalities increases, and as sportsmen and sportswomen become increasingly famous, newspapers and magazines regularly carry stories of stars, both major and minor, struck down by related ailments. In South Africa, the late Springbok rugby captain Joost van der Westhuizen is the most famous of at least four members of the national side to suffer from MND. In the US, American footballer Steve Gleason is another recent victim of MND that, it is thought, was caused by recurrent head injuries from the sport.

What this shows us is simple enough: how quickly even our strongest athletes can be felled once the brain stops working. Pictures of Gleason or van der Westhuizen being pushed in a wheelchair around the sports stadiums in which their formerly powerful bodies once carried them to glory describes this tragedy better than a thousand words. These show how fragile our brain is and that, once the brain is damaged, the body does not last long.

> ## White matter and grey matter
> Most readers will have heard of white matter and grey matter, while those with an Agatha Christie bent might well recall her detective hero Hercule Poirot's insistence on relying on his 'little grey cells' – in other words, his intelligence – to solve his cases. But what is white matter, and how does it differ from grey matter?

9   McKee, A. C. et al. 'TDP-43 Proteinopathy and Motor Neurone Disease in Chronic Traumatic Encephalopathy.' *J Neuropathol Exp Neurol* (2010): 69 (9): 918–29.

White matter is the paler tissue, and comprises most of the brain by weight. Its function is to support the brain's grey matter, and it does this by connecting different areas of grey matter to each other. The long, thin part of the neuron that does this connecting is called an axon, and it is these axons that carry the messages from your brain to your broader nervous system to tell your body what to do. The axons are coated in a white fatty substance called the myelin sheath, whose colour gives white matter its name.

Grey matter is the darker tissue in the brain, and is made up of the mass of neural cells that make you, well, you: memory, language, consciousness and thought, to name just a few. Also within your grey matter are dendrites, which are short extensions of the neural cells, and which pass information between these neural cells.

Not surprisingly, then, the shrewd Poirot was right: grey matter processes information. White matter, on the other hand, connects the different areas of the brain to ensure quick thinking. Between them, they comprise your central nervous system, which is your brain and your spinal cord.

At this point your inner Poirot might be wondering how communication takes place between these cells. That is done by messengers: the hormones serotonin and dopamine. These messengers, or neurotransmitters, can often prove to be a weak link in our system and – as we shall see in this chapter and the next – if we become depressed, anxious or addicted, then it is often these that are to blame.

The final aspect of this part of your body's extraordinary communication apparatus is the peripheral nervous system. This is made up of the nerves that emanate from the spinal cord outwards to the rest of your body. They take and receive messages that, for example, make your muscles move, give you the sensations of touch and taste, or warn you that you have just burned this morning's toast.

For an optimal life, then, an essential goal is to protect our brain. For most of us this will have little to do with managing years of physical punishment in a sports stadium or a boxing ring; instead it means guarding ourselves against the brain-altering effects of stress, lack of sleep and poor diet. As this chapter will show, our brain is plastic – which in medical-speak refers to its ability to change (for better or for worse) throughout our lives: how our brain shrinks in stressful situations, and how it blossoms in optimal circumstances. We will also look at what drives cravings, and what causes forgetfulness and dementia. Harnessing these insights puts us on the road to a healthy brain, a literally vital step towards having a healthy body.

Neuroplasticity

It was not that long ago that the medical profession thought that the brain formed in childhood remained unchanged for the rest of our lives.[10] That meant it did not evolve any further, and that in turn meant you could not recover any of its power after an injury – which is why, fifty years ago, if you suffered a stroke, your doctor would not bother to try to rehabilitate your brain because the medical world did not believe a damaged brain could possibly regenerate.

It was not until the 1970s that the term 'brain plasticity' surfaced. The term refers to a groundbreaking concept: that the adult brain *can* rebuild with positive experiences and, conversely, it can break down with negative experiences. I like to think that the Russian physiologist Ivan Pavlov should be credited as the father of what is now called neuroplasticity. Having become Russia's first Nobel Laureate in 1904, he went on to become famous for his 'Pavlov's dog' experiments. The first step was training a dog to associate the sound of a bell with food; Pavlov showed that a brain pathway would *develop* to cause the dog to salivate merely at the sound of that bell.

It took another eighty years for the concept of 'new brain pathways' to evolve into a better understanding of neuroplasticity. In the 1980s scientists

10   Pascual-Leone, A. 'The Plastic Human Brain Cortex.' *Ann Rev Neurosci* (2005): 28: 377–401.

showed that if a monkey's finger was amputated, the fingers either side of the stump would start to take over the missing digit's function, and would do so in just six weeks.[11] In medical-speak, the brain showed 'adaptive neuroplastic change', presumably to ensure the monkey's continued survival. You might recall from the chapter on adrenal strain how our stress response helps us to adapt and survive; similarly, it seems that neuroplasticity is the mechanism that helps our brain respond to stress, which helps us to adapt and survive.

There are two types of neuroplasticity: type 1 is rewiring the brain after an injury, and is called *structural* neuroplasticity. The monkey study is an example of this. How does it work? Well, it is a bit like what happens with Google Maps when it realises the road ahead is blocked: Google's computers redirect you to your destination using the next best route. Similarly, when your brain needs to rebuild its structure after an injury, it will reorganise neural pathways using the next best route.

Type 2 is learning a new activity, and is called *functional* neuroplasticity. The more we practise something, the better we get at it. Why? Because the brain builds neurons to improve our performance. There is no shortage of examples:

- One famous study looked at the brains of London cab drivers. While bus drivers need to know only a handful of routes, cab drivers have to memorise at least 400 simply to qualify – a test known as 'The Knowledge'. The result of all this studying is that the central part of a cabbie's brain (the hippocampus) is larger and more developed than that of a bus driver, who has no need to develop that skill.[12]
- Another good example involves research on medical students: their brains were scanned while they were studying for exams and compared against those who were not. The former quickly developed larger grey matter as a consequence of their studying.[13]

11   Merzenich, M. M. et al. 'Somatosensory Cortical Map Changes Following Digit Amputation in Adult Monkeys.' *J Comp Neurol* (1984): 224 (4): 591–605.

12   Maguire, E. A. et al. 'London Taxi Drivers and Bus Drivers: A Structural MRI and Neuropsychological Analysis.' *Hippocampus* (2006): 16: 1091–101.

13   Draganski, B. et al. 'Temporal and Spatial Dynamics of Brain Structure Changes during Extensive Learning.' *J Neurosci* (7 June 2006): 26 (23): 6314–17.

- Learning to play a musical instrument results in the grey matter of your brain growing.[14]
- Learning a second language results in a different section of your brain developing.[15]
- Practising a hand-eye coordination sport like juggling, tennis or golf sees a temporary growth in the brain cortex that controls that activity. Rather like a muscle, exercising the brain results in the brain strengthening in that direction. In the same way, if we *stop* practising that sport then the associated grey matter shrinks and our ability once again regresses.[16] This is vital to understand: the useful habits that we practise are reinforced, while any habits we have discarded are considered no longer useful and, like the unneeded branches of a tree, are pruned.

These studies show the adult brain is an active organ that continuously grows larger or smaller depending on how much we use it. This is functional neuroplasticity in action, and it goes on throughout our life. It turns out that the brain is far more than a storage house for memories; it is in a constant state of rebuilding from childhood to adulthood.

What, then, about an elderly person's brain? Is that neuroplastic? Can it generate new tissue? And are elderly people able to generate new brain pathways in their autumn years in the same way that young people can? The traditional answer was that they could not, but recent evidence suggests the answer is yes.

The easiest way to test this is to give someone a difficult task and see if they get better at it. When elderly adults were asked to practise juggling over a ninety-day period, their brains responded with neuroplasticity: new grey matter was formed and they improved at the task.[17] In other words, they

14   Gaser, C. et al. 'Brain Structures Differ Between Musicians and Non-musicians.' *J Neurosci* (2003): 23: 9240–5.

15   Mechelli, A. et al. 'Neurolinguistics: Structural Plasticity in the Bilingual Brain.' *Nature* (2004): 431: 757.

16   Draganski, B. et al. 'Neuroplasticity: Changes in Grey Matter Induced by Training.' *Nature* (2004): 427: 311–12.

17   Boyke, J. et al. 'Training-induced Brain Structure Changes in the Elderly.' *J Neurosci* (2008): 28: 7031–5.

showed functional neuroplasticity. In elderly stroke victims, the part of the brain that allows them to walk might have been profoundly damaged. However, using intensive stimulation, some patients regained the ability to use their hands and legs, and to recover the power of speech.[18] In other words, they showed structural neuroplasticity.

And although mammals typically make fewer new brain cells during their life, recent research suggests humans are different: when doing autopsies on the brains of young and old people, scientists found the number of active cells in the hippocampus was similar in both. The hippocampus is at the centre of the brain and is intrinsic to our ability to learn and remember facts; having fewer cells in the hippocampus is associated with reduced memory function[19]. However, the older people did have a smaller pool of *stem* cells to draw on and at some stage those would run out. In the final chapter we will see how the work being done with stem cells might help.

So, while it is true that we have to work a little harder to rebuild our brain when we are older, it turns out that our potential to benefit from neuroplasticity does not leave us. And that means we should not stop stimulating our brain. In fact, because brain neuroplasticity gets more sluggish as we age, we need to work twice as hard to keep our brain fit in our twilight years.

NEURODEGENERATION

Because our brain gets less flexible as we age, putting the elderly in front of the television, alone, for hours on end, avoiding exercise and with almost no mental stimulation, is a particularly bad idea. Indeed, few things deteriorate the brain faster – and that during a time when it perhaps most needs stimulation.

However, this does not only afflict the elderly. Isolation at any age causes brain tissue to break down in a process called neurodegeneration, as the brain

18   Hara, Y. 'Brain Plasticity and Rehabilitation in Stroke Victims.' *J Nippon Med Sch* (2015): 82: 4–13.
19   Boldrini, M. et al. 'Human hippocampal neurogenesis persists throughout aging.' *Cell Stem Cell* (2018): 22: 589–99.

– quite literally – shrivels away. This process was shown in the work of Dr Nathan Fox, who examined the brains of children left isolated in terrible conditions in orphanages in Romania. Those orphanages, home to thousands of children for years, became notorious in the 1990s.

Fox followed these children for fourteen years and highlighted their plight. Perhaps most poignantly, when he entered infant wards there was an eerie silence. Why? Because nobody picked up the youngsters or showed them love, and so they had learned even at that young age that no one would respond to their cries. They were utterly isolated, and their ceasing to cry was one result. Another was revealed by brain imaging: the neglect, lack of love and lack of stimulation caused their brains to shrink in both volume and in grey matter.[20]

The regions of the brain

The brain not only controls our body's functions and interprets information from the outside world, it is the seat of what makes each of us 'us' – our personality, intelligence, abilities, creativity and much else besides.

As the diagram on page 366 shows, it has three main areas: the forebrain, the brainstem and the hindbrain.

The forebrain is by far the largest, and is our 'evolved' brain: also known as the cerebrum, it is comprised of two nerve-linked hemi-spheres, each of which is divided into four lobes; it is here that higher-level functions such as speech, abstract thought and reasoning take place; it is also where vision, hearing and touch, for example, are processed.

The brainstem is composed of the pons, the medulla and the midbrain. It connects the cerebrum and the cerebellum (the hindbrain) with the spinal cord, and is the brain's relay station

20 Weir, K. 'The Lasting Impact of Neglect.' *American Psychological Association* (2014): 45 (6): 36.

for messages. This is also where a range of automatic functions are performed including breathing, digestion and our waking and sleeping cycle.

The third part of the brain, the hindbrain, is also called the cerebellum, which means 'little brain' in Latin. It is here that our muscle movements are coordinated, as well as our balance and posture.

Figure 1: The three main areas of the brain

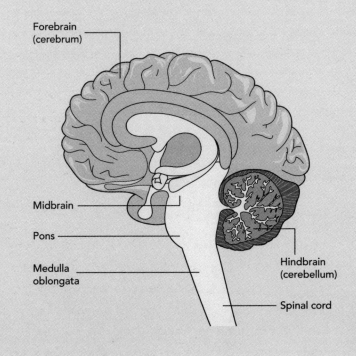

How can I use neuroplasticity?

The takeaway from this is simple: from the cradle to the grave, our brains are plastic and will grow or shrivel depending on how we treat them. Stimulating the brain causes grey matter to expand (neurogenesis), while emotional abuse of the brain causes grey matter to shrink (neurodegeneration), which is devastating for development and health.

Neuroplasticity, then, is the basis of who we are, and our brain is affected positively or negatively every moment of every day. Life happens to us, but *we* retain the power to decide how to react. With that said, I would like you to meet three people who understand the power of positively stimulating the brain.

The first is Stephen Jepson, and he is someone who has done a lot with his life, including getting his masters in ceramics and spending eight years as a professor at the University of Florida. At the time of writing, he is in his mid-seventies and focuses on the art of play. Jepson reckons most of us forget how to play after childhood and so, believing in play over exercise, has devised an educational website called www.neverleavetheplayground. com. He recommends that adults be constantly busy with play to stimulate hand-eye coordination for body and brain. Going for a thirty-minute jog and then sitting on a chair for the rest of the day is, he says, not healthy; and, just like children, we should play in different ways throughout the day. Jepson practises what he preaches: his website shows him juggling, racing down a slide, swimming and even riding a unicycle.

The second is Wang Deshun, nicknamed 'China's hottest grandpa': an artist, DJ, actor and – as of 2015, when he turned seventy-nine – a ramp model. Although nature determines your age, he told *The New York Times*, 'you determine your state of mind'.[21] Wang spends his mornings reading and learning, and his afternoons exercising. He eats what he wants, but these days drinks less alcohol than he used to. As we age, most of us tend to fall into fixed routines and fail to find time to do some of the things we used to enjoy; commonly, we do not try out new experiences. Wang says there is a simple test for how old you are: 'Do you dare to try something you have never done before?'

Another man who practises what he preaches, Wang said his next challenge was to go skydiving.

The third person is my late grandfather, who was fortunate to survive the trenches of World War I (many, and perhaps most, of the men in his battalion

21 'An 80-Year-Old Model Reshapes China's Views on Aging'. *The New York Times* (3 November 2016).

did not). I remember him as someone who recognised the importance of play and of a positive approach to life. Instead of being bitter about his life experiences – and they were difficult, including years spent trying to fend for his family in Canada and Scotland during the Great Depression – he was grateful that he had survived the war, and he remained an optimist. Indeed, science shows that the more grateful we are for our lot, the healthier we become.[22] A lifelong cricket fan, at the age of ninety, with a twinkle in his eye, he bowled me out in a game of backyard cricket. I could not have been more proud of him.

The experiences of these three great men demonstrate important insights into what stimulates the brain's plasticity: exercise and balance, pushing ourselves to try new things (playing music, practising a language or even being a ramp model), and letting go of negative experiences to focus on life's positive aspects.

And we certainly need to abandon the notion that once grandchildren come along or once we reach a certain age we should starting to act like 'old people'. If we want to optimise our health as we age, then science shows we must keep stimulating our brain: never stop playing, regularly embrace new activities, and always *believe* that you can bowl out the young whippersnappers.

Let us take a look at some specific examples of what we can do to continue to stimulate the brain as we age:

- Aerobic exercise: remarkably, exercise has been shown to stimulate the brain and make us more intelligent. It does this by stimulating the release of a protein called brain-derived neurotrophic factor (BDNF) which stimulates new brain tissue. Stroke victims who do regular aerobic exercise rebuild their brain tissue and accelerate their recovery,[23]

---

22   Bhullar, N. et al. 'Dispositional Gratitude Mediates the Relationship Between a Past-Positive Temporal Frame and Well-being.' *Science Direct* (2015): 76: 52–5.
23   Mang, C. S. 'Promoting Neuroplasticity for Motor Rehabilitation After Stroke: Considering the Effects of Aerobic Exercise and Genetic Variation on Brain-Derived Neurotrophic Factor.' *Phys Ther* (2013): 93: 1707–16.

and regular exercise cuts our risk of dementia.[24] No matter what age you are, you should do some exercise every day.

- Play a musical instrument: even if, like me, you are unlikely to head-line at Carnegie Hall, science has shown that the mental dexterity needed to practise playing the piano or the flute, for example, is exceptionally good for neuroplasticity, and has been shown to benefit the brains of the elderly.[25]

- Balancing exercises: practising neurogenesis not only helps our memory, it helps the entire brain. And doing daily balancing exer-cises helps to rebuild the cerebellum. That improves our balance (practice makes perfect, right?), helps to keep us mobile and lessens our chances of falling and breaking a limb.[26]

- Practise a second language: people who speak a second language cut their chance of developing dementia.[27] Speaking more than one language requires coordination through multiple areas of the brain, and has been shown to be extremely beneficial.

- Dance: if you can, then hit the floor like John Travolta or Ginger Rogers; if you are not up to their standard, dance anyway. Elderly people who dance regularly show superior cognitive, motor and perceptual abilities compared to their peers who do not.[28] Dancing stimulates numerous brain activities from rhythm to coordination to socialising, and these are excellent for neurogenesis.

24 Larson, E. B. et al. 'Exercise is Associated with Reduced Risk for Incident Dementia Among Persons 65 Years of Age or Older.' *Ann Intern Med* (2006): 144: 73–81.
25 Seinfeld, S. et al. 'Effects of Music Learning and Piano Practice on Cognitive Function, Mood and Quality of Life in Older Adults.' *Front Psychol* (2013): 4: 810.
26 Sherrington, C. et al. 'Effective Exercise for the Prevention of Falls: A Systematic Review and Meta-analysis.' *J Am Geriatr Soc* (2008): 56: 2234–43.
27 Alladi, S. et al. 'Bilingualism Delays Age at Onset of Dementia, Independent of Education and Immigration Status.' *Neurology* (2013).
28 Kattenstroth, J.-C. et al. 'Superior Sensory, Motor and Cognitive Performance in Elderly Individuals with Multi-year Dancing Activities.' *Front Aging Neurosci* (21 July 2010).

- Variety: it is important to keep stimulating the brain in as many different ways as possible. Try Sudoku, cards, painting, gardening, cooking – anything that adds to your repertoire of skills. If you can combine that with seeing the world through a child's eyes – with wonder – then you have an excellent chance of staying inquisitive about life and keeping your brain in optimal health to the very end.

Before closing this section it is worth mentioning two relatively recent developments that have added to our understanding of the brain and neuroplasticity. The first is that antidepressant medication seems to help the brain – in other words, it accelerates neurogenesis. That is good news and, despite the bad press antidepressants often get, is not as strange as it might seem: after all, we know stress breaks down brain tissue (something we will go into shortly) and we know antidepressants combat stress, which probably explains why they have the opposite effect. Stroke victims, for instance, who were given the anti-depressant Prozac, exhibited much faster recovery times than those who only did rehabilitation exercises.[29] It is thought that Prozac helps to accelerate brain plasticity and speed up recovery.

Another study showed that Prozac-like tablets taken over a lengthy period stimulated new nerves to form and caused those nerves to become healthy adult nerves more quickly in the brain's central memory section, which is called the hippocampus. In other words, the study showed that anti-depressant tablets work by stimulating neurogenesis.[30]

Linked to this, researchers have used rats to see how antidepressants affect the brain, and they showed that, if rats are gradually stressed into depression, they start to run out of BDNF, which is a nerve stimulator. We know that exercise stimulates BDNF, and studies show that giving rats an antidepressant similar to Prozac caused BDNF to increase and brain tissue to

29   Chollet, F. et al. 'Fluoxetine for Motor Recovery After Acute Ischaemic Stroke (FLAME): A Randomised Placebo-controlled Trial.' *Lancet Neurol* (2011): 10: 123–30.
30   Hen, R. et al. 'Chronic Fluoxetine Stimulates Maturation and Synaptic Plasticity of Adult-born Hippocampal Granule Cells.' *J Neurosci* (2008): 1374–84.

rebuild.[31] These three examples suggest to me that Prozac-like medication can accelerate brain-healing after a stroke and can accelerate neurogenesis in depressed people. It seems likely that it achieves this by activating nerve stimulators like BDNF.

The second development is in the area of virtual reality, or VR, which could soon prove to be a powerful contributor to neuroplasticity. When you put on a VR headset, all you can see in any direction is the world you are shown on that wrap-around screen. This fake world becomes your reality, and it makes for a powerful experience. What your eyes see, the brain believes. It is like stepping into James Cameron's movie *Avatar* where paraplegic Jake Sully is transported into the body of a Navi warrior, and can run and jump, lighting up his brain with excitement. VR companies have developed similar realities for stroke victims; the underlying thesis is that if we see our arm moving on command, then the brain should accelerate nerve regeneration for that arm movement.

Companies like MindMaze – tagline: 'mind over matter' – use VR to help patients recover from brain injuries. The company, which was founded by a neuroscientist, claims a 35 per cent improvement in limb function in just four weeks. The Cochrane Library has reviewed the results of companies like MindMaze, and has concluded that VR has a place in rehabilitating stroke victims.[32]

STRESS

We saw earlier that negative experiences shrink the brain and positive experiences enlarge it. In previous chapters we learned that ongoing stress breaks down brain tissue. By way of a reminder, we saw that:

31 Mao, Q. Q. et al. 'Long-term Treatment with Peony-glycosides Reverses Chronic Unpredictable Mild Stress-induced Depressive-like Behaviour via Increasing Expression of Neurotrophins in Rat Brain.' *Behav Brain Res* (2010): 210: 171–7.
32 'Virtual Reality for Stroke Rehabilitation.' *Cochrane* (February 2015): http://www.cochrane.org/CD008349/STROKE_virtual-reality-for-stroke-rehabilitation

- Long-term exposure to the stress hormone cortisol has been shown to cause the nerve endings to break down in the brains of rats.[33] Stress shrinks our brain, leaving us forgetful and depressed.
- Chronic stress causes the grey matter in a rat's brain to shrink, and the white matter to grow. Grey matter is our higher-thinking part of the brain, while white matter is associated with emotional disorders.[34]
- Long-term stress in humans is associated with higher cortisol levels, worsening memory[35] and depression.[36] Long-term stress has also been shown to damage other parts of the body: it causes DNA damage,[37] tumour growth,[38] heart problems[39] and accelerated ageing.[40]
- A 2012 survey from the UK showed that stress not only damages us; it kills us. As our daily stress increases, so too does our chance of dying.[41]

In other words, we ignore the impact of stress at our peril: it not only damages our brain causing depression and memory loss; it kills us.

The section on neuroplasticity showed us that activities like studying and playing hand-eye coordination games build brain tissue, and we know stress

33 Swaab, D. et al. 'Elevated Cortisol in Rats Induces Neuronal Damage.' *Ageing Res Rev* (2005): 4 (2): 141–94.

34 Chetty, S. et al. 'Stress and Glucocorticoids Promote Oligodendrogenesis in the Adult Hippocampus.' *Mol Psychiatry* (2014): 19: 1275–83.

35 Lupien, S. et al. 'The Douglas Hospital Longitudinal Study of Normal and Pathological Aging.' *J Psychiatry Neurosci* (2005): 30: 328–34.

36 Steptoe, A. et al. 'Depression and Elevated Cortisol.' *Am J Epidemiol* (2008): 167 (1): 96–102.

37 Flint, M. S. et al. 'Induction of DNA Damage, Alteration of DNA Repair and Transcriptional Activation by Stress Hormones.' *Psychoneuroendocrinology* (2007): 32 (5): 470–9.

38 Thaker, P. H. et al. 'Chronic Stress Promotes Tumor Growth and Angiogenesis in a Mouse Model of Ovarian Carcinoma.' *Nat Med* (2006): 12: 939–44.

39 Goldstein DS. 'Review: Catecholamines and Stress.' *Endocr Regul* (June 2003): 37 (2): 69–80.

40 Lu, T. et al. 'Gene Regulation and DNA Damage in the Ageing Human Brain.' *Nature* (24 June 2004): 429 (6994): 883–91.

41 Russ, T. C. 'Association Between Psychological Distress and Mortality: Individual Participant Pooled Analysis of 10 Prospective Cohort Studies.' *BMJ* (2012): 345.

breaks down brain tissue. So it makes sense to reduce stress's load and live a more balanced life. One way is to reduce our stress levels; the other is to work to counter its insidious effects, and we can do the latter by embracing brain exercises. One obvious way is through mindful meditation, which to me seems the easiest way to start a meditating programme.

First, though, I will explain *why* mindfulness is so important and then discuss the studies that support meditation in general.

Mindfulness

Like most people, I rarely focus on what is happening inside my body. Most of us are so busy worrying about what we have not done or what we ought to do that we switch off any thoughts about how our body is feeling *right now*. This ability to switch off from, say, pain can be useful in dangerous situations; it is far less so when it allows us to ignore the damage of long-term stress. Add to that the distractions that modern living brings, with Facebook or television keeping our brains constantly occupied, and it is hardly surprising that we rarely, if ever, check in with ourselves. The result is that our body can become exhausted and our brain depressed without us even knowing. Rather like the frog in the pot of water that is slowly heated up until it boils, we accept this state as normal and do not do enough to change it.

Being perpetually busy, lacking the time to listen to how our body is feeling, achieving our goals at all costs – this is known as 'brain-based living' and it means we seldom, if ever, feel the signs of stress, until one day we are surprised that we have developed stress-driven illnesses such as heart disease, cancer, arthritis or one of the auto-immune diseases.

But if we can simply slow our mind each day and listen to what our body is saying, we will be able to feel when we are starting to hurt, and know when we should give our body a rest. *That* is what mindfulness is designed to do: it is the meditative act of being aware (or 'mindful') of every breath we take, of every sound we hear, of how each part of our body feels at this very moment.

Of course, it takes practice to become aware of our five senses – sight, sound, smell, touch and taste – but the benefits of mindfulness are numerous, as we shall shortly see.

The basic idea of mindfulness is that either we control our thoughts or our thoughts control us. But for those who have not tried it, the obvious question is: how to start? Perhaps the easiest way is to sit still and focus calmly on the act of breathing: the rise and fall of the chest, the sensation as we inhale through the nose, drawing the air into the lungs and then exhaling. That is an example of mindfulness: it helps to push away our thoughts and worries. If we notice them intruding, we can dismiss them by focusing again on our breathing. In so doing, we are regulating the incessant chatter of the brain, and allowing the messages from the body to register with the brain.

As it happens, parts of the brain *are* specifically programmed to allow us to connect it to how the body is feeling. Indeed, this is such a basic function that nature has placed these areas in the brain's centre. They come with grand names like the amygdala and the cingulate gyrus, but perhaps the most studied is the insula (Latin for 'island').[42] We saw earlier that our brain is plastic, and we know therefore that if we do not use a function (such as staying in touch with our body) then we will lose it, or at least that function will be less responsive; we also saw that practising a function increases its ability and sensitivity. This applies equally to the insula: studies show that the more we practise mindful meditation, the more the insula grows, helping us to stay better in touch with how our body is feeling.[43] Failing to use it, of course, means we lose that ability, and become at risk of driving our body to the point of exhaustion in pursuit of whatever goal was important at the time.

To my mind this comes to the crux of stress management: we can treat the *effects* of stress by supporting the adrenals with tablets, and we can reduce anxiety by supporting the brain with tablets. But if we continue to run busy schedules without checking how our body is feeling, we will damage ourselves and have no idea that we are doing it. There is no pill that will strengthen the insula, there is no injection that will make the brain listen to how the body is

42   Gu, X. et al. 'Anterior Insula Cortex and Emotional Awareness.' *J Comp Neurol* (2013): 521: 3371–88.
43   Haase, L. et al. 'Mindfulness-based Training Attenuates Insula Response to an Aversive Interoceptive Challenge.' *Soc Cogn Affect Neurosci* (2016): 11: 182–90.

feeling. Only a mindfulness-based meditation practice will achieve this vital part of the stress-management puzzle.

The practice of mindfulness is an easy introduction to meditation: sitting quietly and scanning the different parts of the body, from the sensation of breath to the tingling in our toes. It connects the brain to the body, and is essential to achieving optimal health.

Meditation

There are many techniques in meditation to help us achieve a healthy brain state. Daily meditative practice not only connects the body to the brain via the insula; it has other proven medical benefits too, as Sarah Lazar, a neuroscientist, was one of the first to demonstrate. In 2005 Lazar showed that meditation not only increases healthy brain waves; it actually changes the brain's physical structure. She also found an association between regular meditation and increased brain tissue thickness.[44] In 2017, she demonstrated conclusively that meditation was not only *associated* with healthy brain thickness, but that it had *caused* this healthy brain thickening.[45]

The other area where meditation has been shown to have a positive effect is on our telomeres, the end caps of our chromosomes, which shorten as our cells divide. Stress has been shown to reduce the length of our telomeres and speed up cell-death, while meditation has been shown to counter that: to reduce stress and maintain telomere length.[46]

Summary

We know mental stress is extremely damaging to our health, and it may still prove to be the most important factor in shortening our lives. When someone comes to my clinic with stress-induced fatigue, I might well order blood tests

---

44   Lazer, S. W. et al. 'Meditation Experience is Associated with Increased Cortical Thickness.' *Neuroreport* (2005): 16: 1893–7.

45   See, for example: http://news.harvard.edu/gazette/story/2011/01/eight-weeks-to-a-better-brain/

46   Epel, E. et al. 'Can Meditation Slow Rate of Cell Ageing? Cognitive Stress, Mindfulness and Telomeres.' *Ann N Y Acad Sci* (2009): 1172.

to see how exhausted their DHEA, progesterone, cortisol and testosterone levels are. That said, although I can correct those elements of ill-health, if the patient does not understand that they have switched off so effectively from their body that they have now become ill, then they might not reverse this process and never truly heal. There is plenty of evidence to show that meditation is not some weird cultic practice, but an essential part of health.

Dealing with stress may well be the most important skill we can learn to optimise our health. Viktor Frankl – psychiatrist, neurologist and survivor of the Holocaust – understood the power of the mind when he wrote: 'Everything can be taken from a man, but one thing: the last of the human freedoms – to choose one's attitude in any given set of circumstances, to choose one's own way.'

If Frankl could choose how his brain was going to react while trying to survive a concentration camp, then surely we have the ability to choose how our brain will react in far lesser circumstances: when the boss shouts at us, when work piles up on our desk, when another person cuts us up in traffic or when our kids wind us up as only our kids can. We retain the freedom to choose how we will react in each case.

Deciding that it makes sense to choose how to react to situations is one thing; achieving that is another. How can we do this? That requires understanding a little more about how the brain works, and that brings us to the concept of brainwaves.

BRAINWAVES

At my clinic, we make use of a neuro-feedback machine to help people (like me) with busy brains, who struggle to meditate. The neuro-feedback machine has electrodes that attach to the scalp and measure the electrical activity of the brain. This electrical activity is measured as brainwaves and is the starting point to all of our thoughts and emotions.

In simple terms our brainwaves divide into:

- Delta waves (0.5–3Hz). These are our slowest waves, and are prominent during dreamless sleep.

- Theta waves (3–8Hz). These occur during more active sleep and in the deepest state of Zen meditation.
- Alpha waves (8–12Hz). These are our slow-idling-when-awake waves, and are prominent during daydreaming, meditation and endurance exercise.
- Beta waves (12–30Hz). These are often considered to be the fast waves that cause busy brains, and they dominate when we are trying to get lots of things done.
- Gamma waves (25–100Hz). These are our fastest waves, and they help us to learn and to multitask information from different parts of the brain.

Most of us live with too much stress, which means our brains buzz with an excess of beta waves and not enough alpha waves. This is where zebras are superior – after the beta-wave state of fight or flight, they are able to switch back to an alpha state much more quickly than we could. Interestingly, some of the most successful humans are also able to access their alpha state more easily: professional sportsmen are better than amateurs at attaining a high alpha-wave brain state,[47] and professional golfers sink more putts when their brains are in a high alpha-wave state.[48]

At my clinic, brain training typically focuses on performing relaxing brain exercises; these cause the fast beta waves to reduce and the calm alpha waves to increase. This approach has shown great success in people with high anxiety that causes burnout and exhaustion.[49]

In the last couple of years, scientists have approached brainwaves from another angle: instead of doing relaxing exercises to stimulate the 10Hz alpha brainwaves, they connected the brain to a 10Hz electrical current and sat back to see what would happen. The result was that all twenty participants' alpha

47 Babiloni, C. et al. 'Resting State Cortical Rhythms in Athletes. A High-resolution EEG Study.' *Brain Res Bull* (2010): 81: 149–56.
48 Babiloni, C. et al. 'Intra-hemispheric Functional Coupling of Alpha Rhythms is Related to a Golfer's Performance: A Coherence EEG Study.' *Int J Psychophysiol* (2011): 82: 260–8.
49 Moore, N. 'A Review of EEG Biofeedback Treatment of Anxiety Disorders.' *Clin EEG Neurosci* (2000): 31: 1–6.

brainwaves were enhanced and they experienced a significant increase in their ability for creative thinking.[50]

Most people do not need a neuro-feedback machine and they certainly do not need to put an electrical current through their brain. The point is that when you look at meditation, which helps us attain those 10Hz alpha brain-waves, it benefits the brain in ways that are far more scientific than making us feel good. Indeed, meditation optimises our health by:

- Stimulating the insula to put the brain in touch with what the body is feeling.
- Decreasing the fast beta waves to achieve a healthy balance in brainwaves.
- Stimulating healthy grey matter in the brain.
- Decreasing DNA damage of the brain.

The brain state we want to achieve is the same as a cat experiences when watching a mouse: the cat is calm and still, yet is ready to spring into action at any moment.

THE BRAIN, PART 1: A FINAL WORD

I am a firm believer that unless we optimise our brain health, we will not have a chance of optimising the rest of our health. Our brain is plastic, it is sculpted continuously throughout our life, and we are the artist of this brain-sculpting. Our ambition ought to be a brain that is the cerebral equivalent of the sculptures of Michelangelo, not that of a traffic bollard.

To achieve that takes work throughout our life. When we find ourselves in a stressed or depressed state, we must work to turn that around otherwise we risk damaging our brain.

Exercise, meditation, mindfulness, painting, reading, learning, laughing, loving, socialising – all of these are vital for our health. Allowing stress to dominate is a sure-fire way to undermine what chance we have of a healthy

50 Lustenberger, C. et al. 'Functional Role of Frontal Alpha Oscillations in Creativity.' *Cortex* (2015): 67: 74–82.

brain. Mastering how our brain responds to given situations gives us the chance to master life.

At this point it is worth reflecting on the quote at the start of this chapter that is attributed to the Buddha: 'The mind is everything. What you think, you become.' Or, if you prefer your quotes more up-to-date, here is one from another son of the Asian subcontinent – Gandhi, India's independence hero, who reportedly said: 'Your beliefs become your thoughts, your thoughts become your words, your words become your actions, your actions become your habits, your habits become your values, your values become your destiny.'

Both, it turns out, were right, which is why all of us should practise positive neuroplasticity every day.

Key points

- The brain is a vital and sensitive organ. Repeated concussion can cause irreparable damage.
- Always play: whether you are nine or ninety, the brain is elastic. It is important to throw a ball, balance on a pole, dive under a wave, and dance the tango. Always look to try something new, to go somewhere new, to have a new experience.
- Emotional stress damages the brain and the body, and might be the single biggest driver of poor health.
- Meditation stimulates the insula to tell the brain what the body is feeling. The more we practise mindful meditation, the better we get at being in touch with our body. Science has shown meditation stimulates new brain tissue and reduces DNA damage.
- Stress is your sworn enemy, and ignoring it is not a solution. If you want optimal health, you must master how your brain deals with stress. The good news? It is not that difficult to do.

Chapter 12

―――――

The Brain, Part 2 – Are You Feeling Sleepy?

A good laugh and a long sleep are the best cures in the doctor's book.

Irish proverb

In the previous chapter, we saw that our brain is plastic, and that it can advance or regress depending on the care we take of it. Yet there is much more to the brain than its plasticity, and each passing year science adds to our knowledge of it. In this chapter we will look at addictions, memory and dementia, but I want to start with perhaps the most curious feature of our lives: sleep.

Sleep

We spend around a third of our lives sleeping and, despite extensive research, this habit remains one of life's great mysteries. Science does not quite understand how we fall asleep, and we are only starting to learn about the vital activities that take place when we are sleeping. Sleep, it turns out, is essential for reorganising what we have learned and studied during the day.[1] It is much more than that too.

For a start, sleep is essential to our health. A very small number of people can get by on tiny amounts of sleep each night, but even they cannot go without it entirely. We can try to compel ourselves not to sleep, but our body will

―――――

1 Warmsley, E. et al. 'Memory, Sleep and Dreaming: Experiencing Consolidation.' *Sleep Med Clin* (2011): 6: 97–108.

eventually force it upon us. I view sleep on the same level as breathing and drinking water. If we hold our breath, the brain eventually forces us to breathe. If we go without water, the brain causes us to crave water until its absence dominates our every waking moment and we drink. It takes just a night or two of not sleeping before the brain compels us into slumber.

The magician David Blaine is no stranger to extraordinary achievements: he has (reputedly) caught a bullet in his teeth, was buried alive in a coffin for seven days, and was able to hold his breath underwater for seventeen minutes, a world record. Yet even Blaine, despite extensive training, failed to break the world record for staying awake. Randy Gardner is the holder of that title, managing to go without sleep for a little over eleven days in 1964 when he was a teenager. Indeed, a lack of sleep is so dangerous that the *Guinness Book of World Records* has deemed this particular stunt too risky, and removed it from its records. Blaine described his experience of sleep deprivation as follows: thirty-six hours in, it is like being drunk; after three days paranoia sets in; and by the fourth day you start hallucinating.[2]

But the dangers of a lack of sleep go far beyond Blaine's experience. A rare condition called Fatal Familial Insomnia (FFI) shows in a chilling way the importance of sleep. FFI is a genetic disorder where, around the age of fifty, patients are no longer able to sleep *at all*. They begin to hallucinate, develop dementia and within eighteen months most are dead.[3] The consequences of total insomnia are swift and brutal.

Fortunately, FFI is extremely rare; practically speaking, the real danger for most of us is not total insomnia but sleep deprivation, or a lack of sufficient sleep. So, how much sleep is enough? The US National Sleep Foundation, which knows a thing or two on the subject, recommends between seven and nine hours a night for adults.[4] Many of us appear to get by on much less:

2   See, for example: 'David Blaine Braves Brain Damage to Challenge World Record for Staying Awake' by Richard Simpson. *Mail Online* (5 December 2007).
3   Schenkein, J. et al. 'Self-management of Fatal Familial Insomnia. Part 1: What is FFI?' *MedGenMed* (2006): 8: 65.
4   Ohayon, M. et al. 'National Sleep Foundation's Sleep Quality Recommendations: First Report.' *Sleep Health* (2017): Vol 3, Issue 1: 6–19.

a Gallup poll found 40 per cent of US adults sleep for six hours or less each night.[5] Some readers might consider six hours of sleep normal, but studies show that sleep deprivation has profound health implications:

- In the short term, sleep deprivation impedes our ability to react or to think logically. At least one study found that acute sleep deprivation impairs our ability and judgement as much as alcohol.[6]

- In the long term, people who get six hours or less each night run a greater risk of hypertension, heart attacks and diabetes.[7] Sleep deprivation can shrink the brain and worsen our risk of contracting Alzheimer's – a subject we will tackle in greater depth later in this chapter.

- Researchers have found that even short-term sleep apnoea – a condition in which the airway closes numerous times while the person is asleep – has serious effects, including a spike in blood sugar levels, higher blood pressure, and increased levels of stress hormones.[8]

- Insufficient sleep is also strongly linked to inflammation, cancer, obesity, strokes and any number of ailments. As we shall see in the next section, sleep brings phenomenal restorative benefits to the body, and without those the body is unable to heal itself.[9]

So much for the damaging effects of sleep deprivation; let us turn to the benefits of sleep. Researchers recently reviewed fifty years of data and concluded that middle-aged adults (those aged between thirty and sixty)

---

5   Moore, D. 'Eyes Wide Open: Americans, Sleep and Stress' (12 February 2002). http://www.gallup.com/poll/5314/eyes-wide-open-americans-sleep-stress.aspx

6   Williamson, A. M. et al. 'Moderate Sleep Deprivation Produces Impairments in Cognitive and Motor-performance Equivalent to Legally Prescribed Levels of Alcohol Intoxication.' *Occup Environ Med* (2000): 57: 649–55.

7   Nagai, M. et al. 'Sleep Duration as a Risk Factor for Cardiovascular Disease – A Review of the Recent Literature.' *Curr Cardiol Review* (2010): 6: 54–61.

8   See, for instance: https://www.worldhealth.net/news/sleep-apnea-wreaks-havoc-your-metabolism/

9   Verkasalo, P. K. et al 'Sleep Duration and Breast Cancer: A Prospective Cohort Study'. *Cancer Res* (2005): 65: 9595–600.

Mullington, J. et al. 'Sleep Loss and Inflammation.' *Best Pract Res Clin Endocrinol Metab* (2010): 24 (5): 775–84.

who sleep effectively enjoy better memory and brain functioning in later life.[10]

In other words, every good sleep is a win in our lifelong battle for optimal health. And every occasion that we do not sleep well, our body breaks down just a little. Treating conditions such as fatigue, adrenal insufficiency, weight gain, mood problems or even skin rejuvenation is of limited benefit if we do not have a healthy sleep pattern. Why? Because all of these problems rely on sleep to restore our health.

WHAT HAPPENS IN THE BRAIN WHEN WE SLEEP?

Ariane Lüthi, one of the world's leading mountain bikers, is someone who knows the importance of staying at the peak of her abilities. During a period of underperformance she posted on her Facebook page that her doctor had recommended a top performance-enhancing treatment – SLEEP.

Sleep, it turns out, is not just about reorganising the day's memories. An astonishing amount takes place during the small hours, including:

- *Glymphatic activation*: we can consider this as taking out the brain's trash. In the rest of your body, the main system that carries out this role is the lymphatic system, which drains toxins and excretes them; the lymph nodes are key to your lymphatic system. There are, however, no lymph nodes in your brain, and yet it generates toxins all the time; after all, it is the most energy-hungry organ we have. So how does your brain do this? It turns out that it has an equivalent called the glymphatic system. Its job is also to remove toxins, and it does this when we sleep; that is when the otherwise largely invisible glymphatic pathways expand to do their job. We know this thanks in part to work done by a team led by Maiken Nedergaard when she was a professor of neurosurgery at the University of Rochester Medical

10 Scullin, M. et al. 'Sleep Cognition and Normal Aging: Integrating a Half-century of Multidisciplinary Research.' *Sage Journals* (2015). http://journals.sagepub.com/doi/abs/10.1177/1745691614556680

Center in the US. In 2012, she used a new system of microscopy to observe the brains of mice while they slept, and in so doing discovered that, while the mice slept, their brains' cells opened up allowing cerebrospinal fluid to flow freely through the organ, bringing nutrients to cells and carrying away toxins. Among the substances washed out is beta-amyloid, a protein that builds up in the brain during our awake state, and which is strongly associated with Alzheimer's.[11]

- *Consolidating memory and skills*: there are two main stages of sleep: the first is rapid eye movement (REM) sleep, and the second is non-rapid eye movement (NREM) sleep, which itself consists of four stages of progressively slower brain waves. Both REM and NREM sleep are essential to our health, and they cycle in ninety-minute stretches throughout the night. As the sleep graph on the right shows, NREM sleep dominates the early hours of the night, while REM sleep, during which we dream and our muscles are paralysed, dominates the later hours. (Given that we need both types of sleep, going to bed late or getting up early means we lose out on one or the other, and that comes with a health cost.) Different things happen during NREM and REM sleep. In NREM sleep, the brain moves fact-based information from the day's temporary storage area to more secure, permanent sites; that is why an early night's sleep before an exam is such a good idea. NREM sleep is also the time that the glymphatic system gets to work removing the day's toxins – including amyloid proteins that are associated with Alzheimer's. REM sleep has a more creative bent, as you will know from recalling some of your more outlandish dreams, and brings phenomenal problem-solving capabilities (as the phrase 'sleep on it' suggests); it also helps our emotional IQ and is the time when we consolidate what is known as 'procedural memory', or 'remembering how to do things'. So, if you previously tried and failed to learn a new skill – skiing, surfing,

11 Xie, L. et al. 'Sleep Drives Metabolite Clearance from the Adult Brain.' *Science* (2013): 342: 373–7.

practising a song on a musical instrument – and then found that you miraculously improved overnight, you can thank REM for that. It is not just humans that use REM sleep: other animals do too, including mice. In a 2016 study, researchers showed that the REM stage is where we consolidate what we have learned into a more permanent skill: they gave mice a series of tasks to learn, and those that were allowed to drop into REM sleep remembered it the following day; those that were not had to relearn it.[12]

Figure 1: A sleep graph, or hypnogram, that shows how we cycle through REM sleep and the four stages of NREM sleep as the night progresses

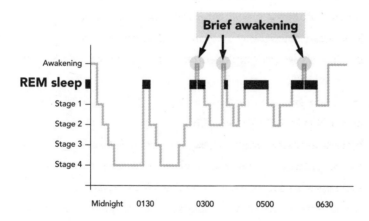

- *Building neurotransmitters*: neurotransmitters are the brain's messenger hormones. We have already encountered serotonin, also known as the 'happy hormone'; it turns out that this hormone gets rebooted during sleep. If you pull an all-nighter, then the following day you will have a low mood and will likely crave junk food. In part, that is

---

12   Boyce, R. et al. 'Causal Evidence for the Role of REM Sleep Theta Rhythm in Contextual Memory Consolidation.' *Science* (2016): 352: 812–16.

due to tired serotonin receptors,[13] and is why it is essential that people dealing with cravings and addictions get enough sleep – as we will see later in this chapter.

• *Rebuilding hormone levels*: this is another key function that takes place when we sleep. Sleep deprivation, on the other hand, causes havoc with our hormones: cortisol levels drop;[14] testosterone levels drop;[15] growth hormone levels drop.[16] Women will experience a decline in their ovary function and lower fertility.[17] I have seen numerous exhausted male executives whose testosterone levels are low and whose libido is shot, and that is largely because they sleep only five hours a night. Giving testosterone to someone like that helps, but not much, and is not the solution. Sleeping eight hours a night is. In short, replacing hormones is often a waste of time unless we correct the patient's inability or unwillingness to get enough sleep.

In other words, an amazing array of essential functions takes place while we sleep. Without sleep our health suffers dramatically; with it we blossom.

Nap time

Humans are wired for two sleeps in each twenty-four-hour cycle – what experts call biphasic sleep. The first of these takes place during the dark hours, when we are meant to get the bulk of our NREM and REM sleep; the second is in the early afternoon, which explains why post-lunch meetings at work are such a bad idea.

13 Eugene, A. R. 'The Neuroprotective Aspects of Sleep.' *MEDtube Sci* (2015): 3: 35–40.

14 Chrousos, G. P. et al. 'Sleep Deprivation Effects on the Activity of the Hypothalamic-pituitary-adrenal and Growth Axes: Potential Clinical Implications.' *Clin Endocrinol* (1999): 51: 205–15.

15 Wittert, G. 'The Relations Between Sleep Disorders and Testosterone in Men.' *Asian J Androl* (2014): 16: 262–5.

16 Davidson, J. R. et al. 'Growth Hormone and Cortisol Secretion in Relation to Sleep and Wakefulness.' *J Psychiatry Neurosci* (1991): 16: 96–102.

17 Kloss, J. D. et al. 'Sleep, Sleep Disturbance and Fertility in Women.' *Sleep Med Rev* (2015): 22: 78–87.

Neuroscientist Matthew Walker has wr[...]
book on sleep called, sensibly enough, *Why We [...]*
it, not least because it covers much more ground tha[...]
in one section of a chapter.

In his book he talks about his visits to Greece as a child in the
1980s, and noticing that shops opened at 9am, closed at 1pm, and
reopened at 5pm for their second stint of trading. Why? Because the
1–5pm slot was reserved for downtime, including napping.

By the beginning of this century, however, that habit started to
fall away, doubtless as economic pressures meant shops needed to
stay open longer. That prompted researchers from Harvard
University to spend six years studying the effect that this
'no-napping' lifestyle had on the cardiovascular health of men and
women between the ages of twenty and eighty-three.

The results were catastrophic: those who no longer napped had a
37 per cent greater risk of dying from heart disease. Men who worked
were worst affected – their risk shot up more than 60 per cent. In
other words, missing out on biphasic sleep means we die earlier.

Walker points out that in places where men continue to nap on a
daily basis, they are far more likely than American men to reach
ninety. As he puts it, 'the practice of biphasic sleep, and a healthy
diet, appear to be the keys to a long-sustained life'.

Why might daytime napping help us? From my perspective the
following explanation seems logical: we know stress is one of our
Three Horsemen, and we know too that many of us work stressed
eight-hour days with adrenalin coursing through our system.
Adrenalin's job is to wire us for survival, but we also know excess
stress (and therefore excess adrenalin) damages our brain, our
arteries and our immune system. If we could fall asleep around
midday, then we would enjoy a stress-free, low-adrenalin state
during our one-hour nap. The result? We would run on four hours
of stress in the morning, enjoy a stress-busting nap, and then run on

some more stress in the afternoon. That would surely be much healthier than what most of us do, which is an eight-hour day (or more) at full tilt.

Something else Walker points out: all adults (barring a fraction of 1 per cent of people who are genetically different) need at least eight hours of sleep each night. Not six, not four, but eight or more, and those who heroically plough on through life living on just five or six hours a night will eventually pay for it. It turns out, too, that you never get back a sleep deficit, which means the effects of one night's bad sleep are marked on you for life. So if you are not getting at least eight hours a night, you must make sure that you do.

SLEEPING AIDS

It is three in the morning, you have to be up at six, and you have not slept. Sound familiar? Fortunately this is only an occasional problem for most of us. But for others the inability to sleep (which in its worst form can be classed as insomnia) is far more serious, and they might well have tried any number of remedies to fix it: meditation, lavender oil, chamomile tea, hot milk, magnesium, calcium, GABA analogues, 5-HTP, alcohol, sedatives like chloral hydrate, antihistamines or progesterone cream. They might even have tried taking scheduled medications such as amitriptyline, quetiapine or gabapentin, or they might have been prescribed a regular sleeping tablet called a benzodiazepine.

Benzodiazepines were made famous by The Rolling Stones on their song 'Mother's Little Helper', in which the woman in the song gets through the stresses of the day by popping pills. Benzodiazepines work by attaching to the brain's GABA receptors, which provide relaxation, and in that way calm the brain.[18]

---

18 GABA is the abbreviation for the neurotransmitter gamma-aminobutyric acid; its job is to reduce activity in those neurons to which it attaches – in other words, in the GABA receptors. In so doing, it relaxes you.

They are a class of medication that my clinic prescribes only occasionally to break the habit of sleeping badly. Why? Because 'benzos' have their dark side:

- They can be addictive.[19]
- They can worsen depression.[20]
- They prevent you from falling into REM sleep.[21]

Most of us can get through any period of sleeplessness without needing such a powerful and dangerous drug. Key to unlocking how to sleep better is to understand more about how this mysterious process happens.

Sleep has two linked aspects: falling asleep and staying asleep. We will start with the first. As you drift off and let go of the day's troubles, your brainwaves slow as you move into and cycle through the REM and NREM sleep states. If you struggle to fall asleep, it is likely that your brain is not sufficiently slowing down its fast beta waves, which are active when we are trying to get things done. Relaxation techniques (making a list of tomorrow's tasks, for instance) can help, as can meditation – we saw in the previous chapter that meditative practices cause more of the slower alpha waves; from there, it is much easier to slip into the slow brainwave state that we recognise as sleep. And while benzodiazepines work by stimulating the calming GABA neurotransmitter, some people prefer GABA supplements (even though the jury is still out on their efficacy). The problem with GABA levels in food is that getting enough would require eating a bucket of spinach a night, which is why some favour the supplements. Other brain-calmers include antihistamines, vitamin B3, hot milk (which contains a protein called casein) and hops.

If you have difficulty *staying* asleep, on the other hand, there is a good chance that you should consider your melatonin-cortisol balance. Melatonin is the night-time sleep hormone, cortisol is the day-time awake hormone, and between

19 Longo, L. P. and Johnson, B. 'Addiction Part 1: Benzodiazepines – Side effects, Abuse Risk and Alternatives.' *Am Fam Physician* (1 April 2000): https://pdfs.semanticscholar.org/725c/babof1060a771d1d5c5d6cf2594e1d8c91be.pdf

20 Parker, G. B. et al. 'Determinants of Treatment-resistant Depression: The Salience of Benzodiazepines.' *J Nerve Ment Dis* (2015): 203: 659–63.

21 Pagel, J. F. et al. 'Medications for the Treatment of Sleep Disorders: An Overview.' *Prim Care Companion J Clin Psychiatry* (2001): 3: 118–25.

them they rule our circadian rhythm. If you keep waking up at night, you are quite possibly either low in melatonin or you are worrying – the latter causes your body to release cortisol, which wakes you up. If you wake up worrying every night, then you must take action. I would suggest cutting out coffee, sugar and alcohol in the evening, and possibly taking natural anti-anxiety remedies such as GABA, kava root, 5-HTP and magnesium. If that does not help, then speak to your doctor – there might be something more serious going on, and as we know good sleep is critical to health. A lack of melatonin, on the other hand, is easily remedied; it is also a fairly common cause of adult sleeplessness because as we age we typically produce less and less melatonin. Adding it can help to reinstate our deep-sleep patterns. Replacing melatonin not only assists sleep; it has also been shown to cut the risk of breast cancer, prostate cancer and depression. Melatonin is also an antioxidant and it might slow ageing.[22]

Naturally enough, you should speak to your doctor if you struggle to sleep. If, after trying the measures above, you still find yourself unable to fall asleep or to stay asleep, your doctor might prescribe medication like amitriptyline or benzodiazepine. But be warned: benzodiazepines do not allow your brain to move into deep sleep, and as a result we do not benefit from the healing activities that take place during this type of sleep. This is why benzodiazepines are suspected of increasing our risk of dying early.[23] Sleep expert Walker is among those who instead favour something called cognitive behavioural therapy for insomnia (CBT-I), which uses a therapist and specific techniques to try to break bad sleeping habits.[24]

Regular sleep is one of our most important activities, and is essential for optimal health. Without it, we will not clear the brain of toxins, we will not rebuild our vital hormones, we will not recharge our neurotransmitters, and we will not consolidate what we have learned. Good sleep *is* good health.

22 Malhotra, S. et al. 'The Therapeutic Potential of Melatonin: A Review of the Science.' *MedGenMed* (2004): 6: 46.
23 Patorno, E. et al. 'Benzodiazepines and risk of all cause mortality in adults: cohort study.' *BMJ* (2017): 358: j2941.
24 CBT-I is strongly recommended by the American College of Physicians as the first-line treatment for people suffering from chronic insomnia – not sleeping tablets.

Happy hormones

I remember one Christmas Day asking my young niece Kirsty how she was enjoying herself. She looked up with her bright, sparkling eyes and, with all her soul, replied: 'It's just *perfect!*'

I was feeling a bit low at the time, and the sheer positivity emanating from this six-year-old made me take notice. I wondered: what happens that we gradually lose the ability to experience such boundless joy? It made me determined to rediscover my joie de vivre.

We have long believed serotonin is at the heart of that. For fifty years, it has been regarded as the brain's primary 'happy hormone' or, to put it more accurately, neurotransmitter. In addition, treatment for depression has commonly been spearheaded by drugs like Prozac, which increase serotonin's availability in the brain. This type of medication, known as SSRI drugs (which stands for selective serotonin re-uptake inhibitors), works by preventing serotonin from leaving the synapses in the brain. The more serotonin, the better the mood.

That is what the medical world has long thought. So is it true?

SSRIs *have* been proven to improve mood and reduce anxiety.[25] However, the belief that depression is simply a lack of serotonin, and that SSRIs perform their function by damming up the brain's serotonin, is considered too simplistic by some. If treatment merely required the damming of our serotonin levels, then why do SSRIs take two months to improve our mood? Surely if it relied only on higher serotonin levels, SSRIs should take no more than a few days?

There are arguments on both sides, and we will start with those in support of serotonin being our primary happy hormone.

- Depression is associated with poor serotonin-functioning in the brain.[26] In other words, people who are depressed tend to have low serotonin levels.

25 Eriksson, E. et al. 'Consistent Superiority of Selective Serotonin Re-uptake Inhibitors Over Placebo in Reducing Depressed Mood in Patients with Major Depression.' *Mol Psychiatry* (2016): 21: 523–30.

26 Owens, M. J. et al. 'Role of Serotonin in Pathophysiology of Depression: Focus on the Serotonin Transporter.' *Clin Chem* (1994): 40: 288–95.

- Tryptophan is an amino acid (which is found in bananas and turkey, among other sources) that the brain uses to make serotonin. If we cut out all tryptophans from the diet, we starve the brain of the food needed to make serotonin. And people who are susceptible to depression do indeed relapse into low moods when tryptophan is removed from their diet.[27]

In other words, people susceptible to depression have low levels of serotonin, and removing the nutrients that help the body to make serotonin worsens their situation. The logical conclusion is that serotonin plays some role in elevating our mood.

When it comes to arguments against, it is worth considering the following:

- The work that SSRIs do is much more complex than simply firing the serotonin button. As we saw in the previous chapter, there is evidence that drugs like Prozac help to improve brain plasticity, that stress breaks down brain tissue,[28] and that SSRIs rebuild brain tissue in people who are depressed.[29] A study on rats explained how that happens: antidepressants increase brain-derived neurotrophic factor (BDNF), which in turns stimulates the formation of new brain cells.[30] In other words, there is plenty of evidence to suggest that at least part of how SSRIs work is by rebuilding brain tissue, not simply by stimulating serotonin receptors.

- Inflammation is the scourge of the body, and there is every reason to believe that its negative effects also harm the brain. Indeed, many brain conditions are now viewed in terms of inflammation including depression, attention deficit hyperactivity disorder (ADHD), schizophrenia

---

27   Smith, K. A. et al. 'Relapse of Depression After Rapid Depletion of Tryptophan.' *The Lancet* (1997): 349: 915–19.

28   Swaab, D. et al. 'Elevated Cortisol in Rats Induces Neuronal Damage.' *Ageing Res Rev* (2005): 4 (2): 141–94.

29   Hen, R. et al. 'Chronic Fluoxetine Stimulates Maturation and Synaptic Plasticity of Adult-born Hippocampal Granule Cells.' *J Neurosci* (2008): 1374–84.

30   Mao, Q. Q. et al. 'Long-term Treatment with Peony-glycosides Reverses Chronic Unpredictable Mild Stress-induced Depressive-like Behaviour via Increasing Expression of Neurotrophins in Rat Brain.' *Behav Brain Res* (2010): 210: 171–7.

and Alzheimer's. All have shown some association with brain inflammation.[31] Take depression, for instance: if we are physically ill – with cancer, arthritis, a heart condition, diabetes or HIV, for example – then that illness can contribute both to inflammation of the brain and to depression.[32] Even if we are not ill and are simply getting older, inflammation (which is easily measured by looking for markers in the blood) can also lead to depression.[33] Later in the section on Alzheimer's we will assess the links to inflammation and see how reducing that could prove important in treating and even reversing many brain conditions.

It looks to me, then, that rediscovering one's joie de vivre is about a lot more than simply pouring serotonin into the brain. A good place to look more closely at happiness is to examine what happens when we are *unhappy*. To do that, we will start with cravings: what is going on in our brain when we crave something?

Cravings

Why is it that I might decide that I do not *want* a coffee, but then – as I stroll past a coffee shop – the aroma draws me in and I end up buying a large cappuccino? What happened to make me suddenly *need* it? And why, after eating healthily for days, does one night of bad sleep make me spend the following morning craving doughnuts and toast? Why is the craving side of our brain so powerful? What is the benefit of having such a guileful temptress? Is there some evolutionary mechanism that means cravings are beneficial?

The answer seems to be that, in the same way that the stress response is designed to help us move away from danger, the craving response is designed to help us move towards that which is advantageous. Daniel Lieberman, a

31   Benicky, J. et al. 'Blockade of Brain Angiotensin II Receptors Ameliorates Stress, Anxiety, Brain Inflammation and Ischaemia: Therapeutic Implications.' *Psychoneuroendocrinology* (2011): 36: 1–18.

32   Dantzer, R. et al. 'Inflammation-associated Depression: From Serotonin to Kynurenine.' *Psychoneuroendocrinology* 36: 426–36.

33   Bremmer, M. A. et al. 'Inflammatory Markers in Late-life Depression: Results from a Population-based Study.' *J Affect Disord* (2008): 106: 249–55.

professor of human evolutionary biology at Harvard, argues that having a sweet tooth allowed our forefathers to find sugar-laden fruit, which helped their survival. It is only in the modern era of sugary excess that this attraction to anything sweet has morphed into an addiction and obesity problem.[34]

For survival, it makes sense that our brain will naturally shy away from discomfort and move towards pleasure. However, the stresses of the modern world confuse that survival message. You might be up all night with the baby, or finishing a twelve-hour late shift, or be studying the night before an exam – in each case you might well find your sleep-deprived brain starts to crave junk food.[35] That is the same survival craving that our ancestors got, but the difference is that, smart as we are, our brain cannot differentiate between the stress of a cold, treacherous winter and the stress of self-inflicted sleep deprivation.

And it can happen in utterly ordinary moments: you might be working away for hours, your brain suddenly tires, and without a second thought you light a cigarette or grab a chocolate from the fridge or pour another cup of coffee . . . without even realising what you are doing. And these days, everything we think we need is brightly wrapped, conveniently close, and constantly available.

Lieberman's theory is intriguing, so let us take a closer look at the key chemical involved in this process, because if we can understand matters from that level then we can work to reverse the problem. The brain hormone that kicks into action when we take our first sip of that delicious cappuccino is dopamine.

And it is not just sugar, coffee, alcohol or cigarettes that cause dopamine to kick into action: the buzz you get from a theme-park ride is dopamine; the alertness you feel after watching a horror movie is dopamine; the high derived from amphetamine slimming tablets or cocaine is dopamine; and the attraction one feels for a new lover – yes that, too, is dopamine.

34 Lieberman, D. E. 'Evolution's Sweet Tooth.' *The New York Times* (5 June 2012).
35 Greer, S. et al. 'The Impact of Sleep Deprivation on Food Desire in the Human Brain.' *Nat Commun* (2013): 4: 2259.

There is plenty of evidence that dopamine is the one to watch. Researchers have shown that when sugar is fed to rats, it triggers their brain to produce dopamine,[36] as does giving them heroin.[37] The simple fact is that dopamine is our most effective excitement hormone, and people will risk everything for its brief rush.

From cravings to addiction

There is probably a pretty clear link in your mind between cravings and addiction – the difference is a matter of degree – and you might wonder how we know when we have moved from craving alcohol, for example, to being *addicted* to it? It comes down to the chemicals. The jump happens when we have triggered our dopamine receptors so much that they burn out.[38] That leaves them ineffectual and leaves us needing more dopamine to get the same brain effect.

Practically speaking, we are addicted to alcohol when we need more alcohol to get the same level of excitement, or when we spend a large amount of time looking for alcohol, or when we are unable to stop using alcohol.[39]

If you are my age, you might recall a famous advert from the 1980s that epitomises what many people still believe to be true about addiction. It showed a rat in a cage with two bottles to choose from – one with water and the other with cocaine-laced water. What happened? As the commentator explained, to a backdrop of plonking piano chords, nine out of ten rats would choose the cocaine, again and again, until they died.

It was gloomy stuff, and so pervasive that many people still believe the underlying dogma: that anyone who takes enough of a drug will become

36   Rada, P. 'Daily Bingeing on Sugar Repeatedly Releases Dopamine in the Accumbens Shell.' *Neuroscience* (2005): 737–44.

37   Tanda, G. et al. 'Cannabinoid and Heroin Activation of Mesolimbic Dopamine Transmission by a Common μ Opioid Receptor Mechanism.' *Science* (1997): 276: 2048–50.

38   Volkow, N. D. et al. 'Imaging Dopamine's Role in Drug Abuse and Addiction.' *Neuropharmacology* (2009): 56: 3–8.

39   'DSM IV Substance Dependence Criteria.' *American Psychiatric Association. Diagnostic and Statistical Manual of Mental Disorders (4th ed.)* American Psychiatric Association (2000).

addicted to it, and that once an addict, always an addict until you die. Because we believe this to be true about addiction, people on rehabilitation programmes still introduce themselves by saying: 'Hello. My name is so-and-so, and I'm an addict/alcoholic.' Even when we have recovered we consider ourselves as, for example, an alcoholic who no longer drinks. In other words, once a drug has sunk its claws into you, you cannot shake it.

Decades later that remains the pervasive wisdom, but – as a professor called Bruce Alexander has shown – it is at least partly wrong. Alexander decided to test out the rat-addict thesis. He started with rats on morphine in solitary confinement cages; later he moved them into a much larger cage with food, sleeping areas, toys and other rats with which they could socialise.

He called the big cage 'Rat Park', and the results of his experiment were nothing short of astonishing. It turned out that the rats in Rat Park typically no longer bothered with morphine-laced water. Why? Because they were *happy*: they had food and toys, they were socialising with other rats, and they therefore had no need to boost their dopamine.[40]

As Alexander notes on his website: 'We ran several experiments comparing the drug consumption of rats in Rat Park with rats in solitary confinement in regular laboratory cages. In virtually every experiment, the rats in solitary confinement consumed more drug solution, by every measure we could devise. And not just a little more. A lot more.' By contrast, the rats in Rat Park consumed 'hardly any morphine solution' at all.

Alexander's work suggests that it is our situation that drives addiction, not the theoretical hooks that drugs drive into our brain. If we are in the equivalent of an empty cage – alone, with no stimulation and no purpose – we will be unhappy and susceptible to addiction. And that brings us back to Lieberman's theory: that we are programmed to move away from the negative and towards the positive. If you are in that empty cage and the only positivity is a bottle of morphine, then that is what you will go for. Again, though, it is not necessarily the drug, but the situation.

---

40 Alexander, B. K. et al. 'The Effect of Housing and Gender on Morphine Self-administration in Rats.' *Psychopharmacology* (1978): 58: 175–9.

Unfortunately, Alexander's work was carried out at a time when support for the War on Drugs in the US was running high, so there was limited appetite for the implications of his findings. But he remains convinced that he is on to something:

'When I talk to addicted people, whether they are addicted to alcohol, drugs, gambling, internet use, sex or anything else, I encounter human beings who really do not have a viable social or cultural life. They use their addictions as a way of coping with their dislocation: as an escape, a pain-killer, or a kind of substitute for a full life,' he writes on his website. 'More and more psychologists and psychiatrists are reporting similar observations. Maybe our fragmented, mobile, ever-changing modern society has produced social and cultural isolation in very large numbers of people, even though their cages are invisible!'

I think he has a point. That is not to deny *some* physical component to addiction (nicotine, for instance, is among the most addictive substances out there), but I am convinced that there are other elements to consider.

Alexander's related finding was that the addicted rats that were put into Rat Park went through a minor withdrawal process before starting to function normally in their new environment. They did not stay addicted forever. Could the same hold true for humans?

Johann Hari, a once-disgraced British journalist, wrote a fascinating book on addictions called *Chasing the Scream: The First and Last Days of the War on Drugs* in which he questions the assertion that all addicts are addicted forever. Hari takes us back to Lee Robins' 1993 study of addiction during the Vietnam War of the 1960s and 1970s, where an estimated 20 per cent of the 2.7 million American soldiers were addicted to drugs.[41] There was widespread fear at that time that the US would be flooded with junkie war veterans when they returned. That did not happen. Instead, and largely as Alexander would have predicted, most of the soldiers transitioned back to normal life. Around 5 per cent were still addicted a year after returning home; however, for the rest it was the situation that made the addiction.

41 Robins, L. 'Vietnam Veterans' Rapid Recovery From Heroin Addiction: A Fluke or Normal Expectation?' *Addiction* (1993): 88: 1041–54.

What we can say about cravings and addiction is that they come freighted with a significant amount of guilt. This is wasted energy. Instead of being overwhelmed by guilt, we would be better-placed to understand what in our life has locked our brain into that cage. Once we have that answer, we can work to change those circumstances, and our brain will no longer need those dopamine hits to cheer it up.

The key message, then, is not to beat oneself up over addiction – whether of drugs, alcohol, cigarettes, food, you name it. Feeling guilty is pointless. It is far better to focus on what causes the brain to crave, and the three most common factors are what I call the three S's:

- Sleep deprivation is probably the single most common trigger for cravings. Why is that? Firstly, because a lack of sleep causes poor serotonin-functioning in our brain,[42] and we know that this is associated with lower moods. And secondly, brain imaging shows that the impulse centres of the brain light up when we are sleep-deprived, and we then crave junk food.[43] As we saw earlier, we will not succeed in our health endeavours unless we sleep properly. Eight hours a night every night is what our brain typically needs to function optimally.

- Stress triggers our cravings,[44] and the more emotional stress we are under, the more our brain shifts towards cravings to escape that cage. Stress also causes the levels of serotonin precursors such as tryptophan[45] to drop, and we know depleted serotonin levels cause low moods in susceptible people.[46]

42   Owens, M. J. et al. 'Role of Serotonin in Pathophysiology of Depression: Focus on the Serotonin Transporter.' *Clin Chem* (1994): 40: 288–95.

43   Walker, M. et al. 'The Impact of Sleep Deprivation on Food Desire in the Human Brain.' *Nat Commun* (2013): 2259.

44   Sinha, R. 'Chronic Stress, Drug Use and Vulnerability to Addiction.' *Ann NY Acad Sci* (2008): 1141: 105–30.

45   Dinan, T. G. 'Glucocorticoids and the Genesis of Depressive Illness. A Psychobiological Model.' *Br J Psychiatry* (1994): 164: 365–71.

46   Smith, K. A. et al. 'Relapse of Depression After Rapid Depletion of Tryptophan.' *The Lancet* (1997): 349: 915–19.

- Sadness: this does not necessarily refer to clinical depression. The fact is that our mood fluctuates all the time, and we are able to recognise a low mood when it hits us. What we ought to do is sit with it until it passes instead of reaching for the dopamine hit. When it comes to clinical depression, however, the sensible option is to treat the low moods before we tackle any craving habits. It would be unreasonable to expect someone in the lonely cage of depression to deal well with having their coffee or sweets or cigarettes or alcohol taken away.

In summary, if you find yourself craving substances then it is worth looking at the three S's and seeing what action you can take. It is far better to see what your brain needs in terms of support than it is to feel guilty.

Memory and forgetfulness

You have surely heard that most of us use just 10 per cent of our brain, a figure that is quickly followed by the 'What If' scenario in which we ponder how much better we would do if we could use, say, 50 per cent of our brain, or perhaps even more. If someone could only develop a pill that gave us the ability to learn a language in a day, to recall every detail of a situation or every word of a conversation – surely that would be something extraordinary?

The movie *Limitless* explores this scenario with actor Bradley Cooper stumbling across a street drug that gives him phenomenal abilities. In a short space of time Cooper's character transforms from down-at-heel writer to financial wizard. But, like any such story, there is a cost to such boundless opportunity: Cooper's character finds that the genie in the bottle is burning up his brain and killing him.

Not surprisingly, the concept of optimising our brain is an attractive one and has led to the development of a medical field in which such drugs – called nootropics – are used to enhance cognition, focus or memory. They are reportedly popular with students, business executives and others who feel they are in a hyper-competitive world.

It remains unclear whether nootropic drugs can safely deliver what they promise. It is just as unclear where the urban myth about using just 10 per cent of your brain came from. The truth is that you need pretty much all of your brain, which is why brain injuries are so damaging. (If you really could do without 90 per cent of your brain, that would also raise the question as to why we have such a large, energy-hungry organ that is so wasteful.)

In any event, it also turns out that, although you might wish to have perfect recall on some occasions, it is extremely important that you are able to forget the bulk of the data your brain processes each day. When you sleep, your brain retains those memories that are important and discards those that are not. Your brain's forgetfulness, to put it one way, also explains the 'use it or lose it' reality that applies to skills such as your golf swing, your language abilities or your piano-playing skills. As the pianist's saying goes: 'If I miss one day of practice, I notice. If I miss two days, the critics notice. If I miss three days, the audience notices.'

This ability to forget might be irritating to concert pianists, but it has the distinct benefit of allowing us to retain only that which is important. For example, there might well be six practical routes home, but we know that one is better than the rest, and our memory of that will be more pronounced than our memory of the other five. When faced with the choice of turning left or right, we know instantly that right is better, and we can probably visualise most of the detail on that route. Had we turned left, we would still make it home; however, the details of that route would not be etched as firmly on our brain.

For most of us, then, our brain parses the mass of information it receives each day, retaining what is important and discarding what is trivial. Some people, however, lack that ability and rank every fact as equally important. One consequence is that they lose the ability of judgement. Perfect recall might be useful in some situations, but our capacity to forget information is essential. Forgetfulness, then, is a normal part of life, though it does vary depending in part on how stressed we are and how well we sleep. Forgetfulness due to dementia, on the other hand, is of an entirely different order.

ALZHEIMER'S

We know by now that our brain is plastic, and that it can grow and shrink depending on how we use it. A quite separate issue arises when parts of the brain die; in that case there is generally no return, and the person moves towards a permanent form of forgetfulness that we call dementia. As dementia worsens, the brain's degeneration causes problems with language, orientation (in other words, getting lost), self-care (not washing) and behavioural issues.

By far the most common form of dementia, and arguably the most feared, is Alzheimer's disease, which:

- Is common – 60–80 per cent of all dementia is Alzheimer's. Around one in nine people have Alzheimer's by the time they reach sixty-five; one in three has it by eighty-five.[47]
- Strips the patient of their dignity, reducing them to a depressed shell of who they once were, and eventually kills them.
- Costs vast amounts of money. In the US, for example, it costs about the same as heart disease or cancer.[48]

Given its importance, you would not be surprised to learn that billions of dollars have been poured into researching this disease. You might be surprised to learn that, so far, it has largely gone in the wrong direction.

November 23, 2016 was Black Wednesday in the world of research into Alzheimer's. The pharmaceutical giant Eli Lilly had spent the previous three years trialling its latest medicine, known as solanezumab, part of its three-decade-long search for a drug to tackle the only fatal condition in the US's top 10 that still cannot be prevented, slowed or cured. On that day, Eli Lilly announced that patients who had received solanezumab 'did not experience a statistically significant slowing in cognitive decline compared to patients treated with placebo'.[49] In other words, solanezumab made no discernible difference.

---

47 Alzheimer's Association – see: https://www.alz.org/documents_custom/2016-facts-and-figures.pdf
48 Hurd, M. et al. 'Monetary Costs of Dementia in the United States.' *N Engl J Med* (2013): 368: 1326–34.
49 Eli Lilly statement: http://lilly.mediaroom.com/index.php?s=9042&item=137604

In the next few paragraphs we will find out why. Firstly, though, we need to look at what causes Alzheimer's – or, at least, what researchers *think* causes it. What certainly *does* happen is that a sticky compound called beta-amyloid plaque starts to cover the memory areas of the brain; the more extensive the plaque, the worse the illness. The logic underpinning Eli Lilly's research was sensible enough: removing the plaque should reverse the disease. That approach has now been debunked.

As is often the case, researchers are a dedicated bunch. Take neurologist Reisa Sperling. Among her numerous achievements, Sperling is co-director of the Harvard Ageing Brain Study; her passion to tackle Alzheimer's began after she lost her grandfather to the disease.

Sperling was concerned that Eli Lilly's study was treating patients too late in their illness. In her Harvard work, she has found that even patients who have a high level of beta-amyloid plaque yet who still function normally tend to decline faster than those with less plaque – implying that beta-amyloid plaque is part of the problem. And yet we cannot ignore ten failed studies that focused on the same solution, nor an eleventh, carried out by Roche, that failed in 2017.

'I do worry, what if we are completely on the wrong track?' Sperling said in a 2017 interview with the *Harvard Gazette*.[50]

By the time beta-amyloid shows up on brain scans, the scarring associated with it has been present for years.[51] Now, you and I know that the best way to deal with scars on the body is to prevent getting them in the first place – if you do not fall off your bike then you will not get that scar. The same principle holds for the brain. In other words, the best way forward is to *prevent* beta-amyloid building up. To do that, we need a deeper understanding about how Alzheimer's evolves.

We will start with a seemingly simple question: what is a memory? When you try to recall someone's name, a nerve impulse needs to be able to travel down a

50 Powell, A. 'Plotting the Demise of Alzheimer's.' *Harvard Gazette* (April 2017). See: https://news.harvard.edu/gazette/story/2017/04/harvard-researchers-plot-early-attack-against-alzheimers/
51 Ibid.

nerve to the very centre of the brain known as the hippocampus. This is the memory area. The nerve impulse then needs to pass successfully across a gap, which is called a synapse. The neurotransmitter acetylcholine (ACh) transports the information across this important gap. It is easy enough to see that having a healthy ACh system is imperative for recalling memories or forming new ones.[52]

Figure 2: The location of the hippocampus

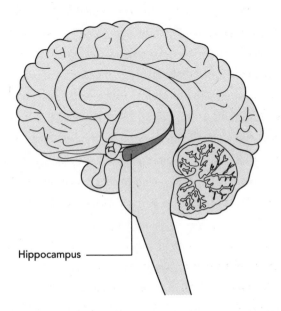

Hippocampus

That is where Alzheimer's research started fifty years ago: with an understanding of the importance of ACh in making memories. From there it progressed as follows:

- *ACh memory receptors:* in the 1980s, researchers looked at how the degeneration of our ACh system causes memory loss and leads to Alzheimer's.[53] The theory was that we could improve

52 Hasselmo, M. E. 'The Role of Acetylcholine in Learning and Memory.' *Curr Opin Neurobiol* (2006): 16 (6): 710–15.
53 Coyle, J. T. et al. 'Alzheimer's Disease: A Disorder of Cortical Cholinergic Innervation.' *Science* (1983): 219: 1184–90.

our memory by increasing the ACh in the synapses. Medicines such as Donepezil helped to improve memory in mild cases of Alzheimer's; however, they have not been able to reverse its progress.[54]

- *Inflammation of the brain*: in the 1990s, research showed that excessive levels of a key brain chemical called glutamate could worsen dementia. Glutamate is useful in the learning process and for brain elasticity; however, too much can give someone the feeling that they have drunk too much coffee and, significantly, it can cause inflammation and oxidative damage in the brain. Linked to that, it has been shown that Alzheimer's sufferers have high levels of brain inflammation and low levels of brain antioxidants.[55] A drug called memantine, which was initially developed to treat diabetes, has been found to counter glutamate's excessive effects in the brain by blocking glutamate receptors and thereby reducing brain inflammation[56]. A separate study has shown that memantine does help people with advanced Alzheimer's by slowing its progress.[57] To date, reducing brain inflammation has proven the most successful way to slow Alzheimer's progress.

- *Tau proteins*: this research, also in the 1990s, helped us better understand the scaffolding that gives our nerve cells their structure. So-called Tau proteins do this job, but if our body does not clear them away properly, the nerve cell can start to look like a messy building site. Tangles of Tau protein accumulate, which makes it difficult for

54 Nieoullon, A. 'Acetylcholinesterase Inhibitors in Alzheimer's Disease: Further Comments on Their Mechanisms of Action and Therapeutic Consequences.' *Psychol Neuropsych Vieil* (2010): 8: 123–31.

55 Moslemnezhad, A. et al. 'Altered Plasma Marker of Oxidative DNA Damage and Total Antioxidant Capacity in Patients with Alzheimer's Disease.' *Caspian J Intern Med* (2016): 7: 88–92.

56 Cacabelos, R. et al. 'The Glutamatergic System and Neurodegeneration in Dementia: Preventive Strategies in Alzheimer's Disease.' *Int J Geriatr Psychiatry* (1999): 14: 3–47.

57 Parsons, C. G. et al. 'Glutamate in CNS Disorders as a Target for Drug Development: An Update.' *Drugs New Perspect. I* (November 1998): 523–69.

the cell to transmit messages.[58] We still have not worked out a good way to remove Tau proteins.

• *The blood-brain barrier*: other research suggests that Alzheimer's patients have problems with the barrier between the body and the brain. The blood-brain barrier is designed to protect the brain from external toxins, and if it becomes scarred then we struggle to bring nutrients into the brain and wash out toxins.[59]

• *Beta-amyloid plaque*: it was not until the mid-1990s when MRI (magnetic resonance imaging) became popular that we started to see what was happening inside the head. MRI images showed us how the brains of Alzheimer's patients accumulate beta-amyloid plaque, and how this sticky substance scars the synapses and nerves in the *memory* areas of the brain.[60] We now know that efforts to remove beta-amyloid plaque do not help Alzheimer's patients.

The question all this research had not answered was this: what causes the brain to accumulate beta-amyloid plaque and Tau proteins in the first place? It now seems that people with Alzheimer's do not necessarily make too *much* amyloid plaque; they are just not very good at clearing it away. Why might that be? One easy answer is poor sleep. We saw earlier how Dr Nedergaard demonstrated that deep NREM sleep is the time when the brain's toxin-removal system awakens and does its job, including clearing beta-amyloid plaque.[61] Poor sleep leads to poor clearance of beta-amyloid plaque, and that means a higher risk for dementia.[62]

58 Goedert, M. et al. 'Tau Proteins and Neurofibrillary Degeneration.' *Brain Pathol* (1991): 1: 279–86.
59 Deane, R. et al. 'The Role of the Blood-brain Barrier in the Pathogenesis of Alzheimer's Disease.' *Curr Alzheimer Res* (2007): 4: 191–7.
60 Hardy, J. et al. 'Amyloid Deposition as the Central Event in the Aetiology of Alzheimer's Disease.' *Trends Pharmacol Sci* (1991): 12: 383–8.
61 Xie, L. et al. 'Sleep Drives Metabolite Clearance from the Adult Brain.' *Science* (2013): 342: 373–7.
62 Spira, A. et al. 'Impact of Sleep on Cognitive Decline and Dementia.' *Curr Opin Psychiatry* (2014): 27: 478–83.

A more important answer into what precedes plaque formation required the application of highly advanced X-ray screening called positron emission tomography, better known as a PET scan. Step one is to swallow some radioactive glucose; step two is the scan, which shows where in the brain the glucose is being used – those areas light up like a Christmas tree. Although the brain accounts for just 2 per cent of our body weight, it uses around 20 per cent of the glucose and oxygen.[63] If the brain is healthy, then the hippocampus – the central memory part – will glow showing a good uptake of glucose. But that is not the case if the patient is developing Alzheimer's: their hippocampus area will look dark and inactive. In practical terms, poor uptake of glucose means the nerve cells do not function properly, and that means poor memory. The memory cells are effectively starving despite being surrounded by a sea of glucose.[64]

A decline in glucose uptake appears to be the earliest sign that our brain is moving towards Alzheimer's, and a PET scan can show a problem years before any symptoms begin – including in twenty-somethings who might be genetically predisposed to develop the disease later in life.[65]

We saw in the chapter on inflammation that a high-sugar diet predisposes us to diabetes. There is increasing evidence that it also predisposes us to Alzheimer's.[66] It is not surprising, then, that diabetics have twice the Alzheimer's risk as the general population.[67] Just as poor insulin-signalling means low glucose-uptake in the body, poor insulin-signalling in the hippocampus leads to low glucose-uptake there too. Without glucose, the memory cells have no fuel, and that means the memory fails.[68]

63 Mergenthaler, P. et al. 'Sugar for the Brain: The Role of Glucose in Physiological and Pathological Brain Function.' *Trends Neurosci* (2013): 36: 587–97.

64 Berti, V. et al. 'PET/CT in Diagnosis of Dementia.' *Ann NY Acad Sci* (2011): 1228: 81–92.

65 Reiman, E. M. et al. 'Functional Brain Abnormalities in Young Adults at Genetic Risk for Late-onset Alzheimer's Dementia.' *Proc Natl Acad Sci USA* (2004): 101: 284–9.

66 Moreira, P. I. 'High-sugar Diets, Type-2 Diabetes and Alzheimer's Disease.' *Curr Opin Clin Nutrit Metab Care* (2013): 16: 440–5.

67 Kiyohara, Y. et al. 'Glucose Tolerance Status and Risk of Dementia in the Community: The Hisayama Study.' *Neurology* (2011): 77 (12): 1126.

68 Feldman, E. et al. 'Insulin-resistance is a Key Link for the Increased Risk of Cognitive Impairment in the Metabolic Syndrome.' *Exp Mol Med* (2015): 47: e149.

Giving Alzheimer's patients insulin (by snorting it up the nose to get it directly into the brain) does improve their brain function.[69] Yet although there is compelling evidence that Alzheimer's starts with poor glucose uptake to the hippocampus, this does not yet explain how that leads to the accumulation of beta-amyloid plaque seen later. So what does the science say about this?

Firstly, we *do* know there is a link, because mice given excessive glucose show worsening dementia and a higher load of beta-amyloid plaque.[70] That link is found in a protein called insulin-degrading enzyme (IDE), whose function is to remove insulin from the body. IDE also, it turns out, removes beta-amyloid plaque from the brain. However, if the system that absorbs glucose into the cells is faulty, then the body will release more insulin in an effort to help the cells to absorb that glucose. That causes IDE to remove this excess insulin, and that means there is less IDE available to remove the beta-amyloid plaque. The result is a build-up of beta-amyloid plaque.[71]

This is why diabetics have a much higher chance of developing Alzheimer's: not only do they struggle to absorb glucose into the hippocampus, but the higher level of insulin they produce also means that their body does not clear enough of the beta-amyloid plaque – because the IDE is focused on removing insulin instead.

Indeed, it is increasingly clear that dealing with Alzheimer's requires tackling the root causes of the issue: inflammation and insulin-resistance.

69   Claxton, A. et al. 'Long-acting Intranasal Insulin Detemir Improves Cognition for Adults with Mild Cognitive Impairment or Early-stage Alzheimer's Disease Dementia.' *J Alzheimers Dis* (2015): 44: 897–906.

70   Cao, D. et al. 'Intake of Sucrose-sweetened Water Induces Insulin Resistance and Exacerbates Memory Deficits and Amyloidosis in a Transgenic Mouse Model of Alzheimer's Disease.' *J Biol Chem* (2007): 282: 36275–82.

71   Pivovarova, O. et al. 'Insulin-degrading Enzyme: New Therapeutic Target for Diabetes and Alzheimer's Disease.' *Ann Med* (2016): 48: 614–24.

Gene-testing for Alzheimer's?

Patients often ask whether they should do a gene test to determine their Alzheimer's risk, and my answer is a cautious yes. I say 'cautious' because one of the genes linked to the risk of developing Alzheimer's is called APOE (it stands for apolipoprotein E) and – depending upon where in the world you come from – you could have the APOE e2, APOE e3 or APOE e4 gene.[72] (And, because you have two copies of these types of genes, or alleles, you might be an e2/e2 person, or an e3/e4 person or some such combination.)

Like most genes, APOE is known as a low-penetrance gene, which means that if you make the correct lifestyle changes you can hugely reduce whatever negative influence the gene might have.

That is not necessarily the case with *high-penetrance* genes, such as the breast cancer gene BRCA. Angelina Jolie tested positive for a mutation in the BRCA1 gene and elected to have a double mastectomy due to the higher risk of breast cancer the mutation confers. However, this simply does not apply to APOE and Alzheimer's; the fact is that low-penetrance genes mean that *how* you live your life (what we call epigenetics) is far more important than whether or not you carry that gene.

And in this case we need to refine that further, because if you have the APOE e2 or APOE e3 gene then you have no increased risk for Alzheimer's whatsoever. However, if you have the APOE e4 gene, then your risk for contracting the disease is between three times greater (if your combination is e3/e4) or fourteen times higher (if it is e4/e4).[73] To reiterate, though, this is a *low-penetrance*

72 Ward, A. et al. 'Prevalence of Apolipoprotein E4 Genotype and Homozygotes (APOE e4/4) among Patients Diagnosed with Alzheimer's Disease: A Systematic Review and Meta-analysis.' *Neuroepidemiology* (2012): 38 (1): 1–17.

73 Chia-Chen, L. et al. 'Apolipoprotein-E and Alzheimer's Disease: Risk, Mechanisms and Therapy.' *Nat Rev Neurol* (2013): 9: 106–18.

gene, and the correct lifestyle choices should make a big difference to that risk. Let us look at how that plays out.

We know our brain constitutes about 2 per cent of our body weight. Much of it is built from cholesterol, and indeed fully 25 per cent of all of our cholesterol can be found in the brain.[74] What that means is that transporting cholesterol to the brain is an important function, and it becomes increasingly important the older we get.

Interestingly, by the time we are elderly – say, in our sixties and above – having higher blood cholesterol levels protects us from mental decline.[75]

So, how does cholesterol get from A to B? The common analogy is that it is transported in boats called lipoproteins. Once the lipoprotein boat reaches its destination, dockworkers called apolipoproteins pull the cargo safely off the boat. There are a number of apolipoproteins that have different docking tasks; the one we are interested in is the E variant.

The way the gene and the dockworker are connected is this: the APOE gene carries the code that makes the apolipoprotein E dockworkers, and depending on whether you carry the e2, e3 or e4 version, your gene will make a slightly different apolipoprotein dockworker with slightly different abilities.

Here is where the connection with Alzheimer's comes in: the apolipoprotein E dockworkers do one of their jobs at the blood-brain barrier; there they take cholesterol off the boat and transport it safely into the brain. Logically enough, then, any damage to this docking system will reduce our ability to supply the brain with cholesterol and essential fatty acids.

74 Dietschy, J. M. 'Central Nervous System: Cholesterol Turnover, Brain Development and Neurodegeneration.' *Biol Chem* (2009): 390: 287–93.
75 West, R. et al. 'Better Memory-functioning Associated with Higher Total and Low-density Lipoprotein Cholesterol Levels in Very Elderly Subjects without the apolipoprotein E4 Allele.' *Am J Geriatr Psychiatry* (2008): 16: 781–5.

Research has shown that eating a high-carbohydrate diet does just that: it creates a perfect storm that damages the brain's apolipoprotein E transport system. And eating a healthy-fat, low-carbohydrate diet, on the other hand, protects it.[76] And what that means is simple: if you have the APOE e4 gene variant, then the sooner (and younger) you start to minimise sugar and starch in your diet and include healthy fats, the better you should be able to neutralise that genetic risk.

A final point: you might recall that at the beginning of the first chapter on the brain I told you that people with the APOE e4 gene tend to scar more easily on the brain if they take a hit to it. Other research shows that, once they contract Alzheimer's, they do not respond as well to treatment.[77]

And that is why I tend to give a cautious yes to people who ask about doing an Alzheimer's gene test:

- 'Cautious' because those who test positive for the APOE e4 gene variant might fear they are fated to get Alzheimer's – and that is *not* the case.

- And 'yes' because, if you do have the APOE e4 gene variant, there is a lot you can do to prevent Alzheimer's. For a start, a healthy lifestyle of exercise and low sugar has been shown to reduce the risk of developing Alzheimer's in APOE e4 carriers.[78] Those who test early and make the lifestyle changes can prevent the onset of Alzheimer's, as we shall see in the next section.

76   Lane-Donovan, C. et al. 'High-Fat Diet Changes Hippocampal Apolipoprotein E (ApoE) in a Genotype- and Carbohydrate-Dependent Manner in Mice.' *PLoS One* (2016): 11 (2): e0148099.

77   Lanctot, C. et al. 'Correlates of Response to Acetylcholinesterase Inhibitor Therapy in Alzheimer's Disease.' *J Psychiatry Neurosci* (2003): 28: 13–26.

78   Head, D. et al. 'Exercise Engagement as a Moderator of the Effects of APOE Genotype on Amyloid Deposition.' *Arch Neurol* (2012): 69 (5): 636–43.

ALZHEIMER'S DIY

A vast amount of time and money has been spent over the years searching for a cure for Alzheimer's, but what if – as Dr Sperling asks – we are on the wrong track? Increasingly it seems as though many of the answers to explaining the Alzheimer's epidemic can be found at home, and that avoiding sugars, enjoying a low-carbohydrate diet, consuming healthy fats and oils, and reducing brain stress could prevent the disease from developing in the first place.

If we want to optimise our brain health, we should consider a path that covers the following areas.

Use ketones for brain energy

Although our brain will use glucose as its energy source, we were not designed for a high-carbohydrate, high-sugar world, and our modern excess damages the body and brain. We saw earlier that PET scans show how Alzheimer's sufferers have lost the ability to absorb glucose into the hippocampus (the memory part of the brain). The good news is that we are designed to survive periodic famines, and during those times our brain will happily use an energy source known as ketones.

Where do ketones come from? Fat. The liver converts fat to ketones, which the brain uses instead of glucose. During times of famine or fasting, ketones can easily contribute 70 per cent of the brain's energy requirements.[79] If people with Alzheimer's harness ketones, they ought to be able to fire up their brain again.

Interestingly, studies have shown significant benefits for adding ketones to the diet of Alzheimer's patients: those who could no longer absorb glucose were able to improve memory performance;[80] while even simply

---

79   White, H. et al. 'Clinical Review: Ketones and Brain Injury.' *Crit Care* (2011): 15: 219.

80   Cunnane, S. et al. 'Can Ketones Help Rescue Brain Fuel Supply in Later Life? Implications for Cognitive Health during Aging and the Treatment of Alzheimer's Disease.' *Front Mol Neurosci* (2016): 9: 53.

adding ketones to the diet (without removing sugar and starch) made a significant difference to the brain over a three-month period.[81]

There are three ways to provide the brain with ketones. The first is to eat healthy oils that the body can easily convert to ketones. This means eating food high in good fats, such as coconut oil, palm oil, olive oil, cheese, butter, eggs and many others. The liver then converts these to ketones. A particularly good source is MCT oil (MCT stands for medium-chain triglycerides; the oil comes from coconut oil and other oils), and you can find it in most health shops.

The second is to eat what are called exogenous ketones, which are simply ketones from outside your body – in other words, ketones that you eat in ketone form. These days you can buy ready-made ketone powder or oil, which bypasses the need for the liver to convert it into ketones, and that means the brain can use it immediately for energy.

And the third is to generate your own ketones from your body's own fat stores. How to do that? By eating a low-carbohydrate diet, which we already know benefits heart health. When it comes to brain health, the medical world has been using this diet for a century to treat head injuries and epilepsy, because it reduces brain inflammation and encourages the brain to heal.[82] If it sounds useful, that is because it is: by removing sugars and starches from the diet, we encourage our body to make energy in the form of ketones, which we know our brain can use. Indeed, Alzheimer's patients on a low-carbohydrate diet exhibit significantly improved memory scores compared to those on a high-carbohydrate diet.[83]

Combine

Consuming MCT oil and eating a low-carbohydrate, healthy-fat (LCHF) diet will, I believe, one day be proven to have the biggest impact on brain

---

81 Henderson, S. T. et al. 'Study of the Ketogenic Agent AC-1202 in Mild to Moderate Alzheimer's Disease: A Randomized, Double-blind, Placebo-controlled, Multicenter trial.' *Nutr Metab (Lond)* (2009): 6: 31.

82 White, H. et al. 'Clinical Review: Ketones and Brain Injury.' *Crit Care* (2011): 15: 219.

83 Krikorian, R. et al. 'Dietary Ketosis Enhances Memory in Mild Cognitive Impairment.' *Neurobiol Aging* (2012): 33: 19–25.

health. Why? Because removing carbohydrates from the diet protects the brain, and adding ketones both protects the brain's cells and improves energy functioning within brain cells.[84] If we add intermittent fasting (not eating between 7pm and 11am), then we create a triple win for brain health, because intermittent fasting is known to boost the production of brain-derived neurotrophic factor (BDNF), which stimulates new brain tissue.[85]

Low-carbohydrate eating and intermittent fasting are increasingly developing into the golden thread of health. In the chapter on the theories of ageing, we saw that our best chance of stimulating our longevity genes is to reduce insulin, and that we can do this by fasting intermittently and by removing carbohydrates. The chapter on inflammation and obesity showed that the best way to lower our heart-attack risk is by reducing insulin through fasting intermittently and by cutting carbohydrates.

Exercise

Being a couch potato is not our natural state, and in the chapter on anabolic versus catabolic hormones we learned how the body needs to be reminded every day to keep our muscles strong. It is the same for the brain – daily exercise stimulates BDNF, which stimulates new brain tissue. Indeed, the more intense the exercise, the more BDNF is released.[86] An added bonus is that exercise has been shown to help reduce levels of beta-amyloid plaque in Alzheimer's patients.[87]

84   Maalouf, M. et al. 'The Neuroprotective Properties of Calorie Restriction, the Ketogenic Diet and Ketone Bodies.' *Brain Res* (2009): 59: 293–315.

85   Li, L. et al. 'Chronic Intermittent Fasting Improves Cognitive Functions and Brain Structures in Mice.' *Plos One* (2013): 8: e66069.

86   Saucedo Marquez, C. M. et al. 'High-intensity Interval Training Evokes Larger Serum BDNF Levels Compared with Intense Continuous Exercise.' *J Appl Physiol* (2015): 119: 1363–73.

87   Heyn, P. et al. 'The Effects of Exercise Training on Elderly Persons with Cognitive Impairment and Dementia: A Meta-analysis.' *Arch Phys Med Rehabil* (2004): 85 (10):1694–704.

Check your vitamin B12

Vitamin B12 is crucial for developing and maintaining the myelin sheath around the nerves – that is, their fatty covering. We absorb vitamin B12 from the stomach, but we get worse at that as we age, which leaves us susceptible to memory loss and nerve degeneration. You can easily check your vitamin B12 level with a blood test, and any deficiency can be reversed with supplements and injections.

Supplements and more

The medication that is currently helping Alzheimer's patients focuses on two things: using tablets like memantine to reduce brain inflammation; and taking ACh medications like donepezil to improve memory. There are ways to get those benefits naturally too.

When it comes to brain inflammation, we saw earlier that excessive glutamate in the brain is one factor that can inflame the brain and lead to degeneration. N-acetylcysteine (NAC) is a supplement we encountered previously, and is widely used to reduce excessive brain glutamate and inflammation.[88] Others worth adding include turmeric, vitamin E and vitamin D. It is easy enough to do a blood test to assess your vitamin D level, and it is sensible too because low vitamin D levels double the risk of dementia.[89] Another good idea is cutting out all foods that you are allergic to – say, grains or dairy – because that might cut inflammation and boost memory.

Improving memory, on the other hand, brings us back to a hormone called pregnenolone that you might recall from the chapter on stress – it is made naturally from cholesterol, and helps us to cope with stress. It pops up here because it is a natural support for memory: in the brain, it stimulates important pathways, safely improving our memory.[90] One of the consequences of

88 Sharipour, R. B. et al. 'N-Acetylcysteine (NAC) in Neurological Conditions: Mechanisms of Action and Therapeutic Opportunities.' *Brain Behav* (2014): 4: 108–22.
89 Littlejohns, T. J. et al. 'Vitamin D and the Risk of Dementia and Alzheimer's Disease.' *Neurology* (2014): 83: 920–8.
90 Sabeti, J. et al. 'Steroid Pregnenolone Sulfate Enhances NMDA-receptor-independent Long-term Potentiation at Hippocampal CA1 Synapses: Role for L-type Calcium Channels and Sigma-Receptors.' *Hippocampus* (2007): 17 (5): 349–69.

high stress is that it can burn out our pregnenolone, which leaves us forgetful. That is why, at times of high stress, it can make sense to supplement pregnenolone in a high dosage (around 120mg daily) to optimise recall. Equally, we must not forget to be mindful of the effect stress has on us – we know that stress and anxiety breaks down brain tissue. We need to minimise stress and treat any anxiety if we want the brain to move back into an anabolic rebuilding state.

Finally, I would reiterate the importance of play. The brain plasticity section of the previous chapter showed how important it is to keep stimulating the brain to generate new tissue. So, learn to speak a new language, start painting, do the crossword, take up juggling or play a musical instrument – those are all great ways to encourage neuroplasticity at any age.

THE BRAIN, PART 2: A FINAL WORD

As I said at the close of the previous chapter, we cannot optimise our general health unless we do the same with the brain. If we are unable to get excited about life, if we are not sleeping well, if we crave sugar, if we feel constantly anxious or if we cannot remember things – these are all indicative of a problem with the brain, and we need to act to prevent long-term problems.

We have seen that our brain is neuroplastic from cradle to grave, and that means whatever negative state the brain is in, it *can* be improved and typically it can return to full health – provided we work at it. If we are irritable day in, day out, then that is what our brain will become. On the other hand, every day that we laugh is a good day for the brain. Every day that we paint or do a crossword or try to master a new language or play an instrument is a day in which our brain gets to work out; the added bonus is that while we sleep, the brain processes what we have learned and, over time, we become better at that task.

By now it is hopefully clear just why our brain is an astonishing organ, and what we can do to help keep it that way. After all, if we do look after it then it could thrive well past our 100th birthday. To that end we should remain grateful for what we have, we should embrace new things, and we should stay inquisitive about life; it is, after all, nothing short of miraculous.

Key points

To keep your brain in optimal health, keep the following in mind:

- Good health starts with sleep. Whether you are an athlete or an academic or something else entirely, you need at least eight hours of sleep a night. It not only consolidates what we have learned in the day; it clears out brain toxins such as beta-amyloid, and rebuilds the hormones we need to ensure we are fabulous tomorrow.

- Choose happiness: there is a big difference between excitement and happiness. We tend to chase excitement, especially when our brain is unhappy. Excitement could be sugar or alcohol or a roller-coaster ride. Happiness on the other hand is time spent with loved ones, playing with children, cuddling a pet and picking up a musical instrument. If you are not happy, then you will seek excitement. So if you find yourself getting cravings then, instead of feeling guilty, consider the three S's that cause it: Sleep, Stress and Sadness. Fix those, and the cravings ought to disappear.

- Cut out sugar; add ketones. Alzheimer's is a common and growing cause of death, and one that many people rightly fear. Decades before it strikes, PET scans can show how the brain's memory centre no longer absorbs glucose for energy, and we know that too much glucose in the brain eventually leads to brain scarring and Alzheimer's. Eating a low-carbohydrate, healthy-fat diet will help the brain to move past its reliance on glucose as fuel. Adding intermittent fasting and daily exercise will help to build new brain tissue. Our brain will happily use ketones, and you can provide it with that alternative energy source. Studies are ongoing to see whether this eating pattern will prevent Alzheimer's.

Chapter 13

THE FUTURE – FROM CRADLE TO . . . WHAT EXACTLY?

> There are two ways to live life. One is as though everything is
> a miracle. The other is as though nothing is a miracle.
>
> *Albert Einstein*

And so we reach the end of the book, which is in a way, I hope, really the beginning for you: the start of your Younger for Longer life. By now it is surely clear that ticking a few health boxes – getting enough sleep, combating stress, doing exercise, eating properly, taking care of our skin – is good, but insufficient. After all, they are part of a whole and, just like an orchestra, the whole really is much greater than the sum of its parts. To do well in *all* areas is the goal.

In this chapter we will pull together the key elements to summarise what healthy ageing means in practice. After that we will look to the future. The research world is packed with extraordinary advances and remarkable possibilities, and examining some of these seems sensible. After all, they might well one day end up being chapters in their own right.

These are the topics that fascinate Silicon Valley, the areas that the likes of British researcher Aubrey de Grey believe will push humans to live far beyond what is thought to be our current scope of 120 years. Some are already in play, while others remain as theoretical maybes – yet all contain elements that make us think differently about health. Understanding the basics of the chapters of this book provides a platform for better assessing what might come next.

How the puzzle fits together

You might be the sort of person who loves reading the last chapter of a book first, in which case you have just started it. I am like that with user manuals: turning straight to the 'quick guide', and ignoring the complicated sections that give a sound understanding of the gadget concerned.

If you are that person, then of course do read on – but, as this chapter is the quick guide and can offer no more than the briefest summary of what came before, I would encourage you to read at least those chapters that most interest you. That way you will have a far deeper understanding as to why what is summarised here is important, and how the parts fit together.

If, on the other hand, you have arrived at the end of the book having read all the way through, then I applaud you. There have been some fun sections, but I am the first to admit that others have been challenging. That is hard to avoid, given that the body is a fundamentally complex thing, and many of its workings remain mysterious even to people who study it for a living.

I remember, many years ago, starting to read the late Stephen Hawking's bestseller *A Brief History of Time*, and feeling pleased that after three chapters I had kept up with his explanations. Not long after that, perhaps in chapter four and certainly by chapter five, the wheels had come off. By chapter six I was lost, lonely and adrift in a sea of explanations of quantum mechanics, and I failed to finish it.

Complexity is the nature of scientific books, and I am no physicist, so being unable to finish Hawking's book was perhaps to be expected. My intention with this book was to ensure that I did not leave anyone behind in a sea of science, and yet that it was sufficiently medical to provide a proper understanding of what is involved. Although few of us are physicists, we are all human – and what is within the covers of this book applies to everyone – so I hope I have succeeded in assembling this orchestra of health for you in a way that is both comprehensive and comprehensible.

So without further ado, let us get to it. First I will summarise the essentials that we must get right if we want to ensure a basic level of health, and then we will look at what we need to do to move us closer to optimal health – that state of being where the zing in our step is ever-present, where we wake every day with purpose and vigour, and where we sleep soundly each night.

Reaching basic health

Sleep

Sleep is the number one aspect of health, and everything else hangs off this factor. Why? Because so much of what we know to be essential happens when we sleep, and probably quite a lot more too that we do not yet know.

Among the things that happen when we sleep are:

- We rebuild our steroid hormones: cortisol, testosterone, DHEA, progesterone and oestrogen. If we do not sleep well then the levels of these hormones dip and, as a result, our energy drops, our immune system is less efficient, and our muscular power and libido drop. Women might well notice that their period becomes irregular.

- We rebuild our neurotransmitters, which are the chemical messengers that carry instructions around the brain and that regulate many of our body's functions, such as appetite and mood. If we do not sleep well then our mood will worsen, we will crave sugar and become more emotional, and our memory will decline.

- We clean the brain via our glymphatic system, which is its toxin removal system. While we sleep, drainage channels open up in the brain removing toxins like amyloid plaque that could otherwise lead to damage. If we do not sleep enough then we will not clean the brain sufficiently, and we run a serious risk of ending up with a toxic, inflamed brain.

- We stimulate neuroplasticity and build new brain pathways. After a good night's sleep we will be better tomorrow at whatever it was we practised today (sport, music, remembering the key facts of this book), and that is because of the brain-building that takes place while we slumber.

At my clinic, the first and most important task is to get people back into a good sleeping habit. Why? Because if we cannot get this factor right then it is highly unlikely we will get much else right.

What helps? Good lifestyle habits are key – exercising, not smoking or drinking alcohol, eating well, de-stressing – while herbal supplements and sleep medications also have a place in rebuilding a healthy sleep routine. Almost everyone needs eight hours of sleep each night, but so important is sleep that many top athletes aim for between nine and eleven hours. Once we have broken the pattern of being unable to sleep, it is much easier to get the rest of our health right.

Energy

Sleeping well at night will ensure that our circadian rhythm is properly aligned, and that will keep us energised during the day and on the road to excellent health. Sleeping better means our daytime energy automatically improves.

But if you still have energy dips during the day then it is wise to look at some other factors:

- Emotions: the brain is a powerful driver of energy, so if you still have slumps then you might be dealing with anxiety and low mood. This does not mean that you are depressed; it simply means that you are under so much stress that your happy hormones are burning out. A stress-induced low mood can also bring sugar cravings or override the desire to exercise, or it can mean you wake up early each day worrying. Most people do not need medicines to correct a low mood, and the chapters on the brain showed that lifestyle activities such as exercise and meditation can help to rebalance low moods, as can taking certain supplements including 5-HTP and saffron flower. As your emotions improve, your joie de vivre and energy should return too.

- Adrenal insufficiency: this is so common that I estimate every second patient I see suffers from some form of it. Ongoing stress is the culprit: it causes our stress hormones to fire continuously from our adrenal glands, which can lead to these hormones burning out. We learned in the stress chapter how zebras are superior to us inasmuch as they rapidly de-stress and relax after being chased by a lion. Humans, on the other hand, can easily run on stress as a daily habit, and that is profoundly unhealthy. Ongoing stress might not leave you with critically low hormone levels that require the help of a hormone specialist, but it could leave you lacking enough of these hormones to ensure a good level of basic health. How would you know? Typically you would have an energy dip in the morning and another in the afternoon. You might notice that you are getting more coughs, colds, aches and pains than normal. What will help are sleep, mindful meditation (which encourages the brain to slow down and to listen to the body when it says it needs to rest) and hormone replacement (cortisol, DHEA, testosterone, progesterone). On that note, we do not always need to supplement with cortisol – simply cutting down on coffee will lower how much cortisol we use, and eating liquorice stops cortisol breaking down as fast, which helps to keep its levels at a healthy level. Adding pregnenolone, another hormone, provides the adrenals with what they need to make all of these hormones, and also gives the brain the means to make acetylcholine, or ACh, a neurotransmitter that sharpens our memory.

- Hormonal weakening: menopause and andropause start to dominate in our forties and fifties, leaving us low in oestrogen, progesterone and testosterone, and feeling tired for much of the day. While adrenal insufficiency often leads to energy dips, menopause leads to continuous fatigue. This hormonal weakening might also be accompanied by an inability to sleep well, irritability, a decreased desire to exercise, muscle weakening, sagging skin and shedding hair. The standard mantra of getting through menopause is to 'halve the sugar and double the exercise', but many women also flush so badly that they need hormonal balancing. Correcting oestrogen and progesterone (by using bio-identical hormones, not synthetic hormones) has been shown to help women live healthier and longer. Supplementing with testosterone has been shown to reduce chronic disease in men, but the jury is still out as to whether or not testosterone extends life. Replacing other hormones, like growth hormone, might make us feel great now, but research shows that long-term use tends to burn us out. Growth hormone does, however, assist in rebuilding bones and cartilage, and there may be a place for it in someone who is recovering from osteoporosis, broken bones or damaged spinal discs.

- Cellular energy: if we have worked on our brain, cut our stress and ensured our hormones are in balance, then the next step would be to look at optimising the energy engines that are found inside every cell in the body. These engines are called mitochondria and we end up with fewer and fewer of them as we age. That means our cellular energy declines as we get older, leaving us flat and fatigued throughout the day. Daily exercise – particularly high-intensity exercise, such as five minutes of burpees and star-jumps – will stimulate the formation of new mitochondria and energise the ones we have. Various supplements will either boost mitochondria or stimulate new ones. My top six supplements to improve mitochondrial energy are: coenzyme Q10, magnesium, the B vitamins, creatine, alpha-lipoic acid, and the amino acid L-arginine.

The whole of the body is far greater than the sum of its parts, and once this extraordinary orchestra is playing together the combined difference in energy these changes bring will make a profound difference: a transformation from a tired, depressed cannot-be-bothered forty-something to a rejuvenated and optimistic person who once again cares about life, their health and their family, and who is eager to discover what new adventures lie ahead.

Once this basic level of health has returned, we can consider those factors that will push us towards optimal health.

REACHING OPTIMAL HEALTH

When it comes to optimal health, which is the goal of this book, I am talking about much more than simply feeling energised. Optimal health has that, of course, but it has more: an extra spark, if you like, all day, every day.

Many things can lead us to this higher plane, yet some stand out. If sugar, stress and toxins are three key things we should avoid, then exercise is the one lifestyle change that is essential to add in.

Exercise

Exercise is to optimal health as sleep is to basic health – it is that important, and we will not attain optimal health without it. And although I encourage my patients to start exercising from the get-go, often they manage it only once they are sleeping better and feel more energised during the day. That reality is the reason I have put exercise into the optimal health section, although I would love for everyone to do more of it when aiming for basic health too, because it makes a big difference.

We have encountered the benefits of exercise all the way through this book:

- Exercise – and particularly high-intensity interval training, or HIIT – reduces insulin resistance every time we get out there. And improved insulin resistance leads to longevity.
- Aerobic exercise (running, swimming, dancing, kickboxing) switches our healthy genes back on as we age.
- Exercise reduces inflammation and in that way lowers the risk of falling victim to the chronic illnesses of inflammation such as heart attacks and strokes.
- As we age we run out of mitochondria; HIIT helps the body to make new mitochondria, which improves the energy in our cells.
- Exercise not only tells our brain to keep building muscle, which is essential, but also to rebuild the nerves that fire up those muscles. Inactive elderly people can lose half of the nerves that activate their muscles, which is one reason it is important to keep moving as we age.
- HIIT naturally increases our testosterone levels, in both men and women. (And some testosterone is essential for women, just as some oestrogen and progesterone are vital for men.)
- Exercise stimulates brain-derived neurotrophic factor (BDNF), which is a protein that stimulates brain rebuilding. This benefits everything from memory to mood, and much more besides.

Inflammation

We have seen throughout this book how inflammation is a major driver of modern illnesses. Heart attacks, strokes, cancers, arthritis, asthma and metabolic syndrome all have one thing in common – inflammation. There is overwhelming evidence that inflammation, not cholesterol, is the primary driver of heart attacks, which on its own would make reducing inflammation an activity well worth pursuing.

There are three key areas where we can take action:

- Nutrition: sugar inflames our arteries and it inflames our body, and contributes to heart attacks, cancers, diabetes and strokes. Whether it is sugar in the form of starchy carbohydrates (such as bread and rice), excessive fruit and fruit juices, beer and wine, or simply the sugar found in fizzy drinks and processed foods, it all turns into excess sugar in our body and inflames us. Cutting out these sugary carbohydrates stops this problem from happening in the first place. Inflammation lurks in other areas too: omega-6 oils (found in sunflower oil, corn or maize, corn syrup, as well as in the meat and dairy products of animals fed on corn) are overly prevalent in our modern diet, and turn into arachidonic acid, which is inflammatory. Exercise burns up arachidonic acid. Omega-3 oils, which are found in fish, neutralise this inflammation.

- Exercise: each time we exercise we do battle with inflammation. Exercise burns off sugar, which is inflammatory; it clears the stress hormone adrenalin from our system (stress has been shown to worsen arterial inflammation, leading to heart attacks); and it uses arachidonic acid to rebuild muscle.

- Gut health: an inflamed gut leads to an inflamed body, and if we bloat after a meal or have wind or feel discomfort then the chances are that we have an inflamed gut. To heal it we should cut out food that is inflaming the gut (wheat is often a culprit), repair the intestinal wall with supplements like glutamine, restore the flora with probiotics, and look at taking supplements that will help to replace stomach acid that we might have run low on.

Toxins

According to the *Lancet* Commission, pollution is responsible for as many as one in four deaths in the world's most severely affected countries.[1] Yet no matter where you live, pollution and other toxins are all around, and we need to be mindful of them.

That is why it makes sense to decide what action we will take to avoid what we believe are toxins, given how long it takes for governments to legislate against them: the US surgeon-general warned in 1964 that smoking caused cancer, yet in the UK, for instance, smoking in public places was not banned for another four decades.

Dealing with toxins means:

- Avoiding toxins: obvious areas include steering clear of cigarettes and excessive alcohol consumption. In addition: eat organic foods, which are free from pesticides, where possible; do not exercise in areas full of car fumes; keep mobile phones and Wi-Fi radiation out of the bedroom; do not drink out of plastic bottles; do not microwave food in plastic containers; do be aware of the toxins that are in many cleaning products and home furnishings, and try to source non-toxic or less toxic alternatives.
- Removing toxins: exercise is important here. So too is avoiding sugars, because they cause a fatty, sluggish liver, which does a worse job of removing toxins from the body. Other tips include taking B vitamins, which boost the liver's methylation pathway, and supplementing with glutathione, because it boosts the glutathione pathway that removes mercury and other heavy metal toxins.

Supplements

We saw in the chapter on theories of ageing that swallowing excessive antioxidants could switch off our own internal antioxidant system, causing more harm than good. That said, and given that modern diets are in danger of lacking some key nutrients, I do advise taking some supplements.

---

1   The *Lancet* Commission on pollution and health (19 October 2017).

My top five are, in reverse order:

- Multivitamins: a good-quality brand taken twice a week only.
- Coenzyme Q10: because it helps our mitochondria to generate energy in every cell.
- Vitamin D3: it strengthens bones, helps to ward off skin cancer, improves the liver, thyroid and brain function, and most importantly boosts our immune system.
- Fish oil: omega-3 is an anti-inflammatory and has key health benefits for the brain, our arteries, our joints, the immune system and for the membrane of every cell in the body.
- Glutathione: my gold medal winner, because it is the brain's favourite anti-inflammatory, and that is good enough for me. Glutathione makes us feel calmer, it counters damage to the brain and it reduces mucous in the lungs. And possibly most importantly, it removes mercury and other heavy metals from the body.

Neuroplasticity

This concept is what drives people like Stephen Jepson, whom we met in the first chapter on the brain. As we now know, the brain is elastic, which means it is in a constant state of building up and breaking down throughout our life, depending on the food we eat, the activities we do and how stressed we are. The slogan that best describes neuroplasticity is 'use it or lose it', and Jepson's idea is that we need to keep playing different games that require different skills each day in order to continue stimulating the brain to rebuild itself. You can see more about him at his website: www.neverleavetheplayground.com.

We know that neuroplasticity does not stop in childhood, and that our brain can rebuild even when we are elderly; it just means we need to work a little harder. As we age we should stimulate our brain in multiple ways: learn to play a musical instrument, get outside and kick a ball, take up dancing, balance on one leg, practise a new language, swim, do a crossword or Sudoku, or find a new path.

As China's so-called 'hottest grandpa' Wang Deshun said, do something new. Coming from someone who was a DJ, actor and ramp model in his retirement years, and whose next ambition was to go skydiving, it seems good advice. The point is that staying inquisitive throughout our life means we will keep stimulating our brain. Once we are wheeled out each day to sit in front of a television, we start to degenerate fast. Even then, though, we can still take action, because until it really *is* too late, it is never too late.

The skin

Modern treatments improve our skin, and having a healthy skin is central to how we feel about ourselves, as well as being important from a health perspective, including helping to prevent cancer. Skin treatments have moved away from relying on surgery and harsh lasers, and focus more on naturally rebuilding the skin.

We have discovered ways of not just stimulating collagen – which is the skin's scaffolding – but of making new skin cells. That is important because, as we age, we run out of skin cells, and that is a key factor in accelerating the ageing of our skin.

Being able to make new skin cells is the ultimate prize, and there are several ways to do this:

- Vitamin creams not only protect us from skin cancer; they also stimulate collagen. In addition, vitamin C serum is the first treatment that has been shown to stimulate the formation of fibroblasts, which are the skin cells that make collagen.
- PRP is a treatment in which a skin specialist draws your blood, spins it to extract growth factors, and then injects those into your skin. This not only improves collagen; it is also the second treatment that has been shown to stimulate new fibroblasts.
- Fat transfer: taking a fat sample from the abdomen and injecting it into the face not only plumps the skin naturally; it also means stem cells are injected that can develop into new fibroblast cells.

- Lastly, stem cells can be injected directly into the skin. Until recently we simply crossed our fingers and hoped they would develop into fibroblasts, but scientists have discovered various peptides and growth factors that stimulate those stem cells to ensure they specifically become new fibroblast cells.

Conclusion

If we can get all of these factors right then we are giving ourselves the best chance of living our best life.

At the beginning of this book we encountered the two paths of life, and saw that the path of excess likely meant we would spend our last decade or two in a state of slow, painful decline. Living a Younger for Longer life might not gain us much in years – our lifespan – but it will surely improve the quality of those years, which we call our Healthspan.

To put it in normal-speak, if we cannot stop the alcohol, stresses or sugar, then we run a significant chance of spending our final years debilitated and in pain. That is not the future I envision for me or for you. My goal is to climb mountains with my family and my dogs for as long possible, and then fade away peacefully.

The point is that once we get these basics right we can look to the future, and to the hope and excitement of the new advances that are heading our way, and that could yet transform our health even further. We will now take a brief look at some of them.

WHAT IS NEXT?

The future of health medicine is indeed bright. Every few months another innovation emerges or researchers work out a better way of doing something remarkable. For example, mid-2018 saw a significant breakthrough in the approach to treating breast cancer when a study demonstrated that gene testing performed on breast cancer samples could show who would benefit from chemotherapy and who would not. It was estimated that this gene testing would save up to 70 per cent of women with the most common form of early stage breast cancer from undergoing the toxic process of chemotherapy.[2]

In this final section of the book, I want to examine some of the key break-throughs that have grabbed the imagination of the world in recent years and that have the potential to boost our health beyond anything that has come before. These are the topics that are generating excitement far beyond the deep-pocketed world of Silicon Valley.

Genetics

Genetics is the study of our heredity – our genes, those double helix hardware packages that drive every cell in our body. But it turns out that we are defined not so much by the DNA we are born with, but by the damage that happens to our DNA during our lives.

Let me explain: in 1990, some of the world's top geneticists collaborated to map out the human genome – the gene that we humans carry as a species. It took a little over a decade, and by 2003 the Human Genome Project was completed. By then, though, interest had shifted from simply discovering the layout of this code to working out what pulls its strings.

By way of an example, every time we eat broccoli, the natural B vitamins that we absorb make what are called methyl groups, and these attach to our DNA and protect it. Every time we inhale car fumes, on the other hand, the toxins we breathe in damage our DNA. These lifestyle triggers, good and bad, are referred to as our epigenetics, and it is this that pulls the strings of our genome. So powerful is this epigenetic influence that some scientists believe it might be more important than the genes that we start out with.

Take identical twins, for instance: at birth they are indeed identical. But as they grow up, different stresses and toxins affect their DNA in different ways, some positive and some negative, and as the years pass they become less identical. By the time they are fifty, identical twins can often look more as though they are from the same family rather than from the same egg and sperm. And

2 Sparano, J. A. et al. 'Adjuvant Chemotherapy Guided by a 21-Gene Expression Assay in Breast Cancer.' *N Engl J Med* (2018): https://www.nejm.org/doi/full/10.1056/NEJMoa1804710

that is because the different stresses and toxins, the positive and the negative effects associated with five decades of life, have changed much about them, even down to their facial features.

The good news is that epigenetics can be harnessed for good, because we can work out which of our genes are inherently weak through a series of gene tests. Often – though not always – there is a lifestyle choice we can make that will reduce the impact of that weak gene. For example, if someone has the FTO gene, which predisposes them to being obese, they can reduce their risk of obesity by about a third simply by exercising each day.[3] There are many other examples of gene tests that track, for example, our genetic heart-attack risk, how well our liver functions, our risk for various cancers or our risk for developing Alzheimer's, and for each of these weak genes there is a supplement or a lifestyle change that we can make that will lower that risk.

This is how genetics applies to our lives today, and much of what I have advised in this book – from exercise to managing stress to cutting out sugar and improving our sleep – will automatically modify the impact of many of those weak genes.

The genetics of tomorrow, however, puts matters into an entirely different sphere. Meet CRISPR, which stands for clustered regularly interspaced short palindromic repeats. Other than being a catchy acronym for a clunky string of words, CRISPR is an important part of your average bacteria's defence mechanism. It works like a pair of scissors at the level of DNA: simply put, CRISPR cuts out a piece of DNA that is not wanted and inserts a piece that is wanted.

DNA messaging – the order that the DNA code is read – is often compared to how we read a book. If one word is wrong, then the sentence conveys a different meaning. For example, 'Twinkle, twinkle big star' does not sound right. But when we substitute the word 'little', the world of nursery rhymes once again feels reassuringly normal. This is how CRISPR works: removing what is wrong on that code and replacing it with something better.

---

3 Kilpeläinen, T. O. et al. 'Physical activity attenuates the influence of FTO variants on obesity risk: A meta-analysis of 218,166 adults and 19,268 children.' *PLoS Medicine* (2011).

But it is no easy task to pop into a cell and swap around different bits of DNA. CRISPR is such a clever system that it is easier to conceive of it as a character in a *Star Wars* movie than something that happens in a petri dish. With a bit of imagination, it could be compared to Luke Skywalker having to destroy the Death Star space station: first, our hero needs a vehicle to get to the Death Star – CRISPR uses a virus to scoot around the body and enter cells; then Luke needs to be guided into dock on the Death Star – CRISPR does this by attaching to RNA, which guides it to the nucleus of the cell and then on to the DNA; lastly Luke needs to hack into the Death Star's motherboard and change the code that wires it – CRISPR does this by cutting out a piece of DNA and replacing it with another.

To date, the research done with CRISPR has been performed successfully on mice, and we humans are the next target. The successes seen so far are very exciting:

- Antibiotic resistance is becoming a growing global problem and we are running out of antibiotics that kill bacteria. CRISPR has been used to enter a bacterium, reprogramme it and kill it off.[4] CRISPR might well be the answer to antibiotic resistance.
- Genetic diseases such as muscular dystrophy, diabetes and cystic fibrosis remain incurable. However, CRISPR is able to cut out bad genes and replace them with healthy genes. Although this is yet to cure any of these diseases, in animal studies it has greatly improved those symptoms. [5]

As exciting as CRISPR promises to be, human trials are in their infancy, and it will be years before we might be able to swallow a CRISPR pill and expect to reverse our genetic deficiencies. Until then it makes sense to follow healthy lifestyle habits in order to optimise the epigenetic influence on our DNA.

4 Reardon, S. 'Modified viruses deliver death to antibiotic-resistant bacteria.' *Nature* (2017): 546.

5 Liao, H. K. et al. 'In Vivo Target Gene Activation via CRISPR/Cas9-Mediated Trans-epigenetic Modulation.' *Cell* (2017): 171: 1495–507.

Sanz, D. J. et al. 'Cas9/gRNA targeted excision of cystic fibrosis-causing deep-intronic splicing mutations restores normal splicing of CFTR mRNA.' *PLoS One* (2017): 12.

Stem cells

Modern medicine is good at treating illness and, as we have seen in this book, we are getting better at preventing damage. However, we are not at all good at reversing the damage that our bodies have accumulated, and this is where stem-cell therapy is starting to make its mark.

A stem cell is a universal cell, which means that it can be turned into whichever organ or piece of tissue is in need of repair. If we cut our skin and a year later can no longer find the scar, that is because stem cells rebuilt that tissue. After a heart attack, stem cells normally migrate to the damaged site and rebuild heart muscle. If stem cells do not do that, then the heart muscle will scar with collagen; this will restrict the heart muscle from recovering fully.

When it comes to stem-cell therapy, there are two key things that we need to ensure happen: after injecting the cells into the body we need to direct them to where they are needed; we then need to tell them what to do, because in that way they will develop into the tissue that needs healing.

Before we get to that stage, though, we need to source the stem cells. Since the late 1950s, stem cells have been extracted from bone marrow and used to treat leukaemia, but that extraction process is painful. The next idea was to use stem cells from human embryos, but that was shelved for ethical reasons.

The good news is that since the millennium we have found a seemingly limitless source of stem cells that are easy to find, relatively painless to harvest, and can be turned into most tissues (or, in medical-speak, are pluripotent): please welcome adipose-derived stem cells, otherwise known as fat.

For the past two decades we have been able to extract fat, process it in a couple of hours to retrieve millions of stem cells, and then inject those back into the body. However, this is where the science largely ends and hope begins. Why? Well, we know stem cells are attracted to areas of inflammation, which means that if you have damaged, inflamed lungs then stem cells should head there and be automatically triggered by the body to turn themselves into new lung tissue. But it is also possible that they could be attracted to your infected sinuses or your inflamed knee and work on that inflamed tissue instead, and at this stage we do not know how to direct them differently. Secondly, those stem cells that *are* attracted to the lungs still need to be told to change into lung tissue in order to rebuild what has been damaged, and the scientific knowledge we currently have means that is not guaranteed. The result is that we can get some good results with stem cells, but there are still too many uncertainties to make it a mainstream treatment.

There are, however, plenty of positive stories, and one of the first involved treating burns victims. For decades, surgeons would take a layer of skin from one part of the body of a burns victim and graft it on to the wound. That works in many cases, but when burns cover more than about one-fifth of the body, the area to be covered might be too large and there might be no unburned skin from which they can take a graft. This is where stem-cell therapy came in. Harvard professor Howard Green, who died in 2015, led the way by starting to grow skin grafts from stem cells. In 1983 his revolutionary technique saved two young brothers from Wyoming who had terrible third-degree burns.

Back then, it took several weeks for laboratory-grown grafts to mature, and that can be too long to save a critically burned patient. But new techniques mean stem cells and fibroblast skin cells are placed much sooner on to the wound, and this lattice of cells is helped by peptide stimulators to grow as skin. Among the most recent beneficiaries is a girl from my country, South Africa. Her name is Pippie Kruger, and she received 80 per cent burns in a barbecue accident in 2011 when she was just two. Her mother, Anice, determined to save her daughter, phoned Green at home, because he was the one person in the world she thought could help. Green did, and a week later Pippie had forty-one living stem-cell grafts applied to her skin.[6] Nearly all of them took, and Pippie survived.

Phenomenal though such outcomes are, there is much more to do. Looking ahead we need to understand better how to trigger stem cells to reach where they are needed and then to turn themselves into the required tissue. Some of that progress is underway: scientists have made exciting progress over the past decade after learning that peptides, which are protein messengers that travel around the body, work well as messengers to direct stem cells. For instance:

6 Powell, A. 'Recalling a lab-led rescue.' *Harvard Gazette* (2013).

- Fifteen insulin-dependent diabetics had peptide-directed stem cells injected into them in 2007, and this procedure allowed fourteen of them to stop all insulin injections for a year. The peptides seemed to guide the stem cells to the pancreas, and then direct them to turn into pancreatic beta-cells, which manufacture insulin. In this case, both of the limitations – getting the stem cells to the right place and converting them into the necessary tissue – were solved.[7]

- Spinal degeneration is a major problem as we age. Scientists have inserted a scaffold into the spines of rats and infused those with growth factors. These growth factors then stimulated the dormant stem cells in the vertebrae to regenerate bone.[8]

- Osteoporosis is another important ageing condition, and causes bones to become brittle. Using peptides, scientists were able to deliver messenger RNA to bones and wake up the DNA that rebuilds bone.[9] That marks a significant improvement on the bisphosphonate medications that are currently used.

- A heart attack often causes the death of part of the heart muscle, which increases the chance of this organ failing. Scientists have found a way to stimulate stem cells to develop into heart muscle with the help of specific peptide growth factors.[10] This new piece of heart tissue is then stitched back on to the heart, making a big difference to the chances of rebuilding a healthy organ.[11]

7   Voltarelli, J. C. et al. 'Autologous Nonmyeloablative Hematopoietic Stem Cell Transplantation in Newly Diagnosed Type 1 Diabetes Mellitus.' *JAMA* (2007): 297: 1568–76.

8   Lee, S. S. et al. 'Gel scaffolds of BMP-2-binding peptide amphiphile nanofibers for spinal arthrodesis.' *Adv Healthcare Mat* (2015): 4: 131–41.

9   Zhang, G. et al. 'A delivery system targeting bone formation surfaces to facilitate RNAi-based anabolic therapy.' *Nat Med* (2012): 18: 307–14.

10 Webber, M. J. et al. 'Development of bioactive peptide amphiphiles for therapeutic cell delivery.' *Acta Biomater* (2010): 6: 3–9.

11 'Heart-muscle patches made with human cells improve heart attack recovery.' *ScienceDaily* (2018).

- Moving up a gear, scientists are now able to take fibroblast skin cells and change them back into stem cells. They can then stimulate those stem cells to turn into healthy muscle cells before injecting those back into rats to treat muscular dystrophy.[12]

- Even more remarkably, scientists can now isolate the stem cells that they want to use and improve the DNA of those stem cells *before using them*. These DNA-enhanced stem cells are then injected back into the patient along with a set of peptides that will direct them to the right place.[13]

- Perhaps most interesting of all is the use of stem cells in the brain, specifically as regards neural stem cells. These cells, the directors of youthfulness, are found mostly in the hypothalamus, which – though only the size of a walnut – is the big communicator between the brain and the body, and which sends numerous hormones into the body that control our health. Neural stem cells decrease in number with age and so, curious to see how important that might be, scientists removed 70 per cent of the neural stem cells in mice to see what would happen. The result – the mice aged rapidly. The scientists then reversed their experiment, injecting neural stem cells into other mice. The result – the second group of mice lived 15 per cent longer.[14]

As matters stand at the time of writing, we have stem cells that can be directed by the right peptides to be able to rebuild bones, rebuild heart muscle, reverse the symptoms of untreatable illnesses like muscular dystrophy, have their DNA optimised and, last but not least, extend healthy life. Although many of these experiments were done on mice, it is clear that we are on the cusp of further significant breakthroughs in the world of stem cells.

12 Filareto, A. et al. 'An ex vivo gene therapy approach to treat muscular dystrophy using inducible pluripotent stem cells.' *Nat Commun* (2013): 4: 1549.

13 Ma, K. et al. 'Synergetic Targeted Delivery of Sleeping-Beauty Transposon System to Mesenchymal Stem Cells Using LPD Nanoparticles Modified with a Phage-Displayed Targeting Peptide.' *Adv Funct Mater* (2013): 23: 1172–81.

14 Zhang, Y. et al. 'Hypothalamic stem cells control ageing speed partly through exosomal miRNAs.' *Nature* (2017): 548: 52–7.

Telomeres

We have encountered telomeres several times in this book – they are the 'shoelace caps' at the end of our DNA that protect the genetic code, but that shorten each time the cell divides. Eventually, after many divisions, they become so short that they no longer offer protection, and the cell is killed.

The enzyme that rebuilds telomeres is called telomerase, and the search has long been on for factors that will enhance telomerase and keep our cells dividing for longer. Meditation, exercise, fish oil and vitamin D have all been shown to increase telomere length and, as long as we follow a healthy life, we should be optimising our telomeres.

Epithalamin is a peptide that is produced in the pineal gland of the brain. It turns out that it naturally boosts telomerase and protects telomere length. Most of this work has been done in Russia, where it has focused on the skin: when a synthetic version of it is added to fibroblast skin cells it stimulates the telomeres to lengthen and it makes the fibroblasts live longer. It also blocks the MMP enzyme, which we know destroys collagen. This peptide, then, allows fibroblasts to live longer and protects our skin's collagen scaffolding. As a tablet or an injectable it could have a big role to play in skin health.

Parabiosis

Typically we use the term 'an injection of fresh blood' to mean providing new ideas, but in science it is being taken more literally: researchers at Stanford University took blood transfusion to dizzying heights by sewing together an old and a young mouse so that they shared the same blood circulation (a somewhat bizarre practice called parabiosis). The result was that the old mouse had improved genes, a rewired brain and improved brain functioning.[15]

Next, they injected old mice with blood from a human umbilical cord, blood from twenty-year-old humans and blood from seventy-year-old humans, having first ensured that the mice would not reject the human blood. The researchers found that the blood from the umbilical cord activated numerous

15 Wyss-Coray, T. et al. 'Young blood reverses age-related impairments in cognitive function and synaptic plasticity in mice.' *Nat Med* (2014): 20: 659–63.

genes that regenerated the brain and improved memory; the blood from young adults stimulated some of these genes; and the blood from the elderly had no beneficial effect at all. It turns out that various peptides in the blood are responsible for these effects, the most promising of which is called TIMP2. Increasing TIMP2 in mice improved their brain health, while removing it worsened their brain health.[16] The next proposed step is a study that will assess the effect of giving older humans the blood from younger humans.

As de Grey was quoted as saying in the chapter on the theories of ageing, it takes 'a certain amount of guts to aim high', and this array of forward-looking studies covering all manner of human health is certainly doing that.

It is also easy to see why Silicon Valley's alchemists are so excited about the future: perhaps one day medicine will be able to use CRISPR technology that splices longevity genes back into our genome, add stem cells with peptides to rebuild damaged organs, produce capsules we could swallow that would protect our telomeres and make our cells live longer, and see us inject fragments of youthful blood to rebuild the brain. It all marks a potent step into a bright, and possibly dangerous, future.

AND FINALLY

Perhaps the best person to inspire us with his take on health is a role model of mine who not only studied healthy ageing, but lived it. The late Dr Shigeaki Hinohara was surely the longest-serving physician and educator in the world. Born in 1911, he died in 2017 aged 105. At the age of 100 he was still practising as superintendent of St Paul's Hospital, Tokyo.

His abilities were legendary: since 1941 he had healed patients at St Luke's International Hospital in Tokyo and taught at St Luke's College of Nursing. After the war he led efforts to develop these institutions into a world-class hospital and, even after turning 100, served as chairman of the board of trustees at both.

16 Wyss-Coray, T. et al. 'Human umbilical cord plasma proteins revitalize hippocampal function in aged mice.' *Nature* (2017): 544: 488–92.

Always inquisitive, Dr Hinohara published about 150 books after turning seventy-five, including one called *Living Long, Living Good* that has sold 1.2 million copies. And, as the founder of the New Elderly Movement, he encouraged others to live a long and happy life, for which he was the ultimate role model.

So if there is one person whose wisdom I choose above all others with which to close this book, it is Dr Hinohara. His philosophies and secrets on life are pleasingly simple. In 2009 he was interviewed by newspaper *The Japan Times* and gave the following pearls of wisdom:

- 'Energy comes from feeling good, not from eating well or sleeping a lot. We all remember how as children, when we were having fun, we often forgot to eat or sleep.'
- 'All people who live long – regardless of nationality, race or gender – (have) one thing in common: none are overweight.'
- 'Always plan ahead.' At ninety-seven, Dr Hinohara's schedule for the next six years was filled with lectures and his hospital work (though he did plan to take time off in 2016 to attend the Tokyo Olympics).
- 'Share what you know. I give 150 lectures a year, some for a hundred elementary-school children, others for 4,500 business people.'
- 'To stay healthy, always take the stairs and carry your own stuff. I take two stairs at a time, to get my muscles moving.'
- 'Find a role model and aim to achieve even more than they could ever do . . . When I am stuck, I ask myself how they would deal with the problem.'

He also knew to expect the unexpected, and to learn from such experiences. In 1970, for instance, he was on a plane that was hijacked by Japanese communists, and spent four days handcuffed to his seat in 40°C; he used the time to observe how his body reacted. At eighty-eight, he wrote the script of a musical titled *The Fall of Freddie the Leaf*, and later acted in it, dancing with the children.

Of all his wise sayings, though, this is my favourite.

'It's wonderful to live long. Until one is sixty years old, it is easy to work for one's family and to achieve one's goals. But in our later years, we should strive to contribute to society. Since the age of sixty-five, I have worked as a volunteer. I still put in eighteen hours, seven days a week and love every minute of it.'[17]

And so, after thirteen chapters and hundreds of references to support numerous points about healthy ageing, I believe Dr Hinohara had a better handle on the subject than anyone: much of our health starts in the brain. Sleep, laughter and play are powerful healers, and while it is exciting to watch the evolution of stem-cell therapy and other medical innovations, the fact remains that our first step is to get the basics right within ourselves, and to enjoy the insights that we gain as our health improves.

After all, nobody wants to reach the end of their life uttering one of my favourite phrases: 'If I had known I was going to live this long, I would have taken better care of myself.'

These days taking better care of ourselves is well within our grasp; indeed, it is literally within your grasp given that what you need to know is contained in the pages of this book.

So let me close by saying that today is the best day to begin creating your Younger for Longer life. Make a start – go back through this chapter's summary right now and jot down the three areas you feel you need to work on first, and then get to work on them. You will not regret it.

17 Kawaguch, J. 'People/Words to Live By: Author/physician Shigeaki Hinohara.' *The Japan Times* (29 January 2009).

Acknowledgements

It seems a little unfair to credit just one person with writing a book. In my experience, it takes an entire village of people: some need to share their thoughts and opinions while others need to sacrifice their time and energy before the story can be wrestled on to the pages and a book is born.

In just this way, *Younger for Longer* was a collaboration of input from many people. Although there is not the space to mention all of them, I am eternally grateful for their assistance along the way. However, I would like to highlight those who have been of the utmost help and at the same time gave the biggest sacrifice, all in order to get this title published.

Firstly, my wife Megan has sacrificed huge tracts of time that we could instead have spent enjoying adventures together. There is a fairly well-known concept of the 'golfing widow', whose husband spends all his time on the fairways of golf courses. I believe that a 'writing widow' suffers more, because during the writing phase, although the author might be physically in the building, they are really far, far away, deep inside the workings of some book. When not writing, they are generally in distant thought, pondering for hours how to transcribe the next concept. With patience, kindness and an unending supply of intuitive love, Megan has helped me, encouraged me, believed in me and constantly fed me through this literary journey.

I would also like to thank Matt and Grant, my two stepsons who put up with my converting the dining-room table into my personal writing bunker, when everybody knows that such a table is far better suited for hosting table-tennis tournaments. I am forever indebted to my parents, Glenda and Duncan. They taught me many things but perhaps their most important lesson was that education has very little to do with exams and everything to do with staying inquisitive. My siblings, Jennifer and her husband Roger, Robert and Beata, Andrew and Yuli, all make sure that I never take myself too seriously, but always feel significantly loved.

Dr Chris Warton was my mentor when I was a junior medical student. He had one profound lesson for me: that I needed to grasp the trunk of the tree before considering looking at the branches, twigs and leaves. In this book, I have followed Dr Warton's advice and explained the big concepts in the first half of each chapter before delivering the detail in the second.

When I was a GP trainee in Bournemouth in the United Kingdom, Dr Jonathan Foulkes was my mentor. He showed me the importance of questioning everything, and that you should never believe what anybody tells you about their medical product until you have thoroughly read the studies behind it. As a result, every big concept in this book has numerous references that you can explore should you wish to examine matters in more detail.

Professor Tim Noakes has been my guide in the last few years. As a firm advocate of low-carbohydrate eating, he has endured more resistance and aggression to his teaching than any scientist should. He has encouraged me to continue to work and stand up for the concepts that I believe in, no matter how difficult. In that lies a greater truth: that in life we should listen to criticism, but never be cowed by it.

I would also like to thank my editors and publishers. Firstly, Duncan Proudfoot at Little, Brown, who despite the fact that I come with no track-record, believed in this book from the get-go. He introduced me to my publishers Nikki Read and Giles Lewis, who broke the rules and embraced this book despite it being way too long. I am grateful to Amanda Keats who coordinated the layout of the book and Una McGovern who did the final edits, both so professionally.

Lastly, I would like to thank my brother Robert Carmichael. Rob is a most talented journalist, author of the book *When Clouds Fell from the Sky* and most importantly to me, the editor-in-chief of this book. Some editors only correct the grammar, others strip out so much of the book that there is nothing left of the author at all. Rob has understood and believed in this project from the start. He has held my hand through my early attempts at writing and encouraged me when I failed. He has taken my clumsy, medical writing style and patiently nudged it closer and closer to something that has started to appear literary. Rob has been much more than an editor and with his unique ability to understand me, medical discussion, and what is needed to construct a book, he has introduced a flow and a confidence that has helped to transform this from a series of medical articles to a great book that I really hope proves useful for you.

Dr Duncan Carmichael
Cape Town, South Africa

Glossary

ACh – acetylcholine, a neurotransmitter.

APOE – apolipoprotein E, a gene that comes in three variants, or alleles: APOE e2, APOE e3 or APOE e4. People with APOE e4 have a higher risk of contracting Alzheimer's but, as this is a low-penetrance gene, lifestyle changes make a big difference.

Apoptosis – the term for cell death, a process that is controlled by the body to remove damaged cells. Compare with senescence.

Atherosclerosis – the thickening of the artery walls.

BCAAs – branch-chain amino acids. Amino acids are the building blocks that make proteins (including muscle); BCAAs are a sub-set of these that we cannot make, and therefore have to consume. The king of BCAAs is glutamine.

BDNF – brain-derived neurotrophic factor, a protein produced in the brain, particularly when we exercise, that improves brain functioning and builds neurons.

Bio-identical hormones – hormone-balancing treatments that have the same molecular and chemical structure as human hormones. Contrast with synthetic hormones.

BPH – benign prostatic hyperplasia is a condition that affects many men in later life. It means they need to get up several times each night to urinate as they are unable to empty their bladder. It is caused by a swollen (though not cancerous) prostate gland, and might be the result of excess DHT production.

CVDs – Cardiovascular diseases. Diseases involving the heart or the circulatory system, for which read heart attacks, heart failure, strokes and related ailments such as hypertension.

CRISPR – clustered regularly inter-spaced short palindromic repeats. A method by which sections of the genetic code can be cut out and replaced.

CRP – C-reactive protein, an inflammatory marker. The higher the level of inflammation in your body, the higher your CRP reading will be in your blood test.

DNA – deoxyribonucleic acid, the helix that is within almost every cell and that contains our genetic code.

DHEA – one of the hormones. It stands for dehydroepiandrosterone.

DHT – dihydrotestosterone, which is one of the hormones that testosterone is metabolised into in the liver.

Epigenetics – the study of how toxins, pollutants and other lifestyle factors influence our genes.

FDA – the US Food and Drug Administration.

Free radicals – atoms or molecules that lack an unpaired electron on their oxygen element. These bounce around the cell like unstable magnets, and cause havoc until neutralised by antioxidants.

Glycation – the sugaring of proteins in the body. See also HbA1c.

HbA1c – a measure of how sugar-coated, or glycated, the red blood cells are.

HDL – high-density lipoprotein, also known as 'good choles-terol'. This is the boat that carries cholesterol from the body back to the liver. Contrast with LDL.

Healthspan – the number of years that we are healthy. Contrast with Lifespan.

HFCS – high-fructose corn syrup, which is bad for our health, as are other sugars such as glucose and alcohol sugars.

HIIT – high-intensity interval train-ing, which is extremely good for our health.

IDE – insulin-degrading enzyme. It removes insulin from the body and beta-amyloid plaque from the brain.

LDL – low-density lipoprotein, also known as 'bad cholesterol'. This is the boat that carries choles-terol from the liver to the body. Contrast with HDL.

Lifespan – the number of years we live. Contrast with Healthspan.

Metabolic syndrome – the array of modern ills in the form of high blood pressure, increased blood sugar levels, excess fat around the waist, and too-high levels of cholesterol and triglycerides that increase the chances of diabetes, heart attacks and strokes.

MMP – matrix metalloproteinase, a type of enzyme that breaks down scar tissue, and therefore colla-gen. MMPs are stimulated by the skin's exposure to the sun, which causes them to attack collagen; this eventually results in saggy skin. Compare with TIMP.

NAC – N-acetylcysteine, an antioxidant that can cross the blood-brain barrier and that is a precursor for glutathione, a key natural antioxidant.

NAFLD – Non-Alcoholic Fatty Liver Disease, a condition that is typically caused by excess sugar, and in which the liver performs poorly, increasing inflammation in the body and increasing the risks of developing chronic diseases.

NER – nucleotide excision repair, a process by which the body cuts out damaged DNA and repairs it.

NHS – the United Kingdom's National Health Service.

NREM sleep – the non-rapid eye movement stage of sleep, during which time the brain moves fact-based information from short-term storage to permanent storage, and the glymphatic system cleans the brain of toxins. Contrast with REM sleep.

REM sleep – the rapid eye movement stage of sleep, during which time we dream, consolidate our memory of how to do things, and build creativity. Contrast with NREM sleep.

SARMs – selective androgen receptor modulators. These are drugs that mimic the effect of testosterone but do not attach to testosterone receptors in doing so; the hope is that they can provide the benefits of testosterone without the side effects and risks.

Senescence – in cellular terms, this refers to biological ageing. Compare with apoptosis.

SOD – superoxide dismutase, the most important intracellular antioxidant that protects cells from inflammatory damage, and is switched on and off by various environmental factors.

Synthetic hormones – hormone-balancing treatments that use chemical compounds that have a different structure to human hormones, but which echo their behaviour. Contrast with bio-identical hormones.

Telomere – the cap-like tags on the ends of our DNA strands that protect the code within. These caps shorten each time our cell divides, and eventually run out of length, resulting in cell death (apoptosis).

Telomerase – an enzyme that stops telomeres from shortening.

TIMP – tissue inhibitor of metallopro-teinase. This blocks the MMP enzyme and therefore helps to build up collagen and scar tissue.

VOCs – volatile organic compounds, which are found in many house-hold items such as carpets, and which are probably carcinogenic.

WHO – World Health Organization.

Index